I0065056

Problem Solving in Interventional Oncology

Problem Solving
in Interventional
Oncology

Edited by

Tze Min Wah, MBChB, PhD, FRCR, EBIR, FCIRSE
Professor of Interventional Radiology, Leeds Institute of Medical Research, University of
Leeds, Leeds; Clinical Lead for LTHT Interventional Oncology Programme, Department of
Diagnostic and Interventional Radiology, Leeds Cancer Centre, St James's University Hospital,
Leeds Teaching Hospitals NHS Trust, Leeds

Séan M. O'Cathail, MBBCh, BAO, BMedSci, MSc, DPhil, MRCPI, MRCP, FRCR
Clinical Senior Lecturer in Clinical Oncology, School of Cancer Sciences, University of Glasgow,
Glasgow; Honorary Consultant Clinical Oncologist, Beatson West of Scotland Cancer Centre,
Glasgow

Dhakshinamoorthy Vijayanand, MBBS, MRCS, FRCS (Ed)
Consultant Liver Transplant and Hepatobiliary Surgeon, and Clinical Lead in Transplant and
Hepatobiliary Surgery, Department of Abdominal Medicine and Surgery, Leeds Cancer Centre,
St James's University Hospital, Leeds Teaching Hospitals NHS Trust, Leeds

Guy Hickson, BSc, MBBS, MRCS, FRCR
Consultant Radiologist, Department of Interventional Radiology, Gloucestershire Royal Hospital,
Gloucestershire Hospitals NHS Foundation Trust, Gloucester

Alison Young, MBChB, MD, FRCP
Consultant Medical Oncologist, Clinical Director Oncology, Leeds Cancer Centre, St James's
University Hospital, Leeds Teaching Hospitals NHS Trust, Leeds

Published in association with the Association of Cancer Physicians

EBN HEALTH

OXFORD, UK

EBN Health
An imprint of Evidence-based Networks Ltd
85 Newland
Witney
Oxfordshire OX28 3JW
UK
Tel: +44 1865 522326
Email: info@ebnhealth.com
Web: www.ebnhealth.com

Distributed worldwide by:
Marston Book Services Ltd
160 Eastern Avenue
Milton Park
Abingdon
Oxfordshire OX14 4SB
UK
Tel: +44 1235 465500
Fax: +44 1235 465555
Email: trade.orders@marston.co.uk

© Evidence-based Networks Ltd 2023

First published 2023

All rights reserved. No part of this publication may be reproduced, stored in a retrieval
system or transmitted in any form or by any means without the prior permission in writing from EBN Health or Evidence-based Networks Ltd.

Although every effort has been made to ensure that all owners of copyright material
have been acknowledged in this publication, we would be glad to acknowledge in subsequent reprints or editions any omissions brought to the attention in writing of EBN
Health or Evidence-based Networks Ltd.

EBN Health and Evidence-based Networks Ltd bear no responsibility for the persistence
or accuracy of URLs for external or third-party internet websites referred to in this publication, and do not guarantee that any content on such websites is, or will remain,
accurate or appropriate.

A catalogue record for this book is available from the British Library.

Print ISBN: 978 099559 548 4
eBook ISBN: 978 173988 149 8

The publisher makes no representation, express or implied, that the dosages in this book
are correct. Readers must therefore always check the product information and clinical
procedures with the most up-to-date published product information and data sheets
provided by the manufacturers and the most recent codes of conduct and safety regula-
tions. The authors and the publisher do not accept any liability for any errors in the text
or for the misuse or misapplication of material in this work.

Series design by Pete Russell Typographic Design, Faringdon, Oxfordshire, UK
Typeset by Thomson Digital, Noida, India
Printed by Hobbs the Printers Ltd, Totton, Hampshire, UK

Contents

Contributors

Dr Omar Abdel-Hadi, Consultant Interventional Radiologist, Department of Diagnostic and Interventional Radiology, Leeds Cancer Centre, St James's University Hospital, Leeds Teaching Hospitals NHS Trust, Leeds

Dr Ewan Mark Anderson, Consultant Radiologist, Surgery and Diagnostics Centre, Churchill Hospital, Oxford University Hospitals NHS Foundation Trust, Oxford

Mr Magdy Attia, Consultant HPB and Transplant Surgeon, Department of Hepatobiliary and Liver Transplant Surgery, Leeds Cancer Centre, St James's University Hospital, Leeds Teaching Hospitals NHS Trust, Leeds

Dr Lawrence Bell, Consultant Radiologist, Department of Radiology, Gloucestershire Royal Hospital, Gloucestershire Hospitals NHS Foundation Trust, Gloucester

Dr Caitlin Bowden, Consultant Clinical Oncologist, Gloucestershire Cancer Centre, Cheltenham General Hospital, Gloucestershire Hospitals NHS Foundation Trust, Cheltenham

Dr Vinson Wai-Shun Chan, Visiting Researcher, School of Medicine, Faculty of Medicine and Health, University of Leeds, Leeds; Honorary Research Assistant, Division of Surgery and Interventional Science, University College London, London; Foundation Year 1 Doctor, Royal Derby Hospital, University Hospitals of Derby and Burton, Derby

Mr Nilanjan Chaudhuri, Consultant and Clinical Lead in Thoracic Surgery, Department of Thoracic Surgery, Leeds Cancer Centre, St James's University Hospital, Leeds Teaching Hospitals NHS Trust, Leeds

Dr Marios P. Decatris, Consultant Medical Oncologist, Gloucestershire Cancer Centre, Cheltenham General Hospital, Gloucestershire Hospitals NHS Foundation Trust, Cheltenham

Mr Henry Delacave, Core Surgical Trainee, Department of Urology, Cheltenham General Hospital, Gloucestershire Hospitals NHS Foundation Trust, Cheltenham

Dr Peter Dickinson, Consultant Clinical Oncologist, Department of Clinical Oncology, Leeds Cancer Centre, St James's University Hospital, Leeds Teaching Hospitals NHS Trust, Leeds

Dr Suraiya Dubash, Consultant Clinical Oncologist, Mount Vernon Cancer Centre, Mount Vernon Hospital, East and North Hertfordshire NHS Trust, Northwood, Middlesex

Mr Jonathan Eyshi, Medical Student, Herbert Wertheim College of Medicine, Florida International University, Miami, FL, USA

Dr Ben Fulton, Consultant Clinical Oncologist, Beatson West of Scotland Cancer Centre, Glasgow

Ms Jacklyn Garcia, Medical Student, Herbert Wertheim College of Medicine, Florida International University, Miami, FL, USA

Dr Amy Greenwood, Consultant Radiologist, Department of Interventional Radiology, Gloucestershire Royal Hospital, Gloucestershire Hospitals NHS Foundation Trust, Gloucester

Dr Derek Grose, Consultant Clinical Oncologist and Honorary Senior Lecturer, Beatson West of Scotland Cancer Centre, Glasgow

Mr Zaed Hamady, Consultant Hepatobiliary, Pancreatic and Laparoscopic Surgeon, Department of General Surgery, University Hospital Southampton NHS Foundation Trust, Southampton

Dr Stephen Harrow, Consultant Clinical Oncologist, Edinburgh Cancer Centre, Western General Hospital, Edinburgh, NHS Lothian

Dr Guy Hickson, Consultant Radiologist, Department of Interventional Radiology, Gloucestershire Royal Hospital, Gloucestershire Hospitals NHS Foundation Trust, Gloucester

Mr Nabil Hussein, Cardiothoracic Surgery Registrar (NTN), Department of Cardiothoracic Surgery, Castle Hill Hospital, Hull University Teaching Hospitals NHS Trust, Cottingham

Dr David Jarosz, Interventional Radiology Fellow, Department of Radiology, Leeds Cancer Centre, St James's University Hospital, Leeds Teaching Hospitals NHS Trust, Leeds

Dr Ruhi Kanani, Clinical Oncology Registrar, Department of Oncology, University College Hospital, University College London Hospitals NHS Foundation Trust, London

Dr Salil Karkhanis, Consultant Interventional Radiologist, Department of Interventional Radiology, Queen Elizabeth Hospital, University Hospitals Birmingham NHS Foundation Trust, Birmingham

Dr Mahaz Kayani, Medical Oncology Registrar, Department of Medical Oncology, Leeds Cancer Centre, St James's University Hospital, Leeds Teaching Hospitals NHS Trust, Leeds

Dr Angus Killean, Specialist Trainee in Clinical Oncology, Edinburgh Cancer Centre, Western General Hospital, Edinburgh, NHS Lothian

Dr James Lenton, Consultant Interventional Radiologist, Department of Diagnostic and Interventional Radiology, Leeds Cancer Centre, St James's University Hospital, Leeds Teaching Hospitals NHS Trust, Leeds

Professor Peter Lodge, Professor of Surgery, Department of Hepatobiliary Surgery, Leeds Cancer Centre, St James's University Hospital, Leeds Teaching Hospitals NHS Trust, Leeds

Professor Fergus Macbeth, Associate Director, Centre for Trials Research, Cardiff University, Cardiff

Mr Declan McDonnell, Clinical Research Fellow/NIHR HPB Surgery, Department of General Surgery, University Hospital Southampton NHS Foundation Trust, Southampton

Dr Jack McKenna, Specialist Registrar in Radiology, Department of Diagnostic and Interventional Radiology, Leeds Cancer Centre, St James's University Hospital, Leeds Teaching Hospitals NHS Trust, Leeds

Miss Faith McMeekin, Consultant Urologist, Department of Urology, Cheltenham General Hospital, Gloucestershire Hospitals NHS Foundation Trust, Cheltenham

Dr Usman Mahay, Consultant Interventional Radiologist, Department of Interventional Radiology, London North West University Healthcare NHS Trust, London

Mr Ashwin Mahendra, Medical Student, Schmidt College of Medicine, Florida Atlantic University, Boca Raton, FL, USA

Mr Richard Milton, Consultant Thoracic Surgeon, Department of Thoracic Surgery, Leeds Cancer Centre, St James's University Hospital, Leeds Teaching Hospitals NHS Trust, Leeds

Dr Sachin Modi, Consultant Interventional Radiologist, Department of Interventional Radiology, University Hospital Southampton NHS Foundation Trust, Southampton

Dr Rebecca Muirhead, Consultant Clinical Oncologist, Department of Oncology, Oxford University Hospitals NHS Foundation Trust, Oxford

Dr Louise J. Murray, Yorkshire Cancer Research Associate Professor in Clinical Oncology, Leeds Institute of Medical Research, School of Medicine, University of Leeds, Leeds; Honorary Consultant in Clinical Oncology, Leeds Cancer Centre, St James's University Hospital, Leeds Teaching Hospitals NHS Trust, Leeds

Dr Arvind Muthirevula, Thoracic Surgery Clinical Fellow, Department of Thoracic Surgery, Leeds Cancer Centre, St James's University Hospital, Leeds Teaching Hospitals NHS Trust, Leeds

Dr Pavan Najran, Consultant Clinical and Interventional Radiologist, Department of Radiology, The Christie NHS Foundation Trust, Manchester

Dr Govindarajan Narayanan, Chief of Interventional Oncology, Miami Cardiac and Vascular Institute, Baptist Health South Florida, Miami, FL, USA

Mr Jeremy Nettleton, Consultant Urologist, Department of Urology, Cheltenham General Hospital, Gloucestershire Hospitals NHS Foundation Trust, Cheltenham

Miss Helen Ng, Medical Student, School of Medicine, University of Leeds, Leeds

Dr Séan M. O'Cathail, Clinical Senior Lecturer in Clinical Oncology, School of Cancer Sciences, University of Glasgow, Glasgow; Honorary Consultant Clinical Oncologist, Beatson West of Scotland Cancer Centre, Glasgow

Dr Praveen Peddu, Consultant Radiologist and Clinical Lead in Interventional HPB, Department of Radiology, King's College Hospital NHS Foundation Trust, London

Dr Adam Peters, Clinical Oncology Registrar, Beatson West of Scotland Cancer Centre, Glasgow

Dr Wai-Yan Poon, Clinical Oncology Registrar, Beatson West of Scotland Cancer Centre, Glasgow; Honorary Clinical Lecturer, School of Medicine, Dentistry and Nursing, College of Medical, Veterinary and Life Sciences, University of Glasgow, Glasgow

Dr Ian Rowe, Associate Professor of Hepatology, Department of Hepatology, Leeds Cancer Centre, St James's University Hospital, Leeds Teaching Hospitals NHS Trust, Leeds

Dr Claire Ryan, Interventional Radiology Fellow, Department of Diagnostic and Interventional Radiology, Leeds Cancer Centre, St James's University Hospital, Leeds Teaching Hospitals NHS Trust, Leeds

Dr Adel Samson, Associate Professor of Medical Oncology, Department of Medical

Oncology, Leeds Cancer Centre, St James's University Hospital, Leeds Teaching Hospitals NHS Trust, Leeds

Dr Shyamal Saujani, Consultant Radiologist, Surgery and Diagnostics Centre, Churchill Hospital, Oxford University Hospitals NHS Foundation Trust, Oxford

Ms Sadhana Shankar, Senior Clinical Fellow in HPB Surgery, Institute of Liver Studies, King's College Hospital NHS Foundation Trust, London

Dr Finbar Slevin, Cancer Research UK Clinical Trial Fellow, Leeds Institute of Clinical Trials Research, School of Medicine, University of Leeds, Leeds; Honorary Consultant in Clinical Oncology, Leeds Cancer Centre, St James's University Hospital, Leeds Teaching Hospitals NHS Trust, Leeds

Dr Jonathan Smith, Consultant Radiologist, Department of Radiology, Leeds Cancer Centre, St James's University Hospital, Leeds Teaching Hospitals NHS Trust, Leeds

Miss Rebecca Smith, Surgical Trainee, Department of Urology, Cheltenham General Hospital, Gloucestershire Hospitals NHS Foundation Trust, Cheltenham

Dr John Spillane, Radiology Registrar, Gloucestershire Royal Hospital, Gloucestershire Hospitals NHS Foundation Trust, Gloucester

Mr Rahul Sreekumar, Senior Clinical Fellow in HPB Surgery, Department of General Surgery, University Hospital Southampton NHS Foundation Trust, Southampton

Dr Brian Stedman, Consultant Interventional Radiologist, Department of Interventional Radiology, University Hospital Southampton NHS Foundation Trust, Southampton

Mr Arjun Takhar, Consultant Laparoscopic and HPB Surgeon, Department of HPB Surgery, University Hospital Southampton NHS Foundation Trust, Southampton

Dr Ashley Thorpe, Radiology Registrar, Gloucestershire Royal Hospital, Gloucestershire Hospitals NHS Foundation Trust, Gloucester

Professor Maxine G. B. Tran, Honorary Consultant Urological Surgeon, Specialist Centre for Kidney Cancer, Royal Free London NHS Foundation Trust, London; Professor of Urology, University College London, London

Professor Tom Treasure, Honorary Professor of Cardiothoracic Surgery, Clinical Operational Research Unit, University College London, London

Mr Dharmadev Trivedi, Consultant Surgeon, Department of Surgery, Warwick Hospital, South Warwickshire University NHS Foundation Trust, Warwick

Dr Ganesh Vigneswaran, Interventional Radiology Fellow, Department of Interventional Radiology, University Hospital Southampton NHS Foundation Trust, Southampton; NIHR Clinical Lecturer, Cancer Sciences, Faculty of Medicine, University of Southampton, Southampton

Mr Dhakshinamoorthy Vijayanand, Consultant Liver Transplant and Hepatobiliary Surgeon, and Clinical Lead in Transplant and Hepatobiliary Surgery, Department of Abdominal Medicine and Surgery, Leeds Cancer Centre, St James's University Hospital, Leeds Teaching Hospitals NHS Trust, Leeds

Professor Tze Min Wah, Professor of Interventional Radiology, Leeds Institute of

Medical Research, University of Leeds, Leeds; Clinical Lead for LTHT Interventional Oncology Programme, Department of Diagnostic and Interventional Radiology, Leeds Cancer Centre, St James's University Hospital, Leeds Teaching Hospitals NHS Trust, Leeds

Mr James Walcott, Senior Clinical Fellow, Department of Hepatobiliary and Liver Transplant Surgery, Leeds Cancer Centre, St James's University Hospital, Leeds Teaching Hospitals NHS Trust, Leeds

Dr Sara Walker, Clinical Oncology Registrar, Beatson West of Scotland Cancer Centre, Glasgow; SABR Clinical Research Fellow, School of Cancer Sciences, University of Glasgow, Glasgow.

Dr Alison Young, Consultant Medical Oncologist, Clinical Director Oncology, Leeds Cancer Centre, St James's University Hospital, Leeds Teaching Hospitals NHS Trust, Leeds

Preface

Our ability to detect, diagnose and treat cancer, often at earlier stages, is increasing thanks to the wider availability of cross-sectional imaging. This presents opportunities for us to rethink how we approach the management of both primary and metastatic disease. In the last decade, interventional oncology has emerged as one of the important pillars of cancer treatment. It complements surgical, medical and clinical oncology to offer minimally invasive cancer treatments via various embolotherapy and ablative technologies that can preserve organ function, avoid or defer systemic treatment, be delivered on an outpatient basis or with a shorter hospital stay, and require a shorter period of convalescence. In 2015 the Interventional Oncology UK (IOUK) specialist group, within the British Society of Interventional Radiology (BSIR), was launched in Leeds. Professor Peter Selby, past president of the Association of Cancer Physicians, led the plenary lecture at the inaugural IOUK meeting titled 'Interventional oncology as one of the pillars of cancer care'.

The Royal College of Radiologists has defined interventional oncology as having two main components: palliative procedures to relieve cancer-related symptoms and disease-modifying treatments to cure cancer. Many aspects of interventional oncology are now embedded in cancer multidisciplinary team discussions to ensure the inclusion of patient-centred, individualized treatment options of benefit.

Surgeons, medical and clinical oncologists have been collaborating to provide and evolve personalized clinical care for many years now. In the spirit of the broadening collaboration involving interventional radiology colleagues seen in many of the best units, IOUK and BSIR were privileged to be invited by the Association of Cancer Physicians to help create a specially curated interventional oncology edition of the award-winning *Problem Solving* series. This collaboration has involved a multidisciplinary panel of editors from around the UK designing and delivering a cross-speciality workshop and subsequently the content of this book.

This book launch has a personal touch thanks to an educational grant awarded by BSIR in memory of Robert Bardsley. Robert sadly passed away in 2019 having been a treasured industry partner in interventional radiology who had championed innovation throughout his career.

This most recent book in the *Problem Solving* series seeks to highlight the role of interventional oncology by providing a broad overview of the topic followed by a multidisciplinary approach to managing a range of cancers. Six chapters written by leading authorities in the field provide a high-level perspective of developments in interventional oncology. Thirty-three individual case histories focusing on oligometastatic, liver, lung, renal and pancreatic-biliary cancers illustrate how interventional oncology may be offered as a complementary treatment option in cancer management alongside surgical, medical and clinical oncology. This rapidly evolving area of cancer care is at the vanguard of bioengineering, medical physics and imaging technologies and will continue to develop apace. Its fundamental principles, however, will endure.

The development of interventional oncology has been driven by the patients who have benefited from these treatments and by the clinicians who have advocated its merits as an important pillar alongside surgery and clinical and medical oncology.

Tze Min Wah, Séan M. O'Cathail, Dhakshinamoorthy Vijayanand,
Guy Hickson and Alison Young, Editors

British Society of Interventional Radiology

Interventional oncology is a rapidly growing field that offers minimally invasive treatment options for people with cancer. Many of the society's members are involved in these treatments and work closely alongside their surgical, medical and clinical oncology colleagues to provide the fourth pillar of cancer care.

While interventional oncology offers many advantages over traditional surgery, it also presents unique challenges. Each patient's case is different, and interventional radiologists must be able to quickly and effectively assess each situation to determine the best course of action. This requires not only technical skill but also a deep understanding of imaging techniques, image interpretation and the biology of cancer. Interventional radiologists are uniquely positioned to provide this.

This book is designed to provide interventional radiologists with the tools they need to successfully navigate the complex landscape of cancer treatment. Its 33 case studies illustrate common challenges faced by interventional radiologists in their oncological practice. Each case study is presented in a step-by-step format, with clear explanations of the decision-making process and the rationale behind each treatment option.

Throughout the book, readers will find practical tips and strategies for optimizing outcomes, as well as insights into emerging technologies and trends in the field. Whether you are an experienced interventional radiologist or a trainee, *Problem Solving in Interventional Oncology* is an essential resource for staying up-to-date with the latest developments in this exciting and rapidly evolving field.

Phil Haslam, President, British Society of Interventional Radiology

Acknowledgements

Editors

The editors and authors are tremendously grateful to their patients for giving permission to share their cancer treatment journey and inspire the trainees and medical students to present their case studies with the aim to improve cancer management. The editors would like to acknowledge the hard work and dedication of the specialist trainees from diverse backgrounds, ranging from medical, surgical, clinical and interventional oncology/radiology, who have contributed to this work. Medical students, our next generation of doctors, have also participated in writing up their case studies, and we hope the experience will equip them well for the next stage of their journey.

The editors warmly acknowledge the generous support they have received in preparing this book. Emeritus Professor Peter Selby kindly introduced and supported the link between the Interventional Oncology United Kingdom (IOUK)/British Society of Interventional Radiology (BSIR) and the Association of Cancer Physicians for the commissioning of the book. Nicole Goldman, executive secretary, coordinated and oversaw the book's preparation and organization in her own time amidst her busy working schedule. The editors, authors and the publisher are grateful to the executive committee of the Association of Cancer Physicians for their support and advice during the development and commissioning of this book. In addition, Dr Chern Lee provided initial input in designing the content for the pancreatic-biliary section before he took up his new role in Singapore.

The editors are grateful to Duncan Enright and Beverley Martin at EBN Health for their expert work, support, goodwill and interest in our purpose in preparing the book.

Professor Tze Min Wah would like to acknowledge the support of Leeds Teaching Hospitals NHS Trust, the University of Leeds, IOUK and BSIR. Dr Séan O'Cathail would like to acknowledge the support of the School of Cancer Sciences at the University of Glasgow, his clinical and academic colleagues at the Beatson West of Scotland Cancer Centre and his collaborators around the UK who have generously contributed their time and effort to this work. Dr Dhakshinamoorthy Vijayanand and Dr Alison Young would like to acknowledge the support of Leeds Teaching Hospitals NHS Trust. Dr Guy Hickson would like to acknowledge the support of IOUK and Gloucestershire Hospitals NHS Foundation Trust.

Tze Min Wah, Séan M. O'Cathail, Dhakshinamoorthy Vijayanand,
Guy Hickson and Alison Young, Editors

Association of Cancer Physicians

As the representative body for medical oncologists in the UK, the Association of Cancer Physicians has a broad set of aims that include a focus on training and education, for its members as well as for other clinicians, healthcare professionals and the public, to support the raising of standards of medical care for cancer patients. The *Problem Solving* series of cancer-related books is developed and prepared by the Association of Cancer Physicians, often in partnership with one or more other specialist medical organizations. The books have been well received and the association is delighted with their standard. The BMA prize for best oncology book of the year was awarded to *Problem Solving in Older Cancer Patients* in 2016, *Problem Solving in Precision Oncology* in 2017, *Problem Solving in Patient-Centred and Integrated Cancer Care* in 2018, and, most recently, *Problem Solving in Cancer and Fertility* in 2022.

This latest publication is a slight departure from the themes of previous titles in the *Problem Solving* series but represents a truly multidisciplinary approach to cancer management. It is the result of close collaboration with colleagues in interventional radiology and will help support education and training in this exciting and rapidly developing field.

The publication has involved considerable work from many contributors, carried out as an educational service and without remuneration. The Association of Cancer Physicians wishes to thank all contributors to this and previous publications as well as those yet to come.

David Cunningham, Chair, Association of Cancer Physicians
Helena Earl, Honorary President, Association of Cancer Physicians

Abbreviations

AFP	Alpha-fetoprotein	IMDC	International Metastatic Renal Cell Carcinoma Database Consortium
ALT	Alanine aminotransferase		
AST	Aspartate aminotransferase	INR	International normalized ratio
ASTRO	American Society for Radiation Oncology	IOERT	Intraoperative electron beam radiotherapy
BCLC	Barcelona Clinic Liver Cancer	IRE	Irreversible electroporation
BED	Biologically effective dose	MDT	Multidisciplinary team
CAPOX	Capecitabine, oxaliplatin	M-PHP	Melphalan percutaneous hepatic perfusion
CEA	Carcinoembryonic antigen		
COPD	Chronic obstructive pulmonary disease	mRECIST	Modified Response Evaluation Criteria in Solid Tumors
CRP	C-reactive protein	mTOR	Mechanistic target of rapamycin
CTLA-4	Cytotoxic T lymphocyte-associated protein 4	MUC-1	Mucin 1 cell surface-associated
		NSCLC	Non-small-cell lung cancer
DEB-TACE	Drug-eluting bead transarterial chemoembolization	OS	Overall survival
		PanIN	Pancreatic intraepithelial neoplasia
DMSA	Dimercaptosuccinic acid	PD-1	Programmed cell death protein 1
DPD	Dihydropyrimidine dehydrogenase	PDAC	Pancreatic ductal adenocarcinoma
DSA	Digital subtraction angiography	PD-L1	Programmed death-ligand 1
EBRT	External beam radiotherapy	PFS	Progression-free survival
EORTC	European Organisation for Research and Treatment of Cancer	PIVKA-II	Protein induced by vitamin K antagonist-II
ERCP	Endoscopic retrograde cholangiopancreatography	PSA	Prostate-specific antigen
		PSMA	Prostate-specific membrane antigen
ESTRO	European Society for Radiotherapy and Oncology	pTA	Percutaneous thermal ablation
		PTC	Percutaneous transhepatic cholangiography
EUS	Endoscopic ultrasound		
FOLFIRI	Fluorouracil, folinic acid, irinotecan	RANKL	Receptor activator of nuclear factor kappa-B ligand
FOLFIRINOX	Folinic acid, fluorouracil, irinotecan, oxaliplatin		
		RCC	Renal cell carcinoma
FOLFOX	Fluorouracil, folinic acid, oxaliplatin	RCR	Royal College of Radiologists
GIST	Gastrointestinal stromal tumour	RCT	Randomized controlled trial
HBsAg	Hepatitis B surface antigen	RTOG	Radiation Therapy Oncology Group
HCC	Hepatocellular carcinoma	SBRT	Stereotactic body radiotherapy
HCV	Hepatitis C virus	SDH	Succinate dehydrogenase
HPF	High-power field	SIRT	Selective internal radiation therapy
HU	Hounsfield units	SRS	Stereotactic radiosurgery
ICPI	Immune checkpoint inhibitor	SUV_{max}	Maximum standardized uptake value
ILD	Interstitial lung disease		

TACE	Transarterial chemoembolization	VEGFR	Vascular endothelial growth factor receptor
TKI	Tyrosine kinase inhibitor		
TLS	Tumour lysis syndrome	VHL	von Hippel–Lindau
VATS	Video-assisted thoracoscopic surgery	VO_{2max}	Maximal oxygen consumption
		WCC	White blood cell count
VCF	Vertebral compression fracture	XELOX	Oxaliplatin, capecitabine
VEGF	Vascular endothelial growth factor		

01 Interventional oncology: past, present and future

Tze Min Wah

Introduction

The current lifetime cancer risk in the UK is 1 in 2, meaning that 50% of the population will be diagnosed with cancer during their lifetime.[1] Although significant progress has been made since the 2000 NHS Cancer Plan[2] and the 2011 national strategy for cancer,[3] there remains a wide variation in access to cancer treatments and regional cancer outcomes in the UK.[2]

In 2019, the NHS Long Term Plan[5] set out further ambitious plans and commitments to improve cancer services and outcomes in England over the next decade. The plan strives to achieve the milestones by 2028 of >55,000 people per annum surviving their cancer for 5 years or more, and most people with cancer (75%) being diagnosed early at stage I or II. The plan also strives to address access variation and inequalities as well as improve quality-of-life outcomes and patient experience.

Our ability to diagnose cancer has improved over the last decade with diagnoses made at an earlier stage, but there are ambitions to improve this further still. Given that cancer is now detected when tumours are smaller, and often incidentally, the cancer treatment strategy does lend itself to a minimally invasive approach such as surgery via keyhole or robotic-assisted approach to remove the tumour while preserving the rest of the organ and avoiding the need for open surgery with radical removal of the organ.

Indeed, the drive for minimally invasive cancer treatment marked the beginning of the interventional oncology era worldwide, since its inception by a team of interventional radiologists in Chicago in 2009.[6] In 2015, the Interventional Oncology United Kingdom specialist group was formally established under the umbrella of the British Society of Interventional Radiology. Interventional oncology is now an established pillar in managing cancer treatments alongside surgical, medical and clinical oncology.

What is interventional oncology?

Interventional oncology has been defined by the Royal College of Radiologists in two main components: supportive (i.e. symptom relieving) and disease modifying. Interventional oncology encompasses the use of image-guided techniques to relieve symptoms caused by cancer as well as treat people with cancer, using a range of innovative technology via a minimally invasive approach. The college has also set out best practice guidance regarding service delivery.[7]

Disease-modifying procedures are defined as those aiming to treat cancer with curative intent or improve oncological durability with loco-regional therapy using an image-guided approach. Image-guided ablation is often used to treat cancer with curative intent, either in primary cancers or in the oligometastatic setting with thermal (e.g. radiofrequency ablation, microwave ablation or cryoablation) or non-thermal (e.g. irreversible electroporation) technology. The vascular approach has included transarterial chemoembolization and selective internal radiation therapy

(SIRT) in the treatment of later stage primary and metastatic liver cancers.[8,9] Supportive and symptomatic procedures are defined as providing relief from cancer-related symptoms or providing diagnosis for subsequent definitive treatment (e.g. diagnostic tests such as image-guided biopsy), as well as palliative procedures such as image-guided drainage of malignant fluid collections (e.g. pleural effusion and ascites) or stent insertion to relieve malignant luminal obstruction.

It is essential to highlight that the decision regarding the best treatment options for cancer patients should be discussed by a multidisciplinary team so that all options, such as interventional oncology and medical, clinical and surgical oncology, are considered to ensure quality and patient-centred cancer care.[10]

Current service provision of interventional oncology in the UK

In 2017, the Interventional Oncology United Kingdom steering committee led a cross-sectional survey to map interventional oncology service provision in the UK. The aim was to evaluate the gap in service delivery and highlight it to various stakeholders to address the need for investment in infrastructures as well as workforce planning.[11] Figure 1.1 highlights the 'inequality' of interventional oncology service provision.

The four major key milestones in the long-term plan for addressing cancer treatment provision and outcomes have included reduction of variation, equity of access and improved patient experience and quality-of-life outcomes. The interventional oncology map produced in 2017 demonstrated the provision gap. In 2022, there remain gaps on the UK map which must be urgently addressed to ensure population equity of access. Patient level feedback (see Further reading) clearly articulates the benefits and quality of care received following various interventional oncology treatments. More quantitative and qualitative clinical research must be conducted to prove this for service commissioning.

In addition, the minimally invasive approaches allow for quicker recovery and shorter hospital stays. Various authors have shown the cost-effectiveness of image-guided ablation in small renal cancer compared with surgical procedures.[12,13] More multicentre studies in the UK would provide better evidence to facilitate service and workforce planning. Furthermore, with the unexpected COVID-19 pandemic in 2020, interventional oncology service delivery has become increasingly sought after as it offers flexibility and greater options for patients. It continued during the challenging period of the pandemic when people with COVID-19 occupied intensive care and high-dependency beds, and major surgical procedures were halted to create bed capacity for acutely unwell patients. Most patients were treated as day case procedures in some institutions or as an overnight stay for cancer treatment, avoiding the need for open surgery.[14]

Future directions

It is well recognized that interventional oncology is a rapidly expanding clinical area. Cancer detection and diagnosis now occur at an earlier stage and are likely to continue to trend in that direction. Given the rapid pace of technological advancement, more innovative ways of treating cancers will continue to be found. One of the most recent innovations in non-thermal ablation technology is image-guided histotripsy in liver cancer treatment, as part of the #Hope4Liver trial (ClinicalTrials.gov NCT04573881), and the successful translation of histotripsy treatment in one of the first UK patients with liver cancer.[15] The COLLISION trial (ClinicalTrials.gov NCT03088150) is providing emerging quantitative level 1 evidence for image-guided ablation

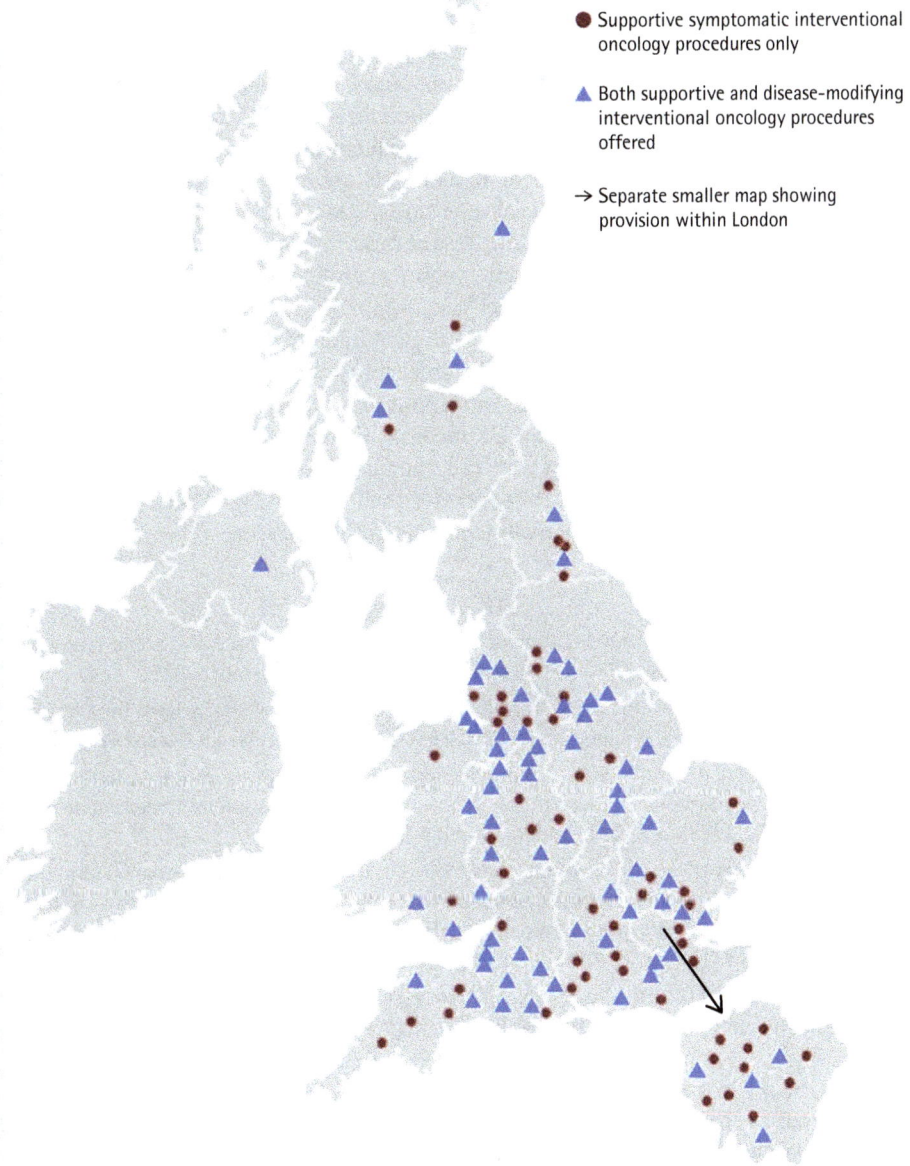

Figure 1.1 A cross-sectional map of interventional oncology service provision in the UK (adapted from Zhong et al.[11]).

in colorectal liver metastasis.[16] The multicentre NEST trial (ISRCTN18156881) is designed to address the level 1 evidence gap in image-guided renal ablation vs robotic partial nephrectomy.[17]

With the emergence of the next generation of academic trainees, the next stage of evidence-based clinical practice in the interventional oncology sphere is likely to go from strength to strength. In 2022, the Barcelona Clinic Liver Cancer staging system showed a clear role of interventional oncology in the treatment strategy for primary liver cancer with the addition of SIRT within the recommendation.[18] There is also an emerging indication for interventional oncology in managing oligometastatic disease, which will be explored in subsequent chapters of this book.

NHS England and the Royal College of Radiologists are currently actively addressing the workforce pipeline in radiology. It is crucial to ensure a sustainable pipeline of doctors and allied healthcare teams to support the changing pace of cancer diagnosis and treatment. Currently, there is a significant workforce shortage in interventional radiology. The lack of visibility of these emerging clinical areas is reflected in the fact that they are not in the UK medical school curriculum.[19] Greater engagement from the Royal College of Radiologists with undergraduate medical schools is therefore crucial at this stage. The excellent wider engagement events from junior doctors' forums (www.irjuniors.com/events) with industry support have helped to provide the much-needed exposure and inspiration for UK medical students to consider and pursue a career in interventional radiology. The future is truly exciting for the next generation of doctors, clinical academics and allied healthcare teams as cancer treatment is evolving at such a pace that minimally invasive interventional oncology treatment is clearly here to stay.

References

1 Cancer Research UK (2022). Cancer risk statistics. Available from: www.cancerresearchuk.org/health-professional/cancer-statistics/risk (accessed 9 December 2022).

2 Department of Health (2000). The NHS Cancer Plan. Available from: www.thh.nhs.uk/documents/_Departments/Cancer/NHSCancerPlan.pdf (accessed 9 December 2022).

3 Department of Health (2011). Improving outcomes: a strategy for cancer. Available from: https://assets.publishing.service.gov.uk/government/uploads/system/uploads/attachment_data/file/213785/dh_123394.pdf (accessed 9 December 2022).

4 Department of Health, NHS England, Public Health England (2015). Progress in improving cancer services and outcomes in England. Available from: www.nao.org.uk/wp-content/uploads/2015/01/Progress-improving-cancer-services-and-outcomes-in-England.pdf (accessed 9 December 2022).

5 NHS England (2019). The NHS Long Term Plan. Available from: www.longtermplan.nhs.uk/wp-content/uploads/2019/08/nhs-long-term-plan-version-1.2.pdf (accessed 9 December 2022).

6 LaTour P (2016). Origins of interventional oncology can be traced to a Chicago pizzeria. Available from: https://rsna2016.rsna.org/dailybulletin/index.cfm?pg=16thu13 (accessed 9 December 2022).

7 Royal College of Radiologists. Interventional oncology: guidance for service delivery. 2nd ed. London: RCR, 2017.

8 Hickey R, Vouche M, Sze DY, et al. Cancer concepts and principles: primer for the interventional oncologist – part II. J Vasc Interv Radiol 2013; 24: 1167–88.

9 Hickey R, Vouche M, Sze DY, et al. Cancer concepts and principles: primer for the interventional oncologist – part I. J Vasc Interv Radiol 2013; 24: 1157–64.

10 Adam A, Kenny LM. Interventional oncology in multidisciplinary cancer treatment in the 21st century. Nat Rev Clin Oncol 2015; 12: 105–13.

11 Zhong J, Atiiga P, Alcorn DJ, et al. Cross-sectional study of the provision of interventional oncology services in the UK. BMJ Open 2017; 7: e016631.

12 Garcia RG, Katz M, Falsarella PM, et al. Percutaneous cryoablation versus robot-assisted partial nephrectomy of renal T1a tumors: a single-center retrospective cost-effectiveness analysis. Cardiovasc Intervent Radiol 2021; 44: 892–900.

13 Wang Y, Chen YW, Leow JJ, et al. Cost-effectiveness of management options for small renal mass: a systematic review. Am J Clin Oncol 2016; 39: 484–90.

14 Shaida N, Alexander A. Re: the impact of COVID-19 on interventional radiology services in the UK: is there an opportunity for service development in interventional oncology? Cardiovasc Intervent Radiol 2021; 44: 1282–3.

15 Jackson J (2021). First UK patients treated for liver cancer using ultrasound technology. Available from: www.nationalhealthexecutive.com/articles/uk-patients-liver-cancer-NHS-ultrasound-technology (accessed 9 December 2022).

16 Puijk RS, Ruarus AH, Vroomen LGPH, et al. Colorectal Liver Metastases: Surgery versus Thermal Ablation (COLLISION) – a phase III single-blind prospective randomised controlled trial. BMC Cancer 2018; 18: 821.

17 Neves JB, Cullen D, Grant L, et al. Protocol for a feasibility study of a cohort embedded randomised controlled trial comparing nephron sparing treatment (NEST) for small renal masses. BMJ Open 2019; 9: e030965.

18 Reig M, Forner A, Rimola J, et al. BCLC strategy for prognosis prediction and treatment recommendation: the 2022 update. J Hepatol 2022; 76: 681–93.

19 Osman FH, Koe JSE, Lau ESW, et al. Study protocol for ELIXIR: an evaluation of learning and exposure to the undergraduate interventional radiology curriculum. J Surg Protoc Res Methodol 2021; 2021: snab006.

Further reading

- Anonymous (2015). Cryoablation versus open surgery. Available from: www.careopinion.org.uk/233603 (accessed 9 December 2022).

- Anonymous (2015). Right renal cryo ablation at St James's University Hospital Leeds. Available from: www.careopinion.org.uk/225096 (accessed 9 December 2022).

02 Oligometastatic disease: definitions, biology and evidence for stereotactic body radiotherapy

Séan M. O'Cathail

Introduction

One of the most enduring truisms of oncology is that disease beyond the primary site is incurable; however, an observation of everyday clinical practice in any oncology centre in the world belies this statement. Surgical resection of pulmonary metastases, in selected patients, has been accepted since the 1960s,[1] while the rate of hepatic resection for colorectal metastases has been increasing consistently.[2] This suggests that as clinicians we believe that there is a population of patients who benefit from intervention despite their metastatic state.

In 1995, Hellman and Weichselbaum coined the termed 'oligometastases' to define an intermediate state in the cancer spectrum that lies between early-stage and widespread metastatic disease.[3] Although lacking a specific definition, this provided a conceptual framework to understand what had become accepted practice in the oncology community; that is, intervening in metastatic disease could result in long-term disease control or cure. More importantly, the acceptance and adoption of the oligometastatic state allowed cancer researchers to coalesce around the idea that metastasis-directed therapies, such as stereotactic body radiotherapy (SBRT) or radiofrequency ablation, might also represent viable treatment options for patients displaying an oligometastatic phenotype.

What is oligometastatic disease?

Although the oncology community has accepted the existence of an oligometastatic disease state, a unifying definition by which patients can be selected for treatment has been lacking. More recently the European Society for Radiotherapy and Oncology (ESTRO) and the American Society for Radiation Oncology (ASTRO) have produced a consensus document which highlighted that oligometastatic disease is typically based on the imaging-detected number of metastases, five being the maximum number outside a trial protocol.[4] Most practising oncologists would recognize the oligometastatic disease 'phenotype' as a low disease burden, young age, good fitness, and an indolent disease pattern often characterized by a long disease-free interval between primary presentation and the development of metastases. These have been referred to colloquially as the 'four aces',[5] the implication being that a 'full house' would have a good prognostic outlook. But how does that reconcile with putting patients with synchronous liver metastases from a colon cancer forward for a liver resection? In an effort to clarify this situation the European Organisation for Research and Treatment of Cancer (EORTC) and ESTRO carried out a Delphi exercise to produce a consensus recommendation on the characterization and classification of oligometastatic disease (Figure 2.1).[6]

From this exercise it is clear the historical understanding of oligometastatic disease represents a limited proportion of what could currently be classified as an 'oligometastatic state'. The importance of the EORTC decision tool is that it creates a comprehensive framework to capture these

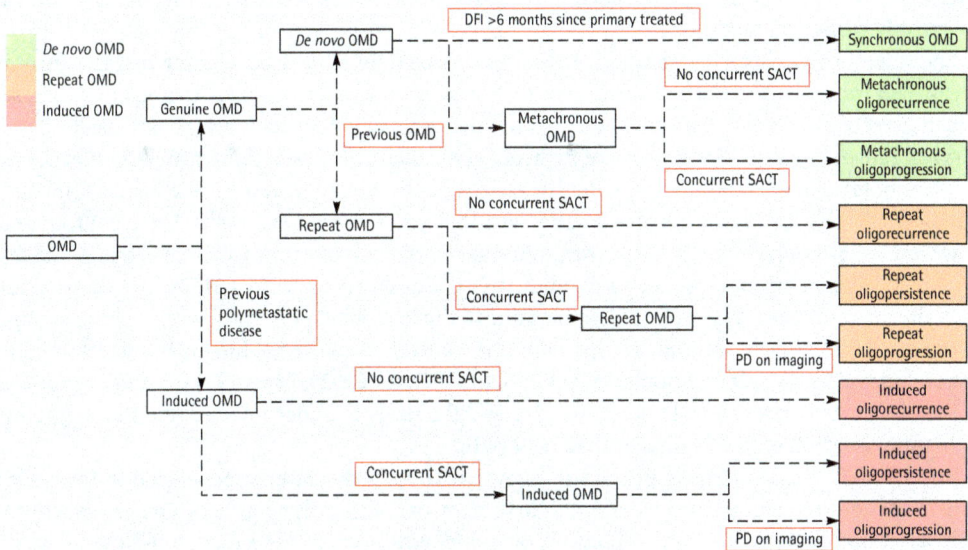

Figure 2.1 EORTC/ESTRO decision tree for the classification of oligometastatic disease (OMD). Differentiation of nine different disease states on the right-hand side is determined by characterization factors including the patient's history of metastases, the number of metastases, the disease-free interval (DFI) since treatment of the primary tumour, the use of concurrent systemic anticancer treatment (SACT), and whether the patient had progressive disease (PD) while receiving SACT (adapted from Guckenberger et al.[6]).

states, define the appropriate research questions, harmonize trial population recruitment and derive an appropriate evidence base to guide future practice.

The biological rationale for ablative therapy in oligometastatic disease

In parallel with the renewed clinical interest in ablative therapies, there has been a surge in scientific understanding of metastases as an evolutionary process.[7] This work is crucial for better use of ablative therapies. Some cancer types, such as colorectal cancer, show very high levels of genetic concordance between the primary site and metastatic sites, suggesting that the classical linear model of metastatic spread is the most relevant.[8] Other tumours, such as renal and prostate, however, demonstrate a parallel branching process where genetically distinct subclones become metastatic, and that different sites can contain different subclones.[9,10] These theories also highlight the importance of routes of metastatic spread. A good example is lymph node dissection, which can alter the development and spread of metastases. SBRT-irradiated lymph nodes have better outcomes compared with treated visceral sites,[11] potentially due to cancer immunoediting.[12] Liver metastases that exhibit an immune phenotype have superior outcomes when resected.[13]

Evidence for treatment in oligometastatic disease

Historically there is very little randomized controlled trial (RCT) evidence to support surgery, ablation or stereotactic radiation use, in spite of the fact that their use has been increasing significantly around the world. Most data supporting any form of ablative treatment are based on single-arm observational studies, whether for pulmonary, hepatic or adrenal metastasectomy, or a variety of organ sites. In some scenarios, the observational data are compelling, but still there is a relatively weak evidence base.

The International Registry of Lung Metastases reported on 5206 cases of lung metastasectomy performed for multiple primary cancer types. Those with the best prognosis, defined as a disease-free interval of more than 36 months and the presence of a single resectable metastasis, had a 10 year survival rate of 34%.[14] In the absence of high-quality randomized data, these better-than-expected survival outcomes in limited metastatic disease led to the incorporation of metastasectomy as a standard of care, as discussed above. The outcome could have reasonably been confounded, however, by 'selection bias' of patients with an indolent disease pattern. An attempt at an RCT to test the added value of lung metastasectomy (PulMiCC; ClinicalTrials.gov NCT01106261) was stopped early due to poor recruitment (N=65), in part due to the loss of belief in equipoise by clinicians and patients.[15] At the time of writing, it is the only current RCT of colorectal lung metastasectomy; the 5 year survival in the intervention arm was 38% (95% CI 23%, 62%) and 29% (95% CI 16%, 52%) in the observation arm. The CIs clearly overlap and the study is underpowered, but the suggestion is that the benefit is probably smaller than believed.[15]

The EORTC 40004 study (ClinicalTrials.gov NCT00043004) attempted to define the added benefit of radiofrequency ablation to systemic therapy in colorectal metastases. Originally a phase III trial, it had to be downsized to phase II owing to slow accrual. At a median follow-up of 9.7 years, it showed an overall survival (OS) benefit,[16] but the median OS of 40.5 months in the systemic therapy arm was better than expected, with a median OS of 45.6 months in the combined modality arm. Both of these studies underline the importance of conducting conclusive late-phase randomized studies, not just to try and demonstrate the superiority of the ablative approach but also to quantify the magnitude of that benefit.

Evidence for SBRT in oligometastatic disease

Fortunately, the radiation oncology community has grasped the opportunity to build an evidence base in support of SBRT in oligometastatic disease, with several notable phase II trials, many of which are referred to in the individual case studies. It should be noted that at the time of writing the phase III data are still awaited.

In 2016, Gomez and colleagues first published the results of their randomized phase II study examining the role of local consolidative therapy with SBRT vs maintenance/observation after first-line therapy in patients with stage IV non-small-cell lung cancer with fewer than four metastases; updated results were published in 2019.[17] The primary outcome was progression-free survival (PFS). The data safety and monitoring committee actually recommended early trial closure after 49 patients were accrued due to the significant benefit seen in the SBRT arm. With an updated median follow-up time of 38.8 months (range 28.3–61.4 months), the PFS benefit was durable (median 14.2 months with SBRT vs 4.4 months with maintenance/observation; $p=0.022$). The authors also noted an OS benefit in the SBRT arm (median 41.2 months with SBRT vs 17.0 months with maintenance/observation; $p=0.017$). Grade 3/4 toxicities were higher in the SBRT arm.

An important study, the SABR-COMET trial (ClinicalTrials.gov NCT01446744), has been seen to be a 'game-changer'. In this randomized phase II study, patients with between one and five metastases and controlled primary disease were randomized in a ratio of 1:2 to standard care alone or SBRT in addition to standard care.[18] The reason why this landmark trial is important is that it defined its primary endpoint as OS. Ninety-nine patients were randomized and, at a median follow-up of 51 months, 5 year OS was 17.7% in the standard care arm vs 42.3% in the SBRT plus standard care arm (stratified log-rank $p=0.006$). Five year PFS was 'not reached' in the standard care arm (3.2% [95% CI 0%, 14%] at 4 years with the last patient censored) and was 17.3% (95% CI 8%, 30%) in the SBRT plus standard care arm (p=0.001).

Some points to note about the study help to understand how important it is. It was designed as a phase II screening trial, where the α-value (type I error rate) is set at a higher value than in a phase III trial. This means that a positive result is not considered definitive and requires a subsequent phase III trial. In spite of randomization there was an imbalance in the number of prostate cancers in the SBRT arm, which may have influenced the magnitude of benefit seen; but, in a sensitivity analysis, it was not found to invalidate the overall result in the context of the study design. Pleasingly, the SABR-COMET-3 trial is currently underway (ClinicalTrials.gov NCT03862911) and should provide a definitive answer in this population.

SABR-COMET also highlighted several important biological insights into oligometastatic disease. There was no significant difference between the arms in time to development of new metastases. A substantial number of patients who were treated with SBRT required further SBRT to new metastases (which was allowed in the protocol). Finally, the relatively short median PFS of 6 months, compared with the longer median OS, would point towards the overall benefit being a result of post-progression treatment benefit rather than initial treatment benefit. These data suggest that the majority of individuals who are deemed to have oligometastatic disease, by the criteria outlined here, have micrometastatic disease at the time of treatment.

Future directions

Looking at the evidence for ablative therapy in the round, there is an emerging tension between 'biology vs burden': are ablative therapies needed to treat a biological phenotype that behaves differently or to simply reduce tumour burden and thus increase survival? We need to better understand the interaction between the site of a treated metastasis, the original tumour biology and the influence of systemic therapy to optimally integrate SBRT into the treatment paradigm. The next generation of SBRT studies aims to address these issues by incorporating high-quality collaborative translational research into their design. This work will go some way towards the urgent need for better prognostic and predictive biomarkers to help tailor an individual ablative treatment course to each patient.

References

1 Wilkins EW, Burke JF, Head JM. The surgical management of metastatic neoplasms in the lung. J Thorac Cardiovasc Surg 1961; 42: 298–309.

2 Morris EJA, Forman D, Thomas JD, et al. Surgical management and outcomes of colorectal cancer liver metastases. Br J Surg 2010; 97: 1110–18.

3 Hellman S, Weichselbaum RR. Oligometastases. J Clin Oncol 1995; 13: 8–10.

4 Lievens Y, Guckenberger M, Gomez D, et al. Defining oligometastatic disease from a radiation oncology perspective: an ESTRO–ASTRO consensus document. Radiother Oncol 2020; 148: 157–66.

5 Palma DA, Louie AV, Rodrigues GB. New strategies in stereotactic radiotherapy for oligometastases. Clin Cancer Res 2015; 21: 5198–204.

6 Guckenberger M, Lievens Y, Bouma AB, et al. Characterisation and classification of oligometastatic disease: a European Society for Radiotherapy and Oncology and European Organisation for Research and Treatment of Cancer consensus recommendation. Lancet Oncol 2020; 21: e18–28.

7   Turajlic S, Swanton C. Metastasis as an evolutionary process. Science 2016; 352: 169–75.

8   Sylvester BE, Vakiani E. Tumor evolution and intratumor heterogeneity in colorectal carcinoma: insights from comparative genomic profiling of primary tumors and matched metastases. J Gastrointest Oncol 2015; 6: 668–75.

9   Brastianos PK, Carter SL, Santagata S, et al. Genomic characterization of brain metastases reveals branched evolution and potential therapeutic targets. Cancer Discov 2015; 5: 1164–77.

10   Hieronymus H, Schultz N, Gopalan A, et al. Copy number alteration burden predicts prostate cancer relapse. Proc Natl Acad Sci 2014; 111: 11139–44.

11   O'Cathail SM, Smith T, Owens R, et al. Superior outcomes of nodal metastases compared to visceral sites in oligometastatic colorectal cancer treated with stereotactic ablative radiotherapy. Radiother Oncol 2020; 151: 280–6.

12   Koebel CM, Vermi W, Swann JB, et al. Adaptive immunity maintains occult cancer in an equilibrium state. Nature 2007; 450: 903–7.

13   Pitroda SP, Khodarev NN, Huang L, et al. Integrated molecular subtyping defines a curable oligometastatic state in colorectal liver metastasis. Nat Commun 2018; 9: 1793.

14   Pastorino U, Buyse M, Friedel G, et al. Long-term results of lung metastasectomy: prognostic analyses based on 5206 cases. J Thorac Cardiovasc Surg 1997; 113: 37–49.

15   Treasure T, Farewell V, Macbeth F, et al. Pulmonary metastasectomy versus continued active monitoring in colorectal cancer (PulMiCC): a multicentre randomised clinical trial. Trials 2019; 20: 718.

16   Ruers T, Van Coevorden F, Punt CJA, et al. Local treatment of unresectable colorectal liver metastases: results of a randomized phase II trial. J Natl Cancer Inst 2017; 109: djx015.

17   Gomez DR, Tang C, Zhang J, et al. Local consolidative therapy vs. maintenance therapy or observation for patients with oligometastatic non-small-cell lung cancer: long-term results of a multi-institutional, phase II, randomized study. J Clin Oncol 2019; 37: 1558–65.

18   Palma DA, Olson R, Harrow S, et al. Stereotactic ablative radiotherapy for the comprehensive treatment of oligometastatic cancers: long-term results of the SABR-COMET phase II randomized trial. J Clin Oncol 2020; 38: 2830–8.

03 Interventional therapy for managing primary hepatic malignancy

Sadhana Shankar, Dhakshinamoorthy Vijayanand

Introduction

Primary liver cancer is the third leading cause of cancer-related mortality worldwide.[1] Hepatocellular carcinoma (HCC) accounts for more than 80% of adult cases. The rest is accounted for by cholangiocarcinoma, mixed hepatocholangiocarcinoma and the rarer malignant mesenchymal tumours.[1] Treatment of these tumours requires walking a tightrope between achieving adequate oncological control and maintaining the liver function as well as the physiological status of the patient. Interventional radiology has introduced an armamentarium of minimally invasive, safe and effective techniques to increase the available treatment options. This chapter discusses some of the technical innovations in interventional radiology that can be applied to the expanding clinical indications for treating primary liver cancers.

HCC

Pathophysiology

HCC is a malignant tumour arising from hepatocytes and is frequently found in a milieu of cirrhosis. Hepatitis B and C infection, alcohol, smoking, aflatoxins, synthetic amines, Thorotrast and radiation, as well as conditions such as haemochromatosis, alpha-1-antitrypsin deficiency and porphyria, are established risk factors which also serve as markers for early screening of HCC. HCCs may be single or multiple. Being hypervascular, they usually present as well-demarcated, encapsulated tumours with typical arterial enhancement and venous washout on contrast-enhanced CT (Figure 3.1). Advanced tumours may present as expansile or infiltrative masses with intrahepatic metastases. Diagnosis is usually based on the typical radiological appearance of the tumour, with or without a cirrhotic liver, and elevated levels of alpha-fetoprotein (AFP) and protein induced by vitamin K antagonist-II (PIVKA-II).

Management

The Barcelona Clinic Liver Cancer (BCLC) staging system is the most widely adopted protocol for treating HCC. It stratifies patients according to their tumour characteristics, underlying degree of cirrhosis and performance status and proposes the most effective holistic treatment approach.[2] Interventional therapies are indicated for BCLC stages 0, A and B; however, as technical and clinical innovations continue, the BCLC staging system has been expanded beyond these formal indications and can benefit carefully selected patients across multiple stages.[2] The interventional radiology techniques used may be broadly classified as ablative therapy or embolotherapy. Ablative treatment can be performed through percutaneous, laparoscopic or open surgical approaches and includes radiofrequency ablation, microwave ablation, cryoablation, high-intensity focused ultrasound, laser ablation, chemical ablation using ethanol, and irreversible electroporation (IRE). Embolotherapy includes transarterial embolization, transarterial chemoembolization (TACE),

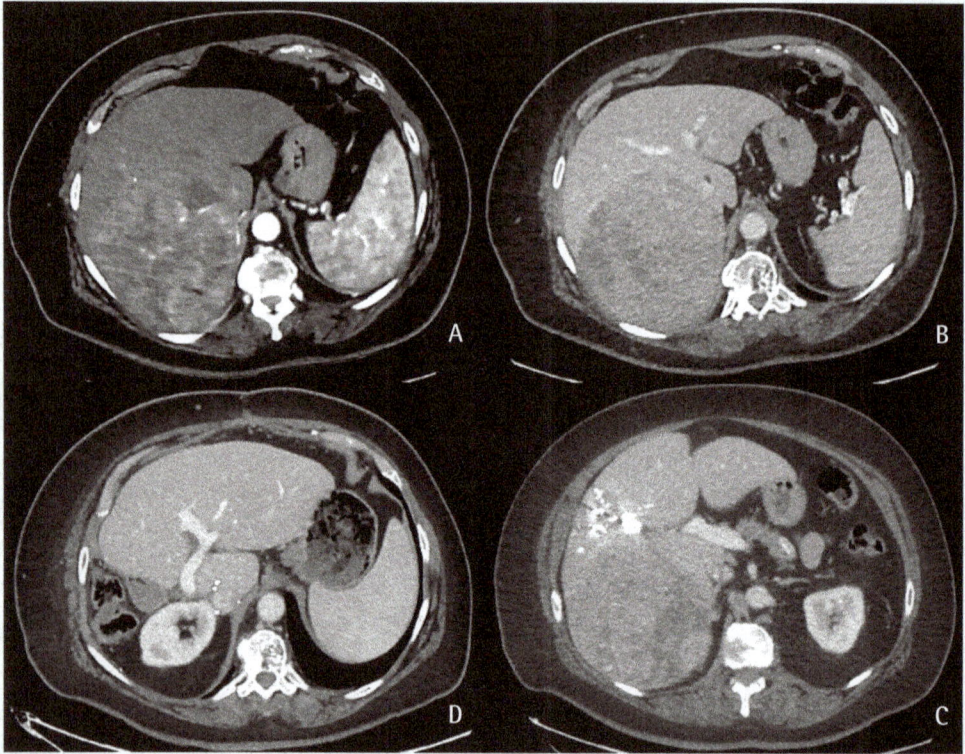

Figure 3.1 CT images of a large HCC in a patient with a non-cirrhotic liver with normal functions and good performance status. (A) Arterial phase showing tumoral enhancement; (B) venous phase showing prompt washout; (C) right portal vein embolization done to induce hypertrophy of remnant liver; embolization coils are visible; (D) remnant liver after right hemihepatectomy.

selective internal radiation therapy (SIRT) and hepatic arterial infusion therapy. Each of these modalities has its merits and demerits and may also be used in combination. How they fit into the HCC treatment paradigm is outlined below.

Interventional therapy for early- and very-early-stage HCC

Although surgery (resection or liver transplantation) is still widely considered for curative treatment of very-early-stage (a single tumour ≤2 cm in size) and early-stage HCC (three or fewer tumours ≤3 cm in size), ablation is recommended for patients precluded from surgery (Figure 3.2). Radiofrequency ablation is the most ubiquitously used ablative technique, and its effectiveness is well established in tumours ≤3 cm.[3] It is performed using a monopolar system; the high-frequency (460–480 kHz) waves generated cause intracellular desiccation and coagulative tissue necrosis. Several randomized controlled trials have shown radiofrequency ablation to be equally effective to surgical resection in terms of disease-free and overall survival (OS), with less morbidity and shorter hospital stays.[4,5] Microwave ablation using 915 MHz or 2.45 GHz causes oscillating water molecules to generate heat and produces a more homogenous ablation area. Therefore, it is now more widely used for the ablation of HCCs as it is less expensive and associated with fewer

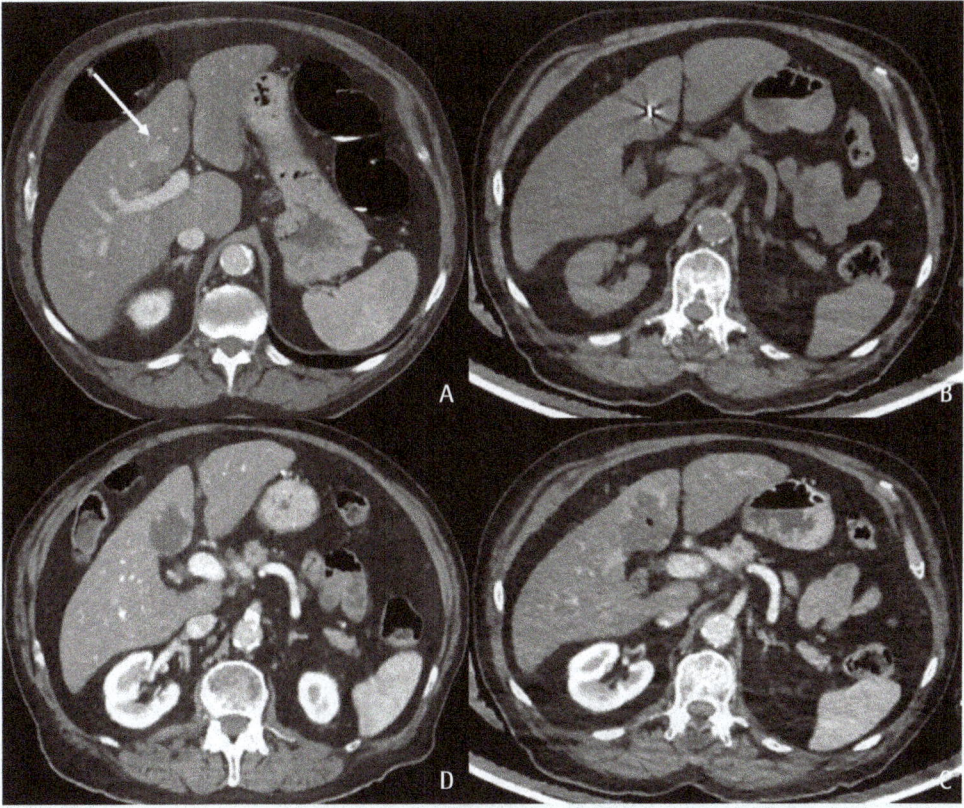

Figure 3.2 CT images of an 81-year-old man with non-alcoholic fatty liver disease and preserved liver function. (A) 2.3 cm HCC in segment IVb of the liver; (B) CT-guided insertion of radiofrequency ablation probe, visible at the site of the tumour; (C) immediate post-ablation scan showing the zone of ablation; (D) 4 weeks post-ablation showing complete response with no residual tumour.

local complications. A meta-analysis comparing the two techniques showed that microwave ablation significantly outperformed radiofrequency ablation in treating larger HCCs up to 4 cm.[6,7] Another advantage of microwave ablation is its technical effectiveness in tumours located <5 mm from major vascular structures.[8] Cryoablation, which causes rapid cooling of tissues to −140°C, causing cell death, is less frequently used because of a higher complication rate and decreased efficacy compared with radiofrequency or microwave ablation. The other techniques, such as high-intensity focused ultrasound, laser and IRE, are backed only by limited evidence and are not routinely used. By contrast, chemical ablation is outdated as it produces inferior results.

Although no formal role exists for TACE and SIRT in patients with early- or very-early-stage HCC, they offer durable control in patients who are unfit or have failed surgery or ablation. When carefully applied to well-selected patients with reasonable hepatic reserve, this concept, called 'tumour stage migration', can provide good long-term survival.[9] Furthermore, a meta-analysis showed that a combination of TACE and radiofrequency ablation produced good overall and recurrence-free survival in solitary HCCs ≤7 cm that were not amenable to curative surgery.[10]

Interventional therapy for intermediate-stage HCC

TACE is the recommended treatment strategy for multinodular tumours outside transplant criteria, without vascular invasion or extrahepatic disease and with preserved liver function. TACE takes advantage of the preferential arterial supply to HCCs and uses it to deliver highly targeted treatment. TACE may be conventional (using lipoidal emulsion) or may use drug-eluting beads or microspheres (DEB-TACE) to provide the chemotherapeutic agent (Figure 3.3). DEB-TACE has gained popularity because of the increased local effect on the tumour and decreased pain and systemic toxicity. In addition, the response to TACE is evaluated 4 weeks later using the modified Response Evaluation Criteria in Solid Tumors.[11] The process can even be effectively repeated in those with partial response or stable disease.

Interventional therapy for bringing or downstaging to liver transplantation

Liver transplantation is the recommended curative therapy for many individuals with early HCC. From an oncological perspective, preoperative tumour burden is the most crucial criterion determining eligibility and benefit from liver transplantation. The Milan criteria are the gold standard transplant criteria for HCC.[12] Several extended measures such as the University of California at San Francisco,[13] up-to-seven[14] and Toronto[15] criteria are also widely followed as selection criteria. However, disease progression while awaiting organ availability precludes a patient from having a transplant. In this scenario, loco-regional therapy in the form of TACE acts as an effective

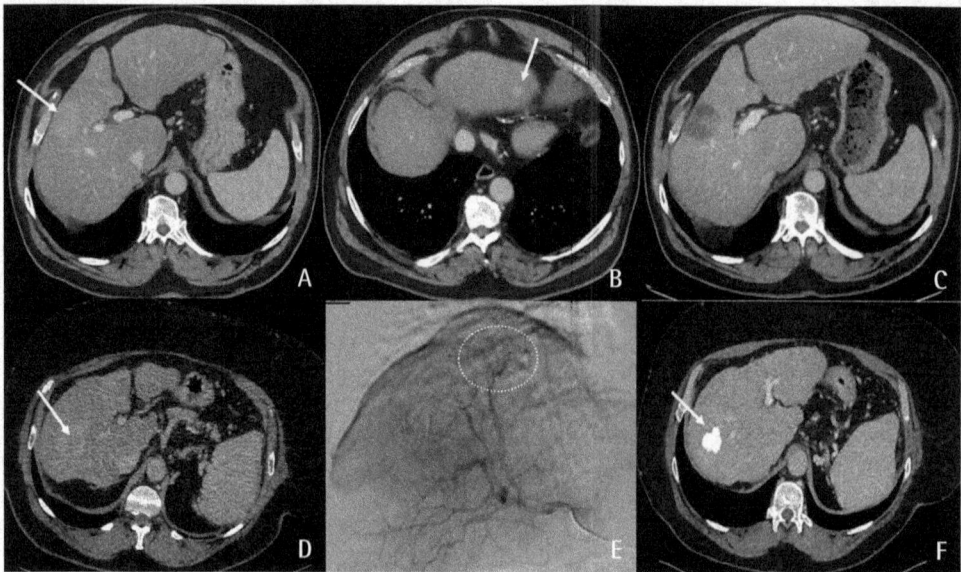

Figure 3.3 CT images of two patients with intermediate-stage HCC who underwent TACE. Top panel: a 67-year-old cirrhotic patient with (A, B) multifocal HCC in segments V and II; (C) post-DEB-TACE scan showing some viable residual tumour. Bottom panel: a 71-year-old cirrhotic patient with (D) HCC in segment VII; (E) conventional TACE with lipoidal done by selective cannulation of the tumoral vessel; (F) post-TACE scan showing uniform uptake of lipoidal emulsion and no viable residual tumour.

bridging therapy to achieve local disease control and reduce waiting list dropouts. The consensus is that patients should receive loco-regional bridging therapy when the estimated waiting time for a liver transplant is more than 6 months.[16] Also, multicentric studies have shown significant improvement in post-transplant HCC recurrence and survival in patients who received bridging therapy before liver transplantation.[17]

Alternatively, when the tumour burden exceeds the regional transplant criteria, evaluation for downstaging therapy is done. For eligible candidates, TACE or SIRT may be offered to reduce the tumour burden to within the transplant criteria. Response to treatment also predicts favourable tumour biology and an improved outcome following transplantation.[18]

Interventional therapy for advanced HCC

For patients with advanced disease, the BCLC staging system recommends systemic chemotherapy. However, for patients with significant tumour-related symptoms who cannot tolerate systemic chemotherapy, interventional therapies such as TACE or transarterial radioembolization can achieve symptom control and improve survival.[19,20] At the other end of the spectrum are patients with advanced HCC and portal vein tumour thrombus with preserved liver and systemic functions. In carefully selected patients, embolotherapy has effectively achieved local disease control and prolonged survival.[21,22] More recently, studies have shown that embolotherapy and radiotherapy can successfully downstage disease in highly selected patients with advanced HCC and macrovascular invasion to proceed to liver transplantation with good survival outcomes.[23,24] Nevertheless, it is essential to remember that a multidisciplinary approach should always be considered for selecting and managing a wide array of patients.

Cholangiocarcinoma

Pathophysiology and management

Cholangiocarcinoma is a malignant tumour arising from the biliary epithelium and may be classified as intrahepatic (peripheral) or extrahepatic (hilar). Unlike HCC, it often occurs in a non-cirrhotic liver. It is usually associated with risk factors such as primary sclerosing cholangitis, hepatolithiasis, biliary parasitic infections, cystic liver diseases, smoking, obesity and chemical carcinogens. Extrahepatic cholangiocarcinoma may be sclerosing, papillary or nodular, whereas intrahepatic cholangiocarcinoma may be mass-forming or infiltrative. Diagnosis is based on clinical features of obstructive jaundice combined with imaging characteristics of a hypovascular lesion alongside dilated bile ducts; tissue biopsy is often required for confirmation.

Interventional therapy as an adjunct to surgery

Surgical resection forms the mainstay of the treatment of cholangiocarcinoma. However, interventional radiology is essential in patients with potentially resectable disease with a small liver remnant and in those with unresectable disease due to advanced stage. Portal vein embolization is commonly used to promote hypertrophy of the remnant liver before primary surgical resection, to prevent liver failure. Recently, venous liver deprivation, which includes embolization of hepatic venous outflow and portal inflow, has gained popularity as it produces marked and rapid hypertrophy of the liver remnant. Another important role of interventional radiology is percutaneous transhepatic cholangiography (PTC) in patients with severe obstructive jaundice and failed endoscopic intervention. PTC may be used for stenting the obstructed biliary system, obtaining tissue diagnosis and improving the presurgical optimization of the patient. In addition, several studies have demonstrated that thermal ablative techniques and embolotherapy may be used as an adjunct to downstage the disease before surgery, to achieve better local control with a marginal improvement in OS.[25,26] However, the rationale for choosing patients is entirely dependent on the individual centre's experience.

Interventional therapy for inoperable or recurrent cholangiocarcinoma

Current evidence suggests that palliative interventional therapy is safe, feasible and effective for control of inoperable or recurrent intrahepatic cholangiocarcinoma after resection.[26–28] TACE and SIRT are the most widely used techniques and are well tolerated even in patients with aggressive invasion. The favourable prognostic factors following TACE include good liver function, objective tumour response and low tumour extent.[29] The major drawback is the risk of ischaemia to the biliary tree, causing necrosis and bilomas with subsequent superinfection, which reaches a frequency of up to 30%.[29] On the other hand, SIRT is rarely associated with biliary complications, and the tumour response depends highly on the radiation dose delivered. So, a good tumour response with improved OS is feasible with SIRT by careful patient selection and individualizing dosing prescriptions.[30] Ablative techniques play a minor role in managing inoperable intrahepatic cholangiocarcinoma. However, a meta-analysis showed that small tumours (≤3 cm) in unfit patients could be reasonable candidates for thermal ablation and provide good OS.[26] Hepatic arterial infusion is yet another novel technique for delivering high-dose chemotherapy directly to the liver through a pump. Several trials (ClinicalTrials.gov NCT05400902 and NCT05290116) are underway to define its efficacy and tolerability as a first-line treatment for inoperable cholangiocarcinoma.

Conclusion

Interventional radiology plays an essential role in the management of primary liver cancers. Techniques such as percutaneous ablation and TACE are often well tolerated and serve as effective therapeutic and palliative options. Careful patient selection, individualized treatment techniques and multidisciplinary management form the crux of successful treatment.

References

1 Ferlay J, Ervik M, Lam F, et al. (2020). Global Cancer Observatory. Cancer today. Available from: https://gco.iarc.fr (accessed 7 February 2023).

2 Reig M, Forner A, Rimola J, et al. BCLC strategy for prognosis prediction and treatment recommendation: the 2022 update. J Hepatol 2022; 76: 681–93.

3 Doyle A, Gorgen A, Muaddi H, et al. Outcomes of radiofrequency ablation as first-line therapy for hepatocellular carcinoma less than 3 cm in potentially transplantable patients. J Hepatol 2019; 70: 866–73.

4 Chen MS, Li JQ, Zheng Y, et al. A prospective randomized trial comparing percutaneous local ablative therapy and partial hepatectomy for small hepatocellular carcinoma. Ann Surg 2006; 243: 321.

5 Feng K, Yan J, Li X, et al. A randomized controlled trial of radiofrequency ablation and surgical resection in the treatment of small hepatocellular carcinoma. J Hepatol 2012; 57: 794–802.

6   Facciorusso A, Di Maso M, Muscatiello N. Microwave ablation versus radiofrequency ablation for the treatment of hepatocellular carcinoma: a systematic review and meta-analysis. Int J Hyperthermia 2016; 32: 339–44.

7   Han J, Fan YC, Wang K. Radiofrequency ablation versus microwave ablation for early-stage hepatocellular carcinoma: a PRISMA-compliant systematic review and meta-analysis. Medicine (Baltimore) 2020; 99: e22703.

8   Huang S, Yu J, Liang P, et al. Percutaneous microwave ablation for hepatocellular carcinoma adjacent to large vessels: a long-term follow-up. Eur J Radiol 2014; 83: 552–8.

9   Chang Y, Jeong SW, Young Jang J, Jae Kim Y. Recent updates of transarterial chemoembolization in hepatocellular carcinoma. Int J Mol Sci 2020; 21: 8165.

10 Guo W, He X, Li Z, Li Y. Combination of transarterial chemoembolization (TACE) and radiofrequency ablation (RFA) vs surgical resection (SR) on survival outcome of early hepatocellular carcinoma: a meta-analysis. Hepatogastroenterology 2015; 62: 710–14.

11 Lencioni R, Llovet JM. Modified RECIST (mRECIST) assessment for hepatocellular carcinoma. Semin Liver Dis 2010; 30: 52–60.

12 Mazzaferro V, Regalia E, Doci R, et al. Liver transplantation for the treatment of small hepatocellular carcinomas in patients with cirrhosis. N Engl J Med 1996; 334: 693–700.

13 Yao FY, Ferrell L, Bass NM, et al. Liver transplantation for hepatocellular carcinoma: expansion of the tumor size limits does not adversely impact survival. Hepatology 2001; 33: 1394–403.

14 Mazzaferro V, Llovet JM, Miceli R, et al. Predicting survival after liver transplantation in patients with hepatocellular carcinoma beyond the Milan criteria: a retrospective, exploratory analysis. Lancet Oncol 2009; 10: 35–43.

15 DuBay D, Sandroussi C, Sandhu L, et al. Liver transplantation for advanced hepatocellular carcinoma using poor tumor differentiation on biopsy as an exclusion criterion. Ann Surg 2011; 253: 166–72.

16 Clavien PA, Lesurtel M, Bossuyt PM, et al. Recommendations for liver transplantation for hepatocellular carcinoma: an international consensus conference report. Lancet Oncol 2012; 13: e11–22.

17 Oligane HC, Xing M, Kim HS. Effect of bridging local-regional therapy on recurrence of hepatocellular carcinoma and survival after orthotopic liver transplantation. Radiology 2017; 282: 869–79.

18 Finkenstedt A, Vikoler A, Portenkirchner M, et al. Excellent post-transplant survival in patients with intermediate stage hepatocellular carcinoma responding to neoadjuvant therapy. Liver Int 2016; 36: 688–95.

19 Vilgrain V, Pereira H, Assenat E, et al. Efficacy and safety of selective internal radiotherapy with yttrium-90 resin microspheres compared with sorafenib in locally advanced and inoperable hepatocellular carcinoma (SARAH): an open-label randomised controlled phase 3 trial. Lancet Oncol 2017; 18: 1624–36.

20 Kalva SP, Pectasides M, Liu R, et al. Safety and effectiveness of chemoembolization with drug-eluting beads for advanced-stage hepatocellular carcinoma. Cardiovasc Intervent Radiol 2014; 37: 381–7.

21 Xue TC, Xie XY, Zhang L, et al. Transarterial chemoembolization for hepatocellular carcinoma with portal vein tumor thrombus: a meta-analysis. BMC Gastroenterol 2013; 13: 1–9.

22 Luo J, Guo RP, Lai EC, et al. Transarterial chemoembolization for unresectable hepatocellular carcinoma with portal vein tumor thrombosis: a prospective comparative study. Ann Surg Oncol 2011; 18: 413–20.

23 Pommergaard HC, Rostved AA, Adam R, et al. Vascular invasion and survival after liver transplantation for hepatocellular carcinoma: a study from the European Liver Transplant Registry. HPB (Oxford) 2018; 20: 768–75.

24 Choi JY, Jeong IY, Park HC, et al. The possibility of radiotherapy as downstaging to living donor liver transplantation for hepatocellular carcinoma with portal vein tumor thrombus. Liver Transpl 2017; 23: 545–51.

25 Butros SR, Shenoy-Bhangle A, Mueller PR, Arellano RS. Radiofrequency ablation of intrahepatic cholangiocarcinoma: feasability, local tumor control, and long-term outcome. Clin Imaging 2014; 38: 490–4.

26 Kim GH, Kim PH, Kim JH, et al. Thermal ablation in the treatment of intrahepatic cholangiocarcinoma: a systematic review and meta-analysis. Eur Radiol 2022; 32: 1205–15.

27 Yang J, Wang J, Zhou H, et al. Efficacy and safety of endoscopic radiofrequency ablation for unresectable extrahepatic cholangiocarcinoma: a randomized trial. Endoscopy 2018; 50: 751–60.

28 Han K, Ko HK, Kim KW, et al. Radiofrequency ablation in the treatment of unresectable intrahepatic cholangiocarcinoma: systematic review and meta-analysis. J Vasc Interv Radiol 2015; 26: 943–8.

29 Vogl TJ, Naguib NN, Nour-Eldin NE, et al. Transarterial chemoembolization in the treatment of patients with unresectable cholangiocarcinoma: results and prognostic factors governing treatment success. Int J Cancer 2012; 131: 733–40.

30 Camacho JC, Kokabi N, Xing M, et al. Modified Response Evaluation Criteria in Solid Tumors and European Association for the Study of the Liver criteria using delayed-phase imaging at an early time point predict survival in patients with unresectable intrahepatic cholangiocarcinoma following yttrium-90 radioembolization. J Vasc Interv Radiol 2014; 25: 256–65.

04 Renal cancer: definitions, biology and management

Maxine G. B. Tran

Introduction

Renal cancer is the 14th most common cancer, representing around 3% of all cancers affecting humans, with more than 430,000 new cases globally each year.[1] The incidence of renal cancer is increasing with associated risk factors of obesity, hypertension and smoking. Inherited genetic predisposition syndromes are thought to account for between 3% and 5% of cases.[2]

The most recent WHO classification describes over 50 histopathological entities, with a new subcategory of molecularly defined renal carcinomas such as fumarate hydratase-deficient renal cell carcinoma (RCC) and succinate dehydrogenase (SDH)-deficient RCC.[3] However, the most common renal cancer types are clear cell, papillary and chromophobe. Up to 30% of renal tumours have benign histology, the most frequent of which are oncocytomas and angiomyolipomas.[2] Longitudinal studies show that small renal cancers (<4 cm) generally exhibit a slow growth rate at an average of 0.19 cm/year. There is notable variability within and between histological subtypes, with clear cell renal carcinoma growing the most rapidly.[4]

Internationally accepted clinical guidelines recommend offering surgery to achieve a cure in localized renal cancer, and that nephron-sparing surgery (partial nephrectomy) should be performed whenever technically possible.[2] Early-stage (cT1, <4 cm) disease has an excellent prognosis with low metastatic potential (1–2%); increasingly, conservative management strategies are being considered, including ablative therapy, active surveillance and watchful waiting.[2] In fact, despite renal cancer being the most lethal of all urological malignancies, death from competing causes of risk outweighs the risk of death due to renal cancer in almost all categories of patient age, comorbidity and tumour size among individuals with cT1 tumours.[5]

Recent developments

The increased use of cross-sectional imaging has led to increased detection of 'renal incidentalomas' and a migration shift in stage of diagnosis to early small renal masses (<4 cm). Earlier diagnosis and an estimated 50% increase in the rate of nephrectomies over the last two decades has, however, had no significant impact on overall kidney cancer mortality,[6] suggesting an element of overdiagnosis and overtreatment. There is therefore mounting interest and clinical need for better disease stratification and treatment options.

The use of renal tumour biopsy has changed from previously being considered of limited value by all the major clinical guidelines to being more acceptable and a useful risk-stratifying tool.[2] This change in practice is clearly evident from a recent update from the DISSRM registry (ClinicalTrials.gov NCT02346435), showing an increase from 5% to 20% of patients having a renal tumour biopsy.[7] The utility of histological diagnosis needs to be balanced, however, with the risks of bleeding and pain as well as the uncertain clinical significance of biopsy tract seeding.[8–10] Clearly, there is space for improvement in the diagnostic pathway for renal masses, and non-invasive alternative approaches to renal tumour biopsy and extirpative surgery are therefore highly pursued. Research into novel imaging techniques such as ^{99m}Tc-sestamibi single-photon emission CT,[11,12] ^{89}Zr-girentuximab PET-CT[12,13] and prostate-specific membrane antigen PET[12,14] have now progressed into clinical trial stage on the pathway to clinical implementation.

A recent multidisciplinary collaboration between clinicians, researchers and patients identified as a research priority exploration of treatment options to minimize side effects and increase effectiveness of therapy and maximize quality of life.[15] Therapeutic approaches such as ablation (cryotherapy, radiofrequency, high-frequency ultrasound and microwave) and non-thermal irreversible electroporation have been generally favourable for cT1a tumours, but the strength of the evidence base has been hindered by non-randomized comparative studies and the absence of randomized controlled trials (RCTs).[2] Current guidelines therefore recommend thermal ablation only for frail and/or comorbid patients with small renal masses.[2] Stereotactic body radiotherapy (SBRT) has also been used as a treatment option for patients with localized renal cancer who are not able to have surgery[2]; however, studies have shown viable tumour cells in post-SBRT biopsies, and persistence of CT visualization of contrast enhancement in tumours following SBRT treatment has limited suitable outcome measures other than non-progression of disease.[2,16] Evidently, well-designed RCTs are required to robustly compare and inform the effectiveness of alternative therapies to surgery in the treatment of renal cancer.[17]

Conclusion

Historically, renal cancer was thought to be one disease, for which surgery was the only curative treatment available. As our understanding of the biology of renal cancers has advanced, so has our management approach, which must continue to evolve. The recognition that not all renal tumours are cancers, that not all cancers need surgery, and that surgery may not necessarily be the only effective treatment option signifies the huge progress that has been made over the last two decades in clinical understanding. Future developments will depend on continued multidisciplinary research collaboration to produce high-level clinical trial evidence. Only then will there be a meaningful impact on clinical practice and improved treatment outcomes for all patients with kidney cancer.

References

1 World Cancer Research Fund International (2020). Kidney cancer statistics. Available from: www.wcrf.org/cancer-trends/kidney-cancer-statistics (accessed 12 September 2022).

2 Ljungberg B, Albiges L, Bedke J, et al. (2022). EAU guidelines on renal cell carcinoma. Available from: https://d56bochluxqnz.cloudfront.net/documents/full-guideline/EAU-Guidelines-on-Renal-Cell-Carinoma-2022.pdf (accessed 12 September 2022).

3 Moch H, Amin MB, Berney DM, et al. The 2022 World Health Organization classification of tumours of the urinary system and male genital organs. Part A: renal, penile, and testicular tumours. Eur Urol 2022; 82: 458–68.

4 Finelli A, Cheung DC, Al-Matar A, et al. Small renal mass surveillance: histology-specific growth rates in a biopsy-characterized cohort. Eur Urol 2020; 78: 460–7.

5 Patel HD, Kates M, Pierorazio PM, et al. Survival after diagnosis of localized T1a kidney cancer: current population-based practice of surgery and nonsurgical management. Urology 2014; 83: 126–32.

6   Welch HG, Skinner JS, Schroeck FR, et al. Regional variation of computed tomographic imaging in the United States and the risk of nephrectomy. JAMA Intern Med 2018; 178: 221–7.

7   Uzosike AC, Patel HD, Alam R, et al. Growth kinetics of small renal masses on active surveillance: variability and results from the DISSRM registry. J Urol 2018; 199: 641–8.

8   Turajlic S, Xu H, Litchfield K, et al. Deterministic evolutionary trajectories influence primary tumor growth: TRACERx renal. Cell 2018; 173: 595–610.

9   Patel HD, Johnson MH, Pierorazio PM, et al. Diagnostic accuracy and risks of biopsy in the diagnosis of a renal mass suspicious for localized renal cell carcinoma: systematic review of the literature. J Urol 2016; 195: 1340–7.

10 Macklin PS, Sullivan ME, Tapping CR, et al. Tumour seeding in the tract of percutaneous renal tumour biopsy: a report on seven cases from a UK tertiary referral centre. Eur Urol 2019; 75: 861–7.

11 Warren H, Boydell AR, Reza A, et al. Use of ^{99m}Tc-sestamibi SPECT/CT for indeterminate renal tumours: a pilot diagnostic accuracy study. BJU Int 2022; 130: 748–50.

12 Roussel E, Capitanio U, Kutikov A, et al. Novel imaging methods for renal mass characterization: a collaborative review. Eur Urol 2022; 81: 476–88.

13 Merkx RIJ, Lobeek D, Konijnenberg M, et al. Phase I study to assess safety, biodistribution and radiation dosimetry for ^{89}Zr-girentuximab in patients with renal cell carcinoma. Eur J Nucl Med Mol Imaging 2021; 48: 3277–85.

14 Muselaers S, Erdem S, Bertolo R, et al. PSMA PET/CT in renal cell carcinoma: an overview of current literature. J Clin Med 2022; 11: 1829.

15 Rossi SH, Blick C, Handforth C, et al. Essential research priorities in renal cancer: a modified Delphi consensus statement. Eur Urol Focus 2020; 6: 991–8.

16 Correa RJM, Louie AV, Zaorsky NG, et al. The emerging role of stereotactic ablative radiotherapy for primary renal cell carcinoma: a systematic review and meta-analysis. Eur Urol Focus 2019; 5: 958–69.

17 Neves JB, Cullen D, Grant L, et al. Protocol for a feasibility study of a cohort embedded randomised controlled trial comparing nephron sparing treatment (NEST) for small renal masses. BMJ Open 2019; 9: e030965.

05 Lung cancers: biology, evidence and management of primary and secondary lung cancers using percutaneous thermal ablation

Ewan Mark Anderson, Shyamal Saujani

Introduction

Lung cancer is the second most common cancer in both men and women and remains a leading cause of cancer death, representing close to 20% of cancer-related deaths.[1] The lung is also a common site of metastases from a range of malignant tumours, particularly sarcoma and colorectal cancer. The introduction of CT screening for early-stage lung cancer and the more widespread use of chest CT in postsurgical follow-up after primary tumour resection potentially allow for the identification of lung tumours at an early stage.

While surgical resection remains the gold standard treatment of early-stage non-small-cell lung cancer (NSCLC), it is also the case that many patients will be considered inoperable because of medical comorbidities. Similarly, while surgery (metastasectomy) has demonstrated efficacy for the treatment of secondary tumours, again medical comorbidity or distribution of disease may render patients inoperable. In both patient groups, minimally invasive techniques have emerged as an option for inoperable patients.

Over the past two decades, there has been increasing evidence that percutaneous thermal ablation (pTA) can provide an effective therapy aimed at radically treating both primary and secondary lung tumours. In selected cases, the outcomes may be similar to those of other localized or ablative techniques.

What techniques are available for pTA?

Currently available modalities for pTA include radiofrequency ablation, microwave ablation and cryoablation. The destruction of tissue is achieved by directly applying extreme temperatures into the tumour via a percutaneously placed applicator.

During radiofrequency ablation, an electric current passes from the applicator tip to grounding pads elsewhere on the patient. The current alternates at a frequency of around 400 kHz causing charged particle agitation and frictional heating close to the applicator. Conduction of initial heating through the target volume can achieve temperatures of between 60°C and 100°C necessary for cellular death.

Microwave ablation uses the propagation of electromagnetic radiation from the applicator through the tissues that varies between 915 and 2450 MHz. This causes water molecules to rotate, gain kinetic energy and cause direct tissue heating. Microwave ablation produces a more uniform ablation zone, and temperature peaks occur much faster than in radiofrequency ablation.[2]

The expansion of gases can cause marked cooling that is used during cryoablation to generate sub-zero temperatures, forming an ice ball to cover the tumour. Cytotoxic cell destruction is achieved at temperatures below −20°C.[3] After the freezing phase, a thawing phase follows by replacing the liquefied gas with helium or internally heating the needle. The whole freeze–thaw process is repeated until effective ablation is obtained.

Whatever ablation modality is used, target identification and needle guidance are achieved using CT or cone beam CT. The inherent contrast between the low-density lung parenchyma and the target lesion facilitates its identification and tracking of the applicator without the need for iodinated contrast.

All procedures may be performed using conscious sedation with local anaesthesia or general anaesthesia. The procedure itself may be painful, particularly when close to the pleura. Under conscious sedation it is necessary for the patient to remain cooperative and able to hold their breath during the procedure, which may be problematic. If general anaesthesia is used, the anaesthetic staff can take care of and monitor the patient while the radiologist can concentrate on the procedure itself. Furthermore, it is possible to minimize respiratory excursion during the procedure, which can help identification of small lesions and facilitate the accurate placement of the applicator. When directly compared, general anaesthesia can reduce the technical challenge of applicator placement without any additional time penalty.[4]

Patient selection for treatment of primary and secondary lung cancers

NSCLC

As pTA techniques can only attempt to control the primary tumour, they are therefore only suitable for treating early-stage NSCLC (stage 1A and 1B) with curative intent. National guidelines would recommend primary surgery for suitable patients, with pTA reserved for those considered medically inoperable[5]; European recommendations would add the caveat that stereotactic body radiotherapy should also be contraindicated ahead of a decision to use pTA.[6] The degree to which patients are considered unfit for surgery may be based on objective assessment (Table 5.1) and the

Table 5.1 Definition of high-risk operable NSCLC used in the American College of Surgeons Oncology Group Z4032 trial (adapted from Fernando et al.[7]).

Major criteria
FEV$_1$ ≤50% predicted
DLCO ≤50% predicted
Minor criteria
Age ≥75 years
FEV$_1$ 51–60% predicted
DLCO 51–60% predicted
Pulmonary hypertension
Poor left ventricular function (ejection fraction ≤40%)
Resting or exercise arterial PO_2 ≤55 mmHg or SpO_2 ≤88%
PCO_2 >45 mmHg

DLCO, diffusing capacity for carbon monoxide; FEV$_1$, forced expiratory volume; PCO_2, partial pressure of carbon dioxide; PO_2, partial pressure of oxygen; SpO_2, peripheral oxygen saturation.

presence of either one major or two minor criteria defining a high-risk population.[7] Overall the proportion of patients unfit for surgery may be around 15%; however, the proportion increases with age and at 75 years may represent as many as 30% of potentially resectable cases.[8]

The decision to treat a patient with pTA should preferably be made by a multidisciplinary team (MDT) including thoracic surgeons, respiratory physicians, medical oncologists, radiation oncologists and radiologists with expertise in lung ablation. The decision is further complicated by the increasing recognition of ground-glass nodules on CT that may represent early-stage lung adenocarcinomas. These preinvasive nodules can progress over time to become invasive lung adenocarcinomas. Lesions in this developmental pathway are termed 'adenocarcinoma spectrum' lesions.

Adenocarcinoma is the commonest lung cancer subtype, accounting for 50% of all lung cancer diagnoses, and its frequency is increasing. It is the predominant subtype found using low-dose CT screening; for example, the experience in European screening was that 60% of screen-detected lesions were adenocarcinoma with 20% squamous cell carcinoma, compared with 44% and 31%, respectively, in a non-screened control group.[9] Pure ground-glass nodules are likely to represent lesions of low malignant potential, either atypical adenomatous hyperplasia or adenocarcinoma *in situ*. As lesions enlarge or develop a small solid component, invasive adenocarcinoma is more likely. For patients considered for lung ablation, it is often not technically possible to seek tissue confirmation of malignancy and it is necessary to consider imaging indicators. Interval growth, defined as an increase in maximal diameter ≥ 2 mm, is strongly predictive of malignancy[10] and may prompt consideration of intervention. Similarly, there are scoring systems, incorporating clinical, morphological and PET-CT features of the nodules, to quantify the risk of malignancy.[11]

Current evidence for use of pTA in NSCLC

The greatest body of evidence is for treatment of NSCLC with radiofrequency ablation. Early, large series reported control of the primary tumour in 47% of patients, with 3 and 5 year survival of 36% and 27%, respectively.[12] Improvements in patient and tumour selection, along with improved ablation procedural techniques, have been reflected in improvements in both tumour control and survival. A more recent large series achieved local tumour control in 79% of 87 patients, with 3 and 5 year overall survival (OS) of 66% and 58%, respectively.[13]

As it is a newer technique, there are fewer mature data on microwave ablation. Similar to the initial experience with radiofrequency ablation, the early reporting series found moderate local tumour control at 3 and 5 years of 64% and 48%, respectively, with OS of 43% and 16% at 3 and 5 years, respectively.[14] More recent reports have shown improved local control in up to 95% of treated cases, with consequently improved survival of 45% at 5 years.[15]

In contrast to the radiofrequency and microwave ablation literature, there are only a handful of studies reporting outcomes after cryoablation. Local control is reported to be similar to that in early reports of radiofrequency or microwave ablation, with recurrence seen in 36% of patients.[16]

Lung metastases

Surgical resection of pulmonary metastases is an accepted standard of care for a number of tumour types.[17] There is a growing consensus that ablative therapies including pTA and radiotherapy along with surgery may offer an effective treatment for suitably selected patients with metastatic disease.[18]

In selecting patients for pTA, it is important that the extent of pulmonary metastatic disease is limited and can be completely treated. This is usually taken to be between five and six lesions ≤ 3.0 cm in diameter. Extrapulmonary disease should similarly be limited to and also completely treatable with ablative techniques. Consideration of disease biology such as interval between primary tumour resection and metastatic occurrence or response to systemic therapy may also influence decisions to treat. Patients with limited life expectancy (less than 12 months) or poor performance status (ECOG ≥2) may be considered unsuitable. Common cancer types suitable for this approach would include colorectal sarcoma, renal cell carcinoma and melanoma. These complex cases require discussion at a suitable site specialty MDT meeting.

Current evidence for use of pTA in lung metastases

The published results of pTA use in the context of oligometastatic lung disease are primarily from cohort studies, and the predominant tumour type is from colorectal primaries. Large cohort studies of more than 200 patients treated with radiofrequency ablation have reported 5 year OS of around 50%,[19,20] with local tumour control of 92%.[19] This is very similar to results reported in the surgical literature. The data on microwave ablation, though less mature than the data on radiofrequency ablation, are encouraging. Local tumour control appears comparable to that of the best published radiofrequency ablation results, with similar OS at 3 years of 60%.[21]

Conclusion and future perspectives

Image-guided pTA has been proven to be a safe and effective treatment for early-stage NSCLC and secondary lung cancer. However, there are limitations including a lack of procedural standardization as well as heterogeneity in the published results, both in control of the treated tumour and how it may influence survival. Studies are often limited to relatively small cohorts from single centres. It is clear that improvements in the planning and execution of pTA have resulted in better published outcomes. As the data mature, it is hoped that lung ablation can achieve equipoise in comparison to surgical resection similar to that seen in other organ systems.

References

1 Siegel RL, Miller KD, Jemal A. Cancer statistics, 2019. CA Cancer J Clin 2019; 69: 7 34.

2 Simon CJ, Dupuy DE, Mayo-Smith WW. Microwave ablation: principles and applications. RadioGraphics 2005; 25 (suppl 1): S69–83.

3 Cazzato RL, Garnon J, Ramamurthy N, et al. Percutaneous image guided cryoablation: current applications and results in the oncologic field. Med Oncol 2016; 33: 140.

4 Chung DYF, Tse DML, Boardman P, et al. High-frequency jet ventilation under general anesthesia facilitates CT-guided lung tumor thermal ablation compared with normal respiration under conscious analgesic sedation. J Vasc Interv Radiol 2014; 25: 1463–9.

5 Ettinger DS, Wood DE, Aggarwal C, et al. NCCN guidelines insights: non-small cell lung cancer, version 1.2020. J Natl Compr Canc Netw 2019; 17: 1464–72.

6 Vansteenkiste J, Crinò L, Dooms C, et al. 2nd ESMO Consensus Conference on Lung Cancer: early-stage non-small-cell lung cancer consensus on diagnosis, treatment and follow-up. Ann Oncol 2014; 25: 1462–74.

7 Fernando HC, Landreneau RJ, Mandrekar SJ, et al. Impact of brachytherapy on local recurrence rates after sublobar resection: results from ACOSOG Z4032 (Alliance), a phase III randomized trial for high-risk operable non-small-cell lung cancer. J Clin Oncol 2014; 32: 2456–62.

8 Mery CM, Pappas AN, Bueno R, et al. Similar long-term survival of elderly patients with non-small cell lung cancer treated with lobectomy or wedge resection within the surveillance, epidemiology, and end results database. Chest 2005; 128: 237–45.

9 de Koning HJ, van der Aalst CM, de Jong PA, et al. Reduced lung-cancer mortality with volume CT screening in a randomized trial. N Engl J Med 2020; 382: 503–13.

10 Callister ME, Baldwin DR, Akram AR, et al. British Thoracic Society guidelines for the investigation and management of pulmonary nodules. Thorax 2015; 70 (suppl 2): ii1–54.

11 Herder GJ, van Tinteren H, Golding RP, et al. Clinical prediction model to characterize pulmonary nodules. Chest 2005; 128: 2490–6.

12 Simon CJ, Dupuy DE, DiPetrillo TA, et al. Pulmonary radiofrequency ablation: long-term safety and efficacy in 153 patients. Radiology 2007; 243: 268–75.

13 Palussière J, Lagarde P, Aupérin A, et al. Percutaneous lung thermal ablation of non-surgical clinical N0 non-small cell lung cancer: results of eight years' experience in 87 patients from two centers. Cardiovasc Intervent Radiol 2015; 38: 160–6.

14 Healey TT, March BT, Baird G, Dupuy DE. Microwave ablation for lung neoplasms: a retrospective analysis of long-term results. J Vasc Interv Radiol 2017; 28: 206–11.

15 Nance M, Khazi Z, Kaifi J, et al. Computerized tomography-guided microwave ablation of patients with stage I non-small cell lung cancers: a single-institution retrospective study. J Clin Imaging Sci 2021; 11: 7.

16 Moore W, Talati R, Bhattacharji P, Bilfinger T. Five-year survival after cryoablation of stage I non-small cell lung cancer in medically inoperable patients. J Vasc Interv Radiol 2015; 26: 312–19.

17 Cheung FPY, Alam NZ, Wright GM. The past, present and future of pulmonary metastasectomy: a review article. Ann Thorac Cardiovasc Surg 2019; 25: 129–41.

18 van Cutsem E, Cervantes A, Adam R, et al. ESMO consensus guidelines for the management of patients with metastatic colorectal cancer. Ann Oncol 2016; 27: 1386–422.

19 de Baère T, Aupérin A, Deschamps F, et al. Radiofrequency ablation is a valid treatment option for lung metastases: experience in 566 patients with 1037 metastases. Ann Oncol 2015; 26: 987–91.

20 Fonck M, Perez JT, Catena V, et al. Pulmonary thermal ablation enables long chemotherapy-free survival in metastatic colorectal cancer patients. Cardiovasc Intervent Radiol 2018; 41: 1727–34.

21 Kurilova I, Gonzalez-Aguirre A, Beets-Tan RG, et al. Microwave ablation in the management of colorectal cancer pulmonary metastases. Cardiovasc Intervent Radiol 2018; 41: 1530–44.

06 Pancreatic cancer: definitions, biology and surgical perspective

Rahul Sreekumar, Declan McDonnell, Zaed Hamady

Introduction

Cancer of the exocrine pancreas accounts for approximately 3% of new cancer diagnoses annually.[1] Although rare in incidence, it is the fourth leading cause of cancer-related mortality. Surgical resection remains the only curative treatment option. The vast majority (>80%) of patients, however, present with metastatic disease and have poor survival outcomes (Figure 6.1).[2] Furthermore, most patients who undergo a curative resection experience disease recurrence within 2 years, with 5 year survival rates of less than 25%. In this chapter we discuss the tumour biology, clinical presentation, diagnostic evaluation, assessment of resectability and role of surgical palliation in pancreatic cancer.

Tumorigenesis and precursor lesions

Pancreatic carcinogenesis follows a multistep process analogous to the adenoma–carcinoma sequence described for colorectal cancer. The precursor lesions are small, asymptomatic and radiologically occult. Pancreatic intraepithelial neoplasia (PanIN), intraductal papillary mucinous neoplasia and mucinous cystic neoplasm are precursor lesions that have a well-described risk of malignant transformation. The commonest of these precursor lesions are PanINs, which account for approximately 80% of lesions identified in resected pancreatic specimens. PanINs are further

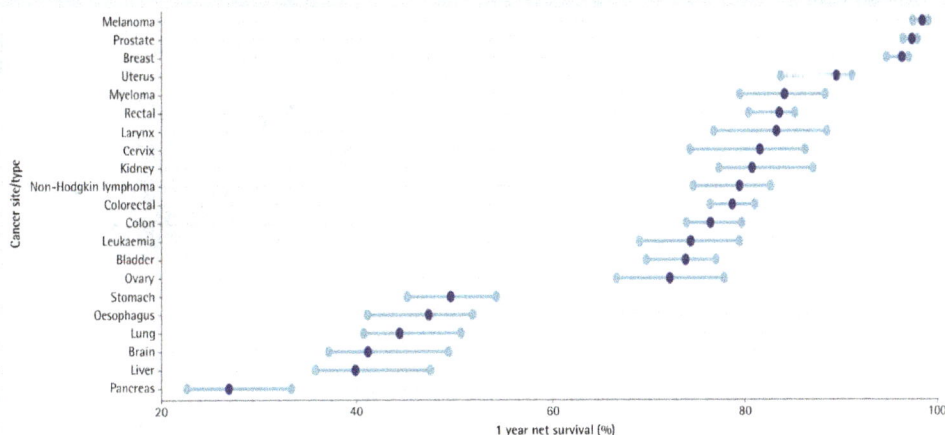

Figure 6.1 Survival outcomes of common malignancies in England (dark blue) and 21 cancer alliances (light blue) (reproduced from NHS Digital[2]).

Table 6.1 Common somatic mutations in PDAC.		
Gene	Chromosome	Cancers with mutation (%)
KRAS	12p	95
CDKN2A	9p	>90
TP53	17p	75
SMAD4	18q	55

pathologically subclassified into low-grade (PanIN-1) and high-grade (PanIN-2/PanIN-3) lesions based on the extent of cellular atypia exhibited.

Evidence that PanINs harbour the capacity to undergo malignant transformation comes from genetic studies that have demonstrated a stepwise accrual of critical mutations (Table 6.1) in precursor lesions, resulting in cellular dedifferentiation and malignant transformation. Critical genes implicated in this process include KRAS, TP53, SMAD4 and CDKN2A (also known as P16) (Figure 6.2).[3] The commonest mutation observed in pancreatic ductal adenocarcinoma (PDAC) is of the KRAS gene, which is found in >90% of PDACs and 45% of low-grade PanINs. Mutations in these critical genes cause aberrant activation of downstream cellular pathways that promote malignant transformation. While a stepwise sequence from PanINs to PDACs has been described, the true genetic profile of these tumours is highly diverse and complex. Whole genome sequencing of PDACs is beginning to shed light on the diverse genetic signatures that drive tumorigenesis,

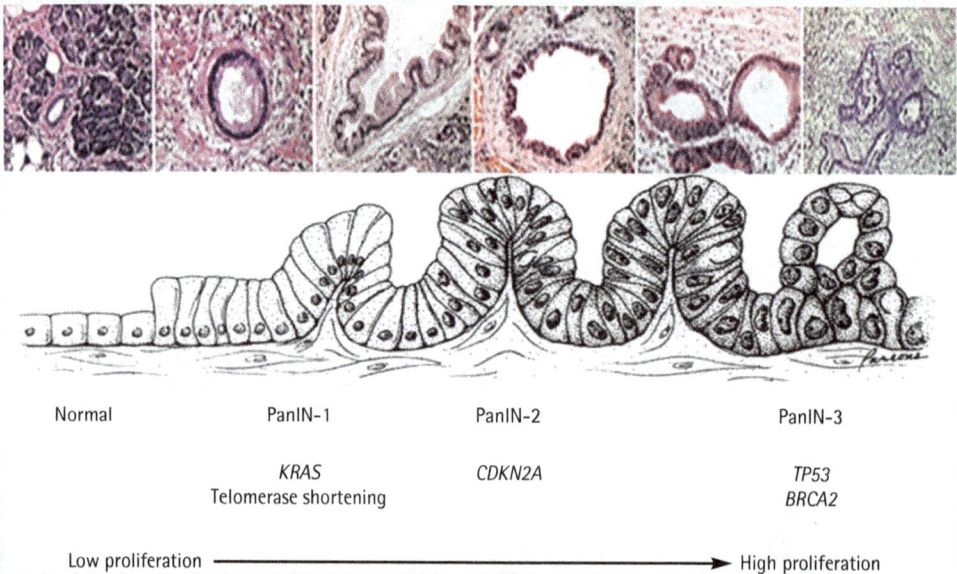

Figure 6.2 Progression from histologically normal epithelium to PanIN and subsequently invasive PDACs. The most critical mutations associated with tumour progression and invasion are also shown (adapted from Hruban et al.[3]).

thus enabling tumour profiling and subtyping. Better delineation of these tumour subtypes and their response to treatment will provide the capacity to develop targeted therapies in future years.

Diagnostic approach

It is not possible to diagnose pancreatic cancer based on signs and symptoms alone. DiMagno et al.[4] demonstrated the lack of specificity and sensitivity of clinical symptoms by reporting that the vast majority of patients (>50%) who presented with classical symptoms associated with pancreatic cancer had an alternative diagnosis on further clinical assessment. Further, the classical teaching associating painless jaundice with a diagnosis of pancreatic cancer is often false, with the majority of patients presenting with the symptom of pain.[5] It is important for clinicians to recognize that acute pancreatitis and new-onset diabetes may be initial presenting symptoms of pancreatic cancer in older people, with studies reporting a 10-fold increase in risk in comparison with age-controlled cohorts. While population screening has not yet been shown to be effective using currently available imaging modalities and biomarkers, a high index of clinical suspicion remains the most useful tool for early diagnosis.

In general, if there is suspicion of an underlying malignancy, the patient will require serological testing including routine blood tests and cross-sectional imaging. There are currently no biomarkers to effectively diagnose PDAC. The serum biomarker most frequently used is the sialylated Lewis body group on mucin 1 cell surface-associated (MUC-1) CA 19-9. This is a cell surface glycoprotein, expressed in both normal and neoplastic pancreatic cells and consequently has poor sensitivity and specificity. Furthermore, 65% of resectable pancreatic cancers do not express CA 19-9, limiting its use as a diagnostic biomarker. Consequently, CA 19-9 is mostly used to assess response to treatment in those who have already been diagnosed by cross-sectional imaging. Sharma et al.[6] recently developed a polygenic risk score by assessing the presence of single nucleotide polymorphisms. The results demonstrated that older patients with high scores and new-onset diabetes had a 10-fold increased risk of pancreatic cancer. The authors suggested that such polygenic scoring systems could highlight target populations for screening. Development of diagnostic strategies to achieve early detection of pancreatic cancer is critical in improving clinical outcomes and survival in future years.

While most patients who present with painful jaundice are investigated with transabdominal ultrasound because of its superiority in detecting cholelithiasis, it is not the imaging modality of choice to detect pancreatic cancer. Inter-user variability and low sensitivity in detecting small tumours (<3 cm) by ultrasound scan make cross-sectional imaging by CT the modality of choice. CT has a sensitivity of >90% for smaller lesions (<2 cm) and can accurately demonstrate the anatomical association between the tumour and closely associated vasculature, making it essential for staging and assessment of surgical resectability. The tumour itself is seen as a hypodense mass that may induce glandular deformity or duct dilation, leading to the classically described double duct sign (dilation of the common bile duct and pancreatic duct). The primary limitation of CT is its inability to detect small liver lesions and peritoneal deposits. Some studies have quoted rates of non-resectability to be as high as 38% in patients considered to have resectable disease after cross-sectional imaging.[7]

MRI and FDG PET are not routinely implemented, but may be used as adjuncts. The use of FDG PET scans in routine diagnostic investigation of patients with pancreatic cancer was assessed in the PET-PANC trial (ISRCTN73852054),[8] which reported a significant improvement in both sensitivity and specificity. Some centres now routinely undertake FDG PET scans on all patients who will undergo treatment as recommended by NICE guidelines, while others use it more selectively. MRI combined with magnetic resonance cholangiopancreatography may be used to detect small iso-dense lesions that are undetectable on multiphasic CT. Endoscopic retrograde cholangiopancreatography (ERCP) is primarily used to stent and decompress the biliary tree of patients who present with biliary obstruction; cytology from brushings may aid in providing a diagnosis in just over 50% of patients.[9] There is also the option for stenting obstructive lesions, which may prove to be the limit of intervention in those deemed for palliation. Endoscopic ultrasound (EUS) is also being increasingly used to stage PDAC, because it is more sensitive than CT at detecting small lesions and possesses the ability to obtain a tissue diagnosis which is not possible with ERCP and is a prerequisite for systemic therapy.

Is biopsy a prerequisite for surgical resection?

After initial diagnosis some patients undergo ERCP and brushings, which might confirm the diagnosis on cytology. In many instances, however, the brushings may prove to be non-diagnostic. The decision-making process then falls to the degree of clinical suspicion of the assessing clinicians. If the evaluating multidisciplinary team (MDT) has a high index of suspicion that the radiological appearances are consistent with an underlying malignancy, the next stage of investigation should be aimed at assessing disease stage and resectability rather than pursuing a definitive pathological diagnosis. Patients who are fit for surgery and appear to have a resectable pancreatic cancer after staging can proceed directly to surgery without pursuing a preoperative biopsy to confirm the diagnosis. However, in instances where the imaging is inconclusive or if the patient has risk factors such as a history of chronic or autoimmune pancreatitis a preoperative biopsy may be recommended. A benign aetiology should be particularly suspected in individuals where imaging reveals multifocal biliary strictures (immunoglobulin G4 disease) or diffuse ductal changes with parenchymal calcification (chronic pancreatitis). A biopsy should only be actively pursued in individuals with a potentially benign diagnosis or in those being considered for systemic chemotherapy. Fine needle aspiration/biopsy should not be routinely pursued when preoperative imaging has confirmed a diagnosis, owing to the risks associated with obtaining a biopsy (2% risk of bleeding and pancreatitis). Concerns have previously been raised with regard to the risk of peritoneal seeding after percutaneous biopsy.[10] This risk has been further removed by most referral centres performing biopsy via an EUS-guided transduodenal approach. When the diagnosis is in doubt, EUS-guided fine needle aspiration has a sensitivity of approximately 90% and a specificity of 96% for the diagnosis of a pancreatic cancer.[11] If specimens obtained by fine needle aspiration are non-diagnostic, EUS-guided core biopsy may be considered where local expertise is available.

Staging and preoperative planning

The preferred TNM staging system for pancreatic cancer may be found in the eighth edition of the cancer staging manual of the American Joint Committee on Cancer.[12] After completion of staging, there are two primary questions that should be addressed in the treatment of pancreatic cancer. First, is biliary decompression by ERCP required? And, second, is the tumour surgically resectable? For patients with obstructive jaundice secondary to a surgically resectable pancreatic head lesion, the use of preoperative biliary drainage is a topic of ongoing debate. Proponents of biliary drainage argue that preoperative stenting is associated with a reduced risk of perioperative sepsis, anastomotic leak and wound infections, while detractors suggest that ERCP in itself presents a risk of cholangitis, ERCP-associated pancreatitis and duodenal perforation. In practice, the decision is also influenced by the time frame within which the patient will have a resection. In general, if a patient is likely to remain on the waiting list for >2 weeks prior to surgery, has bilirubin levels >250 μmol/l, or develops cholangitis or debilitating symptoms (pruritus), biliary decompression would be recommended. Where the disease is not amenable to surgical resection, or neoadjuvant therapy is being considered, stenting is mandatory.

Assessment of resectability

In general, pancreatic cancer may be divided into resectable, borderline and unresectable disease. A patient with evidence of metastatic disease radiologically or at laparotomy should not be considered for resection with curative intent. A tumour may also be considered to be locally advanced and surgically unresectable if it completely encases adjacent critical vascular structures such as the coeliac axis, superior mesenteric artery or portal vein. There is currently less of a consensus on the definition of 'borderline' resectability, often causing confusion in the MDT setting. In reality, this represents a continuum, as demonstrated in Figure 6.3, with some centres more willing than others to consider more radical vascular reconstructive options. The authors, similar to clinicians in other UK centres, consider arterial involvement of the superior mesenteric artery, coeliac trunk or hepatic artery that will require an arterial resection and reconstruction in unresectable disease, while <50% encasement of the superior mesenteric vein–portal vein complex would be considered borderline resectable if reconstructive options were available. However, definitions and practice vary widely within the UK and internationally. Most patients with borderline resectable disease are referred for neoadjuvant chemotherapy prior to surgical exploration. A systematic review of 13 trials studying the role of the folinic acid, fluorouracil, irinotecan, oxaliplatin (FOLFIRINOX) regimen in the neoadjuvant setting reported resection rates of up to 40%, with up to 74% of patients achieving an R0 resection.[13] Cross-sectional imaging modalities are poor at assessing resectability and a trial resection must be considered if the disease is stable or regresses with systemic treatment. Prospective series have reported improved median survival in patients who underwent a successful resection, with the best survival outcomes (25% at 3 years) observed in patients with an R0 resection. As discussed later in this chapter, there is also an evolving case for administration of intraoperative radiotherapy in these patients.

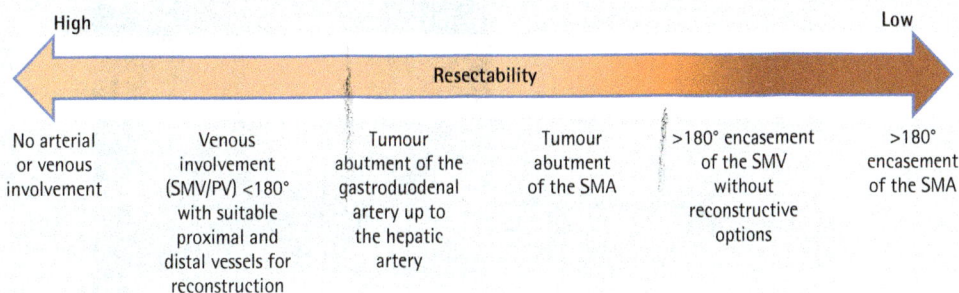

High					Low
No arterial or venous involvement	Venous involvement (SMV/PV) <180° with suitable proximal and distal vessels for reconstruction	Tumour abutment of the gastroduodenal artery up to the hepatic artery	Tumour abutment of the SMA	>180° encasement of the SMV without reconstructive options	>180° encasement of the SMA

Figure 6.3 Factors that determine resectability. PV, portal vein; SMA, superior mesenteric artery; SMV, superior mesenteric vein.

Surgical resection

Lesions in the head of the pancreas require a pancreatico-duodenectomy (Whipple's procedure); pancreatic body and tail tumours require a distal pancreatectomy and splenectomy. Pancreatico-duodenectomy was first described by Kausch in 1912 and later refined by Whipple in 1935.[14] The procedure entails removal of the pancreatic head, duodenum, bile duct, distal stomach, proximal jejunum and surrounding lymph nodes. Resectability of the tumour is dictated by the relationship of the tumour to critical vascular structures described earlier and ability to dissect free or reconstruct the vessels if involved within the tumour. Once resection is complete, the procedure enters a reconstructive phase, during which a pancreatico-jejunostomy, hepatico-jejunostomy and gastro-jejunostomy are performed to re-establish intestinal continuity (Figure 6.4).

The most significant cause of morbidity is secondary to a leak from the pancreatico-jejunal anastomosis, which is encountered in approximately 19.2% of cases.[15] The vast majority of these anastomotic leaks can be managed conservatively, with a very small minority requiring a repeat laparotomy where a total pancreatectomy and splenectomy will have to be performed as a salvage procedure. Curative surgery is associated with a median survival of 21.3 months, with approximately 23% surviving 5 years.[16] Historically, pancreatic resections were associated with high levels of morbidity and mortality; however, with advances in perioperative care, mortality rates of <3% are now reported by most high-volume centres.[17]

Pancreatic cancers of the body and tail can be resected by undertaking a distal pancreatectomy and splenectomy. The procedure entails dissection of the pancreatic neck from the portal vein and mobilization of the splenic flexure to gain optimal access. Distal pancreatectomy for cancer requires an *en bloc* removal of the spleen to achieve optimal tumour clearance. Spleen preservation is only recommended for benign pathology or borderline neoplasm. Patients who undergo a splenectomy are susceptible to overwhelming post-splenectomy sepsis from encapsulated organisms (*Escherichia coli*, *Haemophilus influenzae*, *Neisseria meningitidis* and *Streptococcus pneumoniae*) and ideally must receive prophylactic vaccinations at least 2 weeks before the procedure. Alternatively, the vaccines may be given at least 2 weeks after the procedure. Laparoscopic distal pancreatectomy and splenectomy has evolved to become the standard approach, with accumulating

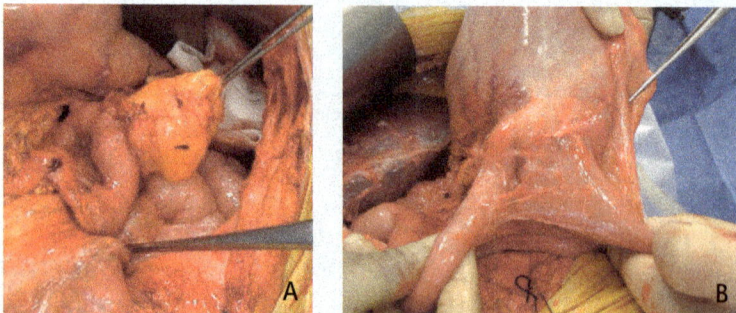

Figure 6.4 Pictures taken during a completion pancreatectomy in a patient who had previously had a Whipple's procedure. Shown are the anastomoses that were constructed during the initial Whipple's procedure. (A) A healed pancreatico-jejunostomy. (B) A healed gastro-jejunostomy.

evidence demonstrating equivocal oncological outcomes and safety profile. Recent systematic reviews have concluded that the laparoscopic approach for distal pancreatectomy is an acceptable treatment modality when performed by skilled surgeons in high-volume centres.[18,19]

Surgery may also play a role in palliation to relieve biliary or gastric outlet obstruction. In the vast majority of cases, biliary obstruction may be relieved by endoscopic intervention. However, in instances where biliary stenting does not produce an optimal outcome, biliary bypass by constructing a hepatico-jejunostomy is a feasible option. Gastric outlet obstruction is experienced by up to 25% of individuals with pancreatic cancer. While endoluminal duodenal stenting is now available in most centres, gastro-jejunostomy provides better long-term outcomes in those expected to have longer survival.[20] Despite improvements in surgical techniques and perioperative care, 5 year survival remains poor even in patients who undergo a curative resection, owing to early disease recurrence. A number of landmark trials have studied the efficacy of adjuvant chemotherapy and reported promising outcomes.[21,22]

Future directions

The last decade has seen significant improvement in the diagnosis and management of pancreatic cancer. Pancreatic surgery, which has historically been associated with significant morbidity and mortality, has evolved into a much safer procedure with excellent perioperative outcomes. Laparoscopic and robotic approaches to the pancreas are also fast evolving, thus further reducing morbidity. Despite these advances, survival remains poor due to the systemic nature of the disease process. The vast majority of patients present late and even in those who undergo a curative resection, 5 year survival is less than 25%. The evolution of biological agents which may be used in combination with traditional DNA-damaging chemotherapeutic agents may aid in expanding boundaries of resectability. Furthermore, basic research into metabolomics, circulating tumour cells and microRNA profiles may provide novel avenues for early detection, thus improving survival outcomes. Thanks to a better understanding of the cancer genomics that drives the disease, a combination of early diagnosis and targeted treatment strategies may revolutionize the management of this lethal malignancy in future years.

References

1 Siegel RL, Miller KD, Jemal A. Cancer statistics, 2016. CA Cancer J Clin 2016; 66: 7–30.

2 NHS Digital (2022). Cancer survival in England: adult, stage at diagnosis, childhood and geographical patterns. Available from: www.cancerdata.nhs.uk/survival/cancersurvivalengland (accessed 14 December 2022).

3 Hruban RH, Maitra A, Goggins M. Update on pancreatic intraepithelial neoplasia. Int J Clin Exp Pathol 2008; 1: 306–16.

4 DiMagno EP, Malagelada JR, Taylor WF, Go VL. A prospective comparison of current diagnostic tests for pancreatic cancer. N Engl J Med 1977; 297: 737–42.

5 Bond-Smith G, Banga N, Hammond TM, Imber CJ. Pancreatic adenocarcinoma. BMJ 2012; 344: e2476.

6 Sharma S, Tapper WJ, Collins A, Hamady ZZR. Predicting pancreatic cancer in the UK Biobank cohort using polygenic risk scores and diabetes mellitus. Gastroenterology 2022; 162: 1665–74.

7   Ta R, O'Connor DB, Sulistijo A, et al. The role of staging laparoscopy in resectable and borderline resectable pancreatic cancer: a systematic review and meta-analysis. Dig Surg 2019; 36: 251–60.

8   Ghaneh P, Hanson R, Titman A, et al. PET-PANC: multicentre prospective diagnostic accuracy and health economic analysis study of the impact of combined modality [18]fluorine-2-fluoro-2-deoxy-D-glucose positron emission tomography with computed tomography scanning in the diagnosis and management of pancreatic cancer. Health Technol Assess 2018; 22: 1–114.

9   Yousaf MN, Ehsan H, Wahab A, et al. Endoscopic retrograde cholangiopancreatography guided interventions in the management of pancreatic cancer. World J Gastrointest Endosc 2020; 12: 323–40.

10 Wang L, Lin N, Xin F, et al. A systematic review of the comparison of the incidence of seeding metastasis between endoscopic biliary drainage and percutaneous transhepatic biliary drainage for resectable malignant biliary obstruction. World J Surg Oncol 2019; 17: 116.

11 Chen G, Liu S, Zhao Y, et al. Diagnostic accuracy of endoscopic ultrasound-guided fine-needle aspiration for pancreatic cancer: a meta-analysis. Pancreatology 2013; 13: 298–304.

12 American Joint Committee on Cancer. Exocrine pancreas. In: Amin MB, Edge SB, Greene FL, et al., eds. AJCC cancer staging manual. 8th ed. New York: Springer, 2017; 337–48.

13 Suker M, Beumer BR, Sadot E, et al. FOLFIRINOX for locally advanced pancreatic cancer: a systematic review and patient-level meta-analysis. Lancet Oncol 2016; 17: 801–10.

14 Are C, Dhir M, Ravipati L. History of pancreaticoduodenectomy: early misconceptions, initial milestones and the pioneers. HPB (Oxford) 2011; 13: 377–84.

15 McMillan MT, Soi S, Asbun HJ, et al. Risk-adjusted outcomes of clinically relevant pancreatic fistula following pancreatoduodenectomy: a model for performance evaluation. Ann Surg 2016; 264: 344–52.

16 Lewis R, Drebin JA, Callery MP, et al. A contemporary analysis of survival for resected pancreatic ductal adenocarcinoma. HPB (Oxford) 2013; 15: 49–60.

17 Panni RZ, Panni UY, Liu J, et al. Re-defining a high volume center for pancreaticoduodenectomy. HPB (Oxford) 2021; 23: 733–8.

18 van Hilst J, Korrel M, de Rooij T, et al. Oncologic outcomes of minimally invasive versus open distal pancreatectomy for pancreatic ductal adenocarcinoma: a systematic review and meta-analysis. Eur J Surg Oncol 2019; 45: 719–27.

19 Ricci C, Casadei R, Taffurelli G, et al. Laparoscopic versus open distal pancreatectomy for ductal adenocarcinoma: a systematic review and meta-analysis. J Gastrointest Surg 2015; 19: 770–81.

20 Jeurnink SM, Steyerberg EW, van Hooft JE, et al. Surgical gastrojejunostomy or endoscopic stent placement for the palliation of malignant gastric outlet obstruction (SUSTENT study): a multicenter randomized trial. Gastrointest Endosc 2010; 71: 490–9.

21 Neoptolemos JP, Palmer DH, Ghaneh P, et al. Comparison of adjuvant gemcitabine and capecitabine with gemcitabine monotherapy in patients with resected pancreatic cancer (ESPAC-4): a multicentre, open-label, randomised, phase 3 trial. Lancet 2017; 389: 1011–24.

22 Conroy T, Hammel P, Hebbar M, et al. FOLFIRINOX or gemcitabine as adjuvant therapy for pancreatic cancer. N Engl J Med 2018; 379: 2395–406.

Further reading

- Hackert T, Sachsenmaier M, Hinz U, et al. Locally advanced pancreatic cancer: neoadjuvant therapy with FOLFIRINOX results in resectability in 60% of the patients. Ann Surg 2016; 264: 457–63.

- Kunzmann V, Siveke JT, Algül H, et al. Nab-paclitaxel plus gemcitabine versus nab-paclitaxel plus gemcitabine followed by FOLFIRINOX induction chemotherapy in locally advanced pancreatic cancer (NEOLAP-AIO-PAK-0113): a multicentre, randomised, phase 2 trial. Lancet Gastroenterol Hepatol 2021; 6: 128–38.

- Moole H, Bechtold M, Puli SR. Efficacy of preoperative biliary drainage in malignant obstructive jaundice: a meta-analysis and systematic review. World J Surg Oncol 2016; 14: 182.

- Neoptolemos JP, Palmer DH, Ghaneh P, et al. Comparison of adjuvant gemcitabine and capecitabine with gemcitabine monotherapy in patients with resected pancreatic cancer (ESPAC-4): a multicentre, open-label, randomised, phase 3 trial. Lancet 2017; 389: 1011–24.

- Riviere D, Gurusamy KS, Kooby DA, et al. Laparoscopic versus open distal pancreatectomy for pancreatic cancer. Cochrane Database Syst Rev 2016; 4: CD011391.

- Zhen DB, Rabe KG, Gallinger S, et al. *BRCA1*, *BRCA2*, *PALB2*, and *CDKN2A* mutations in familial pancreatic cancer: a PACGENE study. Genet Med 2015; 17: 569–77.

01 Pelvic nodal recurrence in prostate cancer

Finbar Slevin, Louise J. Murray

Case history

A 72-year-old man was reviewed after he developed a rising prostate-specific antigen (PSA) level of 0.75 ng/ml. In 2015, he had undergone a robotic-assisted radical prostatectomy for a Gleason 3+4 (International Society of Urological Pathology grade 2) prostate adenocarcinoma with no evidence of extra-prostatic extension and negative surgical resection margins. Postoperative PSA was undetectable at <0.10 ng/ml.

Between 2017 and 2021, PSA became detectable and was observed to have increased from 0.15 to 0.25 ng/ml. In 2022, the PSA level had reached 0.57 ng/ml. [68]Ga prostate-specific membrane antigen (PSMA) PET-CT demonstrated an avid 1.2 cm lymph node in the right obturator region with a maximum standardized uptake value of 12.5. There was no evidence of recurrence in the prostatic fossa or of distant metastatic disease. A decision was taken to treat the pelvic lymph node with stereotactic body radiotherapy (SBRT) at a dose of 30 Gy in three fractions on alternate days. Planning CT was performed with intravenous contrast. The patient was placed in the supine position and immobilized within a vacuum bag. Gross tumour volume encompassed the visible macroscopic disease. Clinical target volume was equal to gross tumour volume. Planning target volume was produced by an isotropic expansion of clinical target volume by 5 mm. Planning target volume was observed to overlap with the right sacral plexus, resulting in some under-coverage (Figure 1.1). Treatment was delivered using daily online cone beam CT verification.

The patient successfully completed treatment with minimal acute toxicity. Response assessment CT at 3 months demonstrated a partial radiological response with an associated decrease in PSA. The patient returned to clinical follow-up guided by serial measurement of PSA.

What evidence is there to support the use of SBRT in this setting?

What alternative treatment options could be considered?

When planning SBRT in the setting of pelvic nodal recurrence, which organs at risk are of importance and for which early and late radiation toxicities would you obtain the patient's consent?

How would your treatment plan change if the patient had received prior postoperative radiotherapy to the prostatic fossa?

What is the role of PET–CT in the management of recurrent prostate cancer?

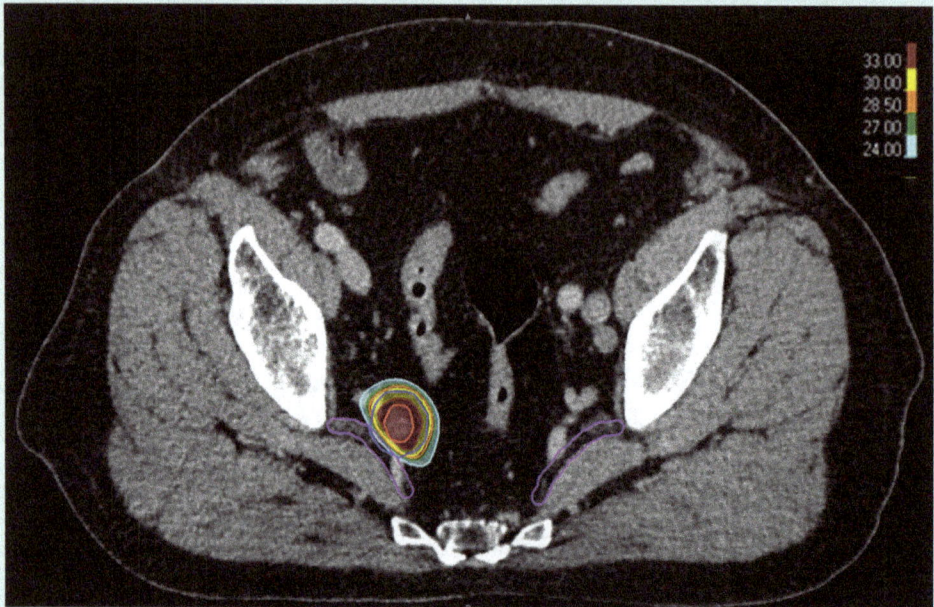

Figure 1.1 Radiotherapy plan. Isodose levels (in Gy) are indicated by the key. The aim was to prescribe 30 Gy in three fractions to the right-sided lymph node. Planning target volume (blue outline) under-coverage was present postero-laterally given the overlap between the planning target volume and sacral plexus (purple outline), also resulting in some antero-lateral and postero-medial spread of the intermediate isodoses; 95% of the planning target volume received 29.1 Gy. Dose escalation towards the centre of the planning target volume is apparent, encompassing the gross tumour volume (red outline). (With thanks to Mr Christopher Pagett for producing this treatment plan. Patient consent for reproduction obtained.)

What evidence is there to support the use of SBRT in this setting?

SBRT is ultra-hypofractionated radiation therapy delivered using tight treatment margins and highly conformal delivery techniques with steep dose gradients. Robust patient immobilization, management of organ motion throughout the radiotherapy pathway and daily online image guidance are required for the safe and effective delivery of pelvic SBRT. Recently, SBRT has increasingly been used to treat limited sites of disease recurrence (so-called oligorecurrence) after primary treatment.[1] It is hypothesized that SBRT has the potential to improve outcomes or even provide a second opportunity for cure beyond first relapse. In addition to the SABR-COMET trial (ClinicalTrials.gov NCT01446744)[2] (discussed in chapter 2), two randomized phase II trials of SBRT for oligorecurrent prostate cancer have also published results which suggest that SBRT might delay further disease progression and the time to commencing androgen deprivation therapy compared with surveillance. In the STOMP trial (ClinicalTrials.gov NCT01558427), median androgen deprivation therapy-free survival was 21 vs 13 months for the metastasis-directed therapy (SBRT or salvage pelvic lymph node dissection) vs surveillance arms, respectively (HR 0.60; 80% CI 0.40%, 0.90%; $p=0.11$).[3] In the ORIOLE trial (ClinicalTrials.gov NCT02680587), disease progression at 6 months occurred in 19% vs 61% in the SBRT vs surveillance arms, respectively ($p=0.005$).[4] Whether androgen deprivation therapy should be given alongside SBRT remains uncertain. In these trials, SBRT was used to defer use of androgen deprivation therapy and its associated potential toxicities and impact on quality of life. SBRT appears to be generally well tolerated, with no grade 3 toxicities reported in STOMP or ORIOLE after median follow-up durations of 36 and 19 months, respectively.[3,4] Despite these promising data, to date no phase III evidence exists to support the use of SBRT in this setting.

What alternative treatment options could be considered?

No clear standard of care exists for pelvic nodal recurrence in prostate cancer, and there is an absence of phase III evidence as to the optimal approach. Potential options include androgen deprivation therapy, docetaxel chemotherapy, androgen receptor-targeted agents such as enzalutamide or abiraterone/prednisolone, SBRT, extended nodal irradiation (elective treatment of pelvic nodal regions at risk of harbouring micrometastatic disease, in addition to the macroscopically involved lymph node) or a combination of the above. In a recent European multicentre observational study, extended nodal irradiation was associated with promising outcomes compared with SBRT, with approximately a 10% improvement in 3 year metastasis-free survival observed in patients treated with extended nodal irradiation vs SBRT, respectively (77% vs 68%; $p=0.01$).[5] The randomized phase II STORM trial (ClinicalTrials.gov NCT03569241), currently in recruitment, compares extended nodal irradiation with SBRT (or salvage pelvic lymph node dissection), with a primary endpoint of 2 year metastasis-free survival.

When planning SBRT in the setting of pelvic nodal recurrence, which organs at risk are of importance and for which early and late radiation toxicities would you obtain the patient's consent?

The UK SABR Consortium guidelines recommend that any organs at risk traversed by a treatment beam should be contoured 2 cm superiorly and inferiorly to the planning target volume.[6] For treatment of a pelvic nodal recurrence, the following organs at risk should be considered as a minimum: bladder, bowel (individual loops or use of a single bowel bag with careful outlining of bowel loops closest to the target if the latter method is used), cauda equina, femoral heads, rectum and sacral plexus. Published optimal and mandatory dose constraints in three and five fractions exist for most organs at risk.[7,8] Patient consent should be obtained for potential early and late SBRT toxicities. Potential early toxicities include, but are not limited to, fatigue, pain, skin erythema, nausea, vomiting, diarrhoea, urinary urgency, frequency and dysuria. Potential late toxicities include, but are not limited to, gastrointestinal haemorrhage, fistulation, obstruction or perforation, sacral plexopathy, skeletal fracture or necrosis and urinary haemorrhage or fistulation.

How would your treatment plan change if the patient had received prior postoperative radiotherapy to the prostatic fossa?

There is increasing use of SBRT as a re-irradiation treatment for pelvic disease recurrence after previous delivery of definitive, neoadjuvant or adjuvant radiotherapy. The use of five fraction SBRT (i.e. 30 Gy in five fractions) may be more appropriate. It is important to review the previous radiotherapy treatment plan and to take account of the previously delivered dose to organs at risk. Broadly, approaches comprise either use of a maximum cumulative constraint (that includes the dose from both the original and re-irradiation courses) or subtraction of the previously delivered dose from a traditional SBRT constraint, with or without allowance for recovery. However, no clear consensus exists regarding the optimum cumulative constraints for most organs at risk, or whether allowance for recovery from the previously delivered treatment should be permitted.[9] In the current scenario, the planning target volume overlapped with the sacral plexus. If, for example, this region of sacral plexus received about 30% of the prescription dose during the previous course of radiotherapy to the prostatic fossa (this would, of course, be confirmed by reviewing the previous plan), in order to meet a cumulative sacral plexus constraint of 32 Gy in five fractions to 0.1 cc, it would likely be necessary to assume 25% recovery from the previously delivered dose to facilitate improved target coverage at re-irradiation.[7] This approach would appear to be acceptable if extrapolating from the data that support some recovery of spinal cord from radiotherapy after a 6 month interval has elapsed.[10]

What is the role of PET-CT in the management of recurrent prostate cancer?

Conventional imaging techniques, such as CT, MRI or bone scintigraphy, have low detection rates for recurrent disease during early biochemical failure. By contrast, use of molecular imaging with PET-CT may identify patients with small-volume recurrent disease who may be eligible for salvage therapies. There are several PET-CT tracers, including isotopes of choline, fluciclovine and PSMA; detailed reviews regarding the role of these in recurrent prostate cancer are available.[11] It is considered that PSMA PET-CT is superior to other PET-CT tracers for the detection of disease recurrence, especially at the low PSA levels (e.g. <2 ng/ml) that characterize post-prostatectomy early biochemical failure. PET-CT also has the potential to guide the approach to salvage radiotherapy. In the phase II/III EMPIRE-1 trial (ClinicalTrials.gov NCT01666808), 3 year event-free survival (defined as biochemical or clinical failure) was evaluated in patients with biochemical recurrence post-prostatectomy randomized to fluciclovine or conventional imaging-directed salvage radiotherapy.[12] Three year event-free survival was significantly improved in the fluciclovine PET-CT arm (76% vs 63%; p=0.0028) and fluciclovine PET-CT led to a change in pre-PET-CT decision making in 35% of patients (addition of extended nodal irradiation to prostatic fossa radiotherapy, change to prostatic fossa radiotherapy alone or avoidance of radiotherapy where distant metastatic disease was identified). A phase III trial of PSMA-directed salvage radiotherapy with a primary endpoint of biochemical progression-free survival is in progress (ClinicalTrials.gov NCT03582774). However, the impact on overall survival (OS) from identifying and treating small-volume recurrent disease at low PSA levels, or changing management decisions based on PET-CT findings, remains uncertain.

Conclusion and learning points

- The optimal management of patients with pelvic nodal recurrence from prostate cancer is unknown.
- There is increasing interest in the use of SBRT in the management of patients with oligometastatic cancer.
- Phase II evidence to support SBRT is promising and suggests high levels of local control with low levels of high-grade toxicity.
- Phase III evidence regarding any OS benefit from SBRT is awaited.

References

1 Tree AC, Khoo VS, Eeles RA, et al. Stereotactic body radiotherapy for oligometastases. Lancet Oncol 2013; 14: e28–37.

2 Palma DA, Olson R, Harrow S, et al. Stereotactic ablative radiotherapy for the comprehensive treatment of oligometastatic cancers: long-term results of the SABR-COMET phase II randomized trial. J Clin Oncol 2020; 38: 2830–8.

3   Ost P, Reynders D, Decaestecker K, et al. Surveillance or metastasis-directed therapy for oligometastatic prostate cancer recurrence: a prospective, randomized, multicenter phase II trial. J Clin Oncol 2018; 36: 446–53.

4   Phillips R, Shi WY, Deek M, et al. Outcomes of observation vs stereotactic ablative radiation for oligometastatic prostate cancer: the ORIOLE phase 2 randomized clinical trial. JAMA Oncol 2020; 6: 650–9.

5   De Bleser E, Jereczek-Fossa BA, Pasquier D, et al. Metastasis-directed therapy in treating nodal oligorecurrent prostate cancer: a multi-institutional analysis comparing the outcome and toxicity of stereotactic body radiotherapy and elective nodal radiotherapy. Eur Urol 2019; 76: 732–9.

6   UK SABR Consortium (2019). Stereotactic ablative radiotherapy (SABR): a resource. Version 6.1. Available from: www.sabr.org.uk/wp-content/uploads/2019/04/SABRconsortium-guidelines-2019-v6.1.0.pdf (accessed 9 March 2022).

7   American Association of Physicists in Medicine (2010). Stereotactic body radiation therapy: the report of AAPM Task Group 101. Available from: www.aapm.org/pubs/reports/detail.asp?docid=102 (accessed 9 March 2022).

8   Diez P, Hanna GG, Aitken KL, et al. UK 2022 consensus on normal tissue dose-volume constraints for oligometastatic, primary lung and hepatocellular carcinoma stereotactic ablative radiotherapy. Clin Oncol (R Coll Radiol) 2022; 34: 288–300.

9   Slevin F, Aitken K, Alongi F, et al. An international Delphi consensus for pelvic stereotactic ablative radiotherapy re-irradiation. Radiother Oncol 2021; 164: 104–14.

10 Kirkpatrick JP, van der Kogel AJ, Schultheiss TE. Radiation dose-volume effects in the spinal cord. Int J Radiat Oncol Biol Phys 2010; 76 (3 suppl): S42–9.

11 Slevin F, Beasley M, Cross W, et al. Patterns of lymph node failure in patients with recurrent prostate cancer postradical prostatectomy and implications for salvage therapies. Adv Radiat Oncol 2020; 5: 1126–40.

12 Jani AB, Schreibmann E, Goyal S, et al. ^{18}F-fluciclovine-PET/CT imaging versus conventional imaging alone to guide postprostatectomy salvage radiotherapy for prostate cancer (EMPIRE-1): a single centre, open-label, phase 2/3 randomised controlled trial. Lancet 2021; 397: 1895–904.

02 Adrenal oligometastasis treated with stereotactic body radiotherapy

Angus Killean, Stephen Harrow

Case history

A 56-year-old man initially presented with an 8 month history of cough and weight loss. He was a non-smoker with a medical history of hypertension only. Chest X-ray showed a right upper zone opacification; a subsequent CT scan of the chest and abdomen revealed a 6 cm spiculated lesion in the right upper lobe. PET-CT showed no other sites of disease. CT-guided biopsy of the right apical lesion confirmed the diagnosis of lung adenocarcinoma, with the presence of an *EGFR* exon 21 mutation. The patient underwent a right upper lobectomy, with final pathological staging confirming pT3N0M0 disease. The patient suffered postoperative complications of a pulmonary embolism and pneumonia but eventually made a full recovery and was discharged home. As this patient was treated before osimertinib had been approved for adjuvant treatment in *EGFR*-positive patients, no adjuvant systemic treatment was given.

Twelve months after completion of surgery, a CT scan of the chest and abdomen showed a new 2.8 cm right adrenal lesion. PET-CT confirmed a right adrenal lesion with high FDG avidity in keeping with a metastasis but with no other disease sites. The patient was asymptomatic and had a WHO performance status of 0. CT-guided biopsy of the lesion confirmed metastatic adenocarcinoma with an *EGFR* exon 21 mutation. Owing to his previous postoperative complications, the patient did not wish to consider an adrenalectomy.

The patient was offered stereotactic body radiotherapy (SBRT) to the adrenal metastasis. He received 40 Gy in five fractions daily. Treatment was well tolerated, with no significant side effects.

What is the goal of treatment for this patient?

What is the evidence base behind the treatment of oligometastatic disease in this setting?

What is the evidence base behind radical treatment for adrenal metastases?

How should this patient be followed up and monitored?

What other treatment options are available if the patient progresses?

What is the goal of treatment for this patient?

This patient has oligometastatic disease, which could be treated surgically or with ablative therapy such as SBRT. There are no strict criteria for defining oligometastases in terms of the site of disease or number of lesions; oligometastatic disease is an intermediate state of limited metastatic spread, with a disease burden greater than localized cancer but less than disseminated malignancy. Patients with oligometastatic disease who have undergone surgery or local ablative therapies to treat all sites of disease may achieve better-than-expected survival and, possibly, cure.[1,2] Therefore, a reasonable aim of treatment for this patient is long-term disease control and prolonging survival while also delaying the need for systemic treatment.

What is the evidence base behind the treatment of oligometastatic disease in this setting?

Until recently, randomized evidence underpinning the management of oligometastatic disease was derived from studies assessing the treatment of patients with limited intracranial metastases and those with malignant spinal cord compression. Improved overall survival (OS) was seen in patients treated with local ablative therapies or surgery.[1] Most evidence otherwise came from single-centre or pooled experiences demonstrating better-than-expected survival, with retrospective studies demonstrating that long-term survival can occur in patients with a variety of primary cancers who have undergone surgery for metastatic disease.[1]

In the last 3 years, more randomized evidence supporting the radical treatment of oligometastatic disease has been published. In a multi-institutional phase II randomized trial, Gomez et al.[3] evaluated the addition of high-dose radiotherapy or surgery (or a combination of the two) vs maintenance therapy or observation in patients with stage IV non-small-cell lung cancer who had three or fewer metastases and had completed first-line systemic treatment. Median progression-free survival (PFS) and OS were significantly longer in the radiotherapy and surgery arm: 14.2 vs 4.4 months ($p=0.022$) and 41.2 vs 17.0 months ($p=0.017$), respectively.

In 2015, NHS England launched the Commissioning through Evaluation scheme for SBRT,[4] where patients participated in a prospective, registry-based clinical effectiveness and safety evaluation study. Included patients had three or fewer sites of metachronous extracranial metastases and a maximum of two spinal metastases. A total number of 1422 patients were recruited, with a preponderance of individuals with prostate cancer (28.6%). With a median follow-up time of 13 months, OS at 1 and 2 years was 92.3% and 79.2%, respectively, with a variance across tumour sites (60.5% 2 year survival in melanoma vs 94.6% in prostate cancer).

What is the evidence base behind radical treatment for adrenal metastases?

Prolonged survival following adrenalectomy for isolated adrenal metastasis, along with active management of the primary cancer, has been documented since at least the early 1980s.[5] However, the clinical evidence supporting this approach is limited to retrospective studies and meta-analyses.

A systematic review carried out by Tanvetyanon et al.[5] included 114 patients who underwent adrenalectomy for synchronous and metachronous metastases, in addition to surgery to their primary lung cancer. The median OS for the synchronous and metachronous groups was 12 and 31 months, respectively. The metachronous group saw 1 and 2 year survival rates of 80% and 52%, respectively. Survival rates at equivalent time points for patients with synchronous metastases were 45% and 30%, respectively.

With the continued adoption of ablative therapies for oligometastatic disease, SBRT is increasingly being offered as an alternative to adrenalectomy. Arcidiacono et al.[6] carried out a single-centre retrospective analysis of 37 patients who received SBRT to adrenal metastases. The cohort had a median OS of 16 months; however, a greater proportion of patients had oligoprogressive disease, which may account for the poorer survival rate compared with the results reported in the systematic review of Tanvetyanon et al.[5]

König et al.[7] retrospectively studied 28 patients who received SBRT to oligoprogressive adrenal metastases. Patients could have up to five additional metastases and the study included a range of primary tumours. Treatment achieved good 1 and 2 year local control (86% and 84.8%, respectively); however, most patients were diagnosed with distant relapse, leading to 1 and 2 year survival rates of 46.6% and 32.0%, respectively, with most patients dying because of systemic tumour progression.

How should this patient be followed up and monitored?

There is no standardized follow-up protocol for patients who have undergone ablative treatment for oligometastatic disease. Regular imaging would allow for the identification of low-volume disease that may be amenable to further radical treatments such as surgery or radiotherapy. In the updated survival data of the SABR-COMET trial (ClinicalTrials.gov NCT01446744), nine patients in the original SBRT arm underwent subsequent salvage SBRT, with three of these patients surviving more than 5 years.[2] The authors argued that the relatively short median PFS in the context of longer median OS in the entire cohort indicated the benefits of salvage SBRT.

Patients who have new, limited disease potentially amenable to radical treatment identified on CT should undergo PET-CT to exclude more disseminated disease that is not visible on CT; biopsy should be considered if there is suspicion of a new primary.

What other treatment options are available if the patient progresses?

Further treatment options depend on the site and extent of progressive disease. Patients who receive treatment for further sites of limited oligometastases may still expect a reasonable prognosis,[2] so further surgery or ablative therapies such as radiotherapy may be offered if appropriate.

If the extent of progression is such that surgery, SBRT or other ablative therapies are unsuitable, then systemic treatment may be offered. This patient's initial molecular pathology had demonstrated an exon 21 *EGFR* mutation, making him eligible for tyrosine kinase inhibitor (TKI) therapy. If a significant period had passed between the primary diagnosis and the development of further metastases, then a repeat biopsy could be considered. NICE guidance currently recommends osimertinib, afatinib, erlotinib or gefitinib as first-line treatment in patients with *EGFR* mutations.[8] Patients who progress after first-line TKI therapy, who were not treated with osimertinib, should be tested for the presence of the *T790M* mutation, either by analysis of plasma-circulating DNA or tumour tissue, and then offered osimertinib if present. If treatment is offered following progression on osimertinib (or in patients where a *T790M* mutation is not detected), platinum doublet chemotherapy is indicated, with the option of maintenance pemetrexed if there is no immediate progression. Patients who progress further are then eligible for immunotherapy, docetaxel plus nintedanib or docetaxel alone.[8]

Conclusion and learning points

- Patients with oligometastatic disease have a limited number of metastases that are potentially treatable with more radical therapy such as surgery or SBRT.
- Observational data in the case of surgery and ablative therapies, as well as growing randomized data in the case of SBRT, show that patients who have radical treatment for oligometastases achieve better-than-expected survival and long-term control of disease.

- Patients unwilling or unable to undergo adrenalectomy may be offered SBRT for adrenal metastases.
- Patients should be monitored with regular imaging following SBRT, as they may be suitable for further surgery or ablative therapies for subsequent new oligometastatic disease.
- In patients with *EGFR* mutations requiring systemic treatment, TKI therapy should be offered first line.

References

1 Palma DA, Salama JK, Lo SS, et al. The oligometastatic state – separating truth from wishful thinking. Nat Rev Clin Oncol 2014; 11: 549–57.

2 Palma DA, Olson R, Harrow S, et al. Stereotactic ablative radiotherapy for the comprehensive treatment of oligometastatic cancers: long-term results of the SABR-COMET phase II randomized trial. J Clin Oncol 2020; 38: 2830–8.

3 Gomez DR, Tang C, Zhang J, et al. Local consolidative therapy vs. maintenance therapy or observation for patients with oligometastatic non-small-cell lung cancer: long-term results of a multi-institutional, phase II, randomized study. J Clin Oncol 2019; 37: 1558–65.

4 Chalkidou A, Macmillan T, Grzeda MT, et al. Stereotactic ablative body radiotherapy in patients with oligometastatic cancers: a prospective, registry-based, single-arm, observational, evaluation study. Lancet Oncol 2021; 22: 98–106.

5 Tanvetyanon T, Robinson LA, Schell MJ, et al. Outcomes of adrenalectomy for isolated synchronous versus metachronous adrenal metastases in non-small-cell lung cancer: a systematic review and pooled analysis. J Clin Oncol 2008; 26: 1142–7.

6 Arcidiacono F, Aristei C, Marchionni A, et al. Stereotactic body radiotherapy for adrenal oligometastasis in lung cancer patients. Br J Radiol 2020; 93: 20200645.

7 König L, Häfner MF, Katayama S, et al. Stereotactic body radiotherapy (SBRT) for adrenal metastases of oligometastatic or oligoprogressive tumor patients. Radiat Oncol 2020, 15: 30.

8 NICE (2019). Lung cancer: diagnosis and management. NICE guideline NG122. Available from: www.nice.org.uk/guidance/ng122 (accessed 7 December 2022).

03 Oligometastatic disease: liver metastasis

Wai-Yan Poon, Derek Grose

Case history

An 81-year-old woman was treated 7 years ago for a locally advanced colon cancer (T3N1M1) with a right hemicolectomy and a synchronous resection of a solitary liver metastasis. She had originally presented with persistent abdominal pain and weight loss of 12 kg.

Her medical history included an aortic valve replacement, hypertension and chronic obstructive pulmonary disease. Despite her comorbidities, as she had an ECOG performance status of 1 it was felt that she was fit for treatment. Adjuvant chemotherapy was discussed with her. She was treated with two cycles of adjuvant oxaliplatin and capecitabine (XELOX) chemotherapy but had to stop owing to toxicities including enteritis, nausea and palmar–plantar erythema.

The patient remained stable on follow-up. Five years after diagnosis, however, a CT scan showed an enlarged liver lesion in segment III, consistent with a liver metastasis; a PET scan confirmed a metabolically active lesion in the left lobe (Figure 3.1). An MRI scan of her liver confirmed the diagnosis. Her case was discussed at a multidisciplinary team (MDT) meeting and she was referred for potential surgical resection. She was referred for thermal ablation as there were some concerns about her fitness for resection. The interventional radiology team, however, felt that the lesion would not be suitable for ablation owing to the proximity of the stomach. The colorectal MDT discussed her case again and it was felt that as she was clinically well and had a long history of oligometastatic disease, there was no need to rush into treatment.

The patient had an interval scan 2 months later which showed that unfortunately the hepatic metastasis had increased in size (previously 2×2.5 cm, now 4×3 cm), but there was no evidence of extrahepatic disease. Hepatic metastasectomy was once again discussed with her, but she did not wish to have surgery. She consented to start palliative single-agent capecitabine. Her fourth cycle was complicated by diarrhoea and rectal bleeding, but she quickly recovered. A follow-up CT scan showed a partial response to chemotherapy, with cytoreduction in her isolated liver metastasis from 4×3.3 cm to 2.3 cm. Her carcinoembryonic antigen level had also dropped from 289 µg/l to 23.6 µg/l.

The patient was subsequently discussed by the stereotactic radiotherapy MDT, who felt she would be a suitable candidate for treatment. She had a PET scan to rule out extrahepatic disease. Owing to the proximity to the stomach, a dose of 45 Gy in five fractions was chosen. She tolerated her treatment well. A CT scan 3 months

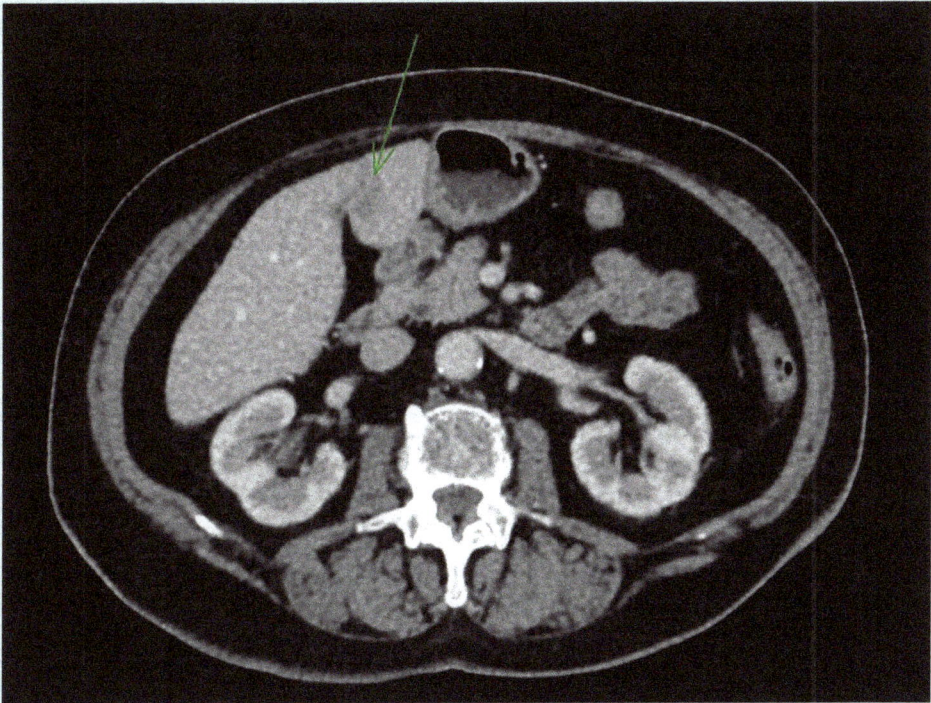

Figure 3.1 CT scan image of the chest, abdomen and pelvis showing the liver metastasis (arrow).

after treatment showed a slight increase in her hepatic lesion, but, on review, it was thought to be treatment-related rather than disease progression. A further CT scan 3 months afterwards showed a partial response to treatment and no further evidence of metastases. A scan 1 year after treatment showed ongoing stable disease in her liver.

What was the goal of cancer treatment in this patient?

What is the evidence base for her treatment options?

What is the toxicity of chemotherapy?

What is the management of liver metastasis in colorectal cancer?

What is the role of stereotactic body radiotherapy (SBRT) in oligometastatic disease?

What was the goal of cancer treatment in this patient?

Despite having metastatic disease at diagnosis, 20–50% of colorectal cancer patients who have oligometastatic disease confined to one organ can achieve long-term survival or even cure if they undergo a complete R0 resection metastasectomy.[1] The patient's wishes should be addressed and their comorbidities and performance status properly assessed before discussion at an MDT meeting. This patient had had a long history of treated oligometastatic disease and, despite being elderly, she was deemed fit for ongoing curative treatment.

What is the evidence base for her treatment options?

Fluorouracil comprises the backbone of systemic treatment for metastatic colorectal cancer and is used in combination with irinotecan or oxaliplatin. de Gramont et al.[2] showed that fluorouracil combinations obtained much higher response rates and progression-free survival than fluorouracil and leucovorin alone. The oral fluoropyrimidine alternative (capecitabine) may be used as an alternative.

Older patients are underrepresented in clinical trials. XELOX and fluorouracil, folinic acid and oxaliplatin (FOLFOX) are the standard adjuvant chemotherapy regimens in stage III colon cancer, but their benefit remains uncertain for people aged 70 years and above. Papamichael et al.[3] drew up consensus recommendations for these patients: for adjuvant treatment, the use of fluorouracil monotherapy or capecitabine was felt to be appropriate for those aged 70 and above. In view of toxicity, combination chemotherapy regimens for older patients are at the discretion of the prescribing oncologist.

As our patient had had an aortic valve replacement, she was offered XELOX rather than FOL-FOX, because for the latter she would require a peripherally inserted central catheter line. XELOX would also reduce the risk of endocarditis toxicity.

What is the toxicity of chemotherapy?

Other than immunosuppression, each chemotherapy drug has its own individualized side effects. The main toxicities of fluorouracil are diarrhoea, myelosuppression, nausea and vomiting, mouth ulcers, fatigue, palmar–plantar syndrome, hair loss and coronary vasospasm. Oxaliplatin can cause similar side effects, as well as peripheral neuropathy and laryngopharyngeal dysaesthesia.

Prior to receiving fluorouracil, all patients must have a dihydropyrimidine dehydrogenase (DPD) enzyme blood test. The DPD enzyme is the initial and rate-limiting enzyme in the degradation of fluorouracil through hepatic metabolism. Approximately, 3% of the population have a DPD deficiency and can develop rapid-onset and life-threatening or fatal chemotherapy toxicity.[4]

Despite not having a DPD deficiency, our patient still suffered from quite severe toxicity from her adjuvant chemotherapy. She required admission for grade 3 diarrhoea (defined by the Common Terminology Criteria for Adverse Events as an increase of seven or more stools per day over baseline) and colitis requiring intravenous fluids, antibiotics and antiemetics. Appropriately, chemotherapy was stopped after this admission. She later demonstrated further sensitivity to capecitabine monotherapy, suggesting that she may not tolerate prolonged durations of systemic anticancer treatment.

What is the management of liver metastasis in colorectal cancer?

The aim for patients with colorectal liver metastases should be complete resection if possible, either through 'surgical' or 'oncological' means. The definition of what is resectable has evolved over time; the current consensus suggests that macroscopic resection should be feasible while maintaining at least 30% of the liver.[5] Often neoadjuvant chemotherapy is used to downstage the disease if the patient's tumour is not deemed technically resectable upfront. Only 10–25% of patients will be suitable for surgery.[6]

Technically resectable upfront

The aim for these patients is to have an R0 resection with upfront surgery with or without peri-operative chemotherapy (3 months of FOLFOX or XELOX before and after surgery).[7] If the patient's tumour is clearly resectable and has good prognostic criteria, perioperative treatment may not be required. In patients with technically resectable disease where the prognosis is unclear, perioperative chemotherapy should be offered. For patients who have not received perioperative chemotherapy, there is no evidence for the use of adjuvant chemotherapy, but there are suggestions that patients with unfavourable prognostic criteria may benefit from adjuvant chemotherapy.[8]

Unresectable disease but with possibility of becoming resectable

In these patients, systemic therapy should be offered to try and downstage the tumour and convert the patient's tumour to resectable. Resectability is reviewed after 2 months of systemic treatment and then again at 4 months. After resection, 75% of patients are reported to relapse, with the majority of relapses occurring in the liver.[9] In these cases, if there is no extrahepatic disease, radiofrequency ablation, cryoablation or SBRT may be used. Radiofrequency ablation is most effective when treating patients with three or fewer lesions measuring <3.5 cm in diameter and not in close proximity to large blood vessels.

What is the role of SBRT in oligometastatic disease?

Oligometastatic disease is defined as five or fewer lesions outside the primary tumour.[10] In synchronous disease, lesions are detected at the time of diagnosis of the primary tumour, and, in metachronous disease, after treatment of the primary tumour. About 20–40% of newly diagnosed patients with metastatic colorectal cancer present with synchronous disease. There is no consensus as to what the standard of care should be for these patients, but, in general, preoperative chemotherapy is usually recommended.

Previously, systemic treatment was used to delay progression but was found not to eradicate the disease completely. The oligometastatic paradigm that was formed in the 1990s suggested that, in some patients, metastatic disease was confined to a small number of areas owing to anatomical and physiological factors.

SBRT aims to achieve high local control rates. There have been multiple retrospective studies and eight prospective studies to date looking at SBRT in liver metastases in various primaries. There has been no comparison between radiofrequency ablation and SBRT, as trials have failed owing to poor recruitment. However, what can be gathered from these trials are certain inclusion criteria that would render a patient a good candidate: between one and three liver metastases seen on CT/MRI in histologically diagnosed carcinoma; ECOG performance status ≤2; unresectable metastases or not fit/declines surgery; discussion in an hepatobiliary MDT; life expectancy >6 months; Child–Pugh class A cirrhosis; adequate organ function, defined as >700 cc normal liver. There have yet to be any trials comparing dose and fractionation in liver metastases. However, it was felt a dose of 46–52 Gy in three fractions would be required to achieve local control of 90% at 1 year.[11] For palliative regimens, 10 fractions may be more useful for larger volume disease and appear to be well tolerated.

For this older patient, who had had previous surgery and had no wish to undergo further surgery, SBRT was the recommended treatment for local control.

Conclusion and learning points

- Where possible, liver metastases should be resected with or without perioperative or adjuvant chemotherapy.

- A thorough comorbidity assessment is required to inform decision making and choice of appropriate chemotherapy agents.
- DPD enzyme should be tested prior to administration of fluorouracil-based chemotherapy.
- Patients with liver metastases and good performance status who either refuse or are not candidates for surgery should be considered for local control with SBRT or local ablative treatments.

References

1 Weiser M, Jarnagin W, Saltz L. Colorectal cancer patients with oligometastatic liver disease: what is the optimal approach? Oncology 2013; 27: 1074–8.

2 de Gramont A, Figer A, Seymour M, et al. Leucovorin and fluorouracil with or without oxaliplatin as first-line treatment in advanced colorectal cancer. J Clin Oncol 2000; 18: 2938–47.

3 Papamichael D, Audisio RA, Glimelius B, et al. Treatment of colorectal cancer in older patients: International Society of Geriatric Oncology (SIOG) consensus recommendations. Ann Oncol 2015; 26: 463–76.

4 Wigle TJ, Tsvetkova EV, Welch SA, Kim RB. DPYD and fluorouracil-based chemotherapy: mini review and case report. Pharmaceutics 2019; 11: 199.

5 Clavien PA, Petrowsky H, DeOliveira ML, Graf R. Strategies for safer liver surgery and partial liver transplantation. N Engl J Med 2007; 356: 1545–59.

6 Adam R, Avisar E, Ariche A, et al. Five year survival following hepatic resection after neoadjuvant therapy for non-resectable colorectal liver metastases. Ann Surg Oncol 2001; 8: 347–53.

7 Nordlinger B, Sorbye H, Glimelius B et al. Perioperative FOLFOX4 chemotherapy and surgery versus surgery alone for resectable liver metastases from colorectal cancer (EORTC 40983): long-term results of a randomised, controlled, phase 3 trial. Lancet Oncol 2013; 14: 1208–15.

8 Kemeny N, Capanu M, D'Angelica M, et al. Phase I trial of adjuvant hepatic arterial infusion (HAI) with floxuridine (FUDR) and dexamethasone plus systemic oxaliplatin, 5-fluorouracil and leucovorin in patients with resected liver metastases from colorectal cancer. Ann Oncol 2009; 20: 1236–41.

9 Van Cutsem E, Cervantes A, Nordlinger B, Arnold D. Metastatic colorectal cancer: ESMO clinical practice guidelines for diagnosis, treatment and follow-up. Ann Oncol 2014; 25 (suppl 3): iii1–9.

10 Palma DA, Olson R, Harrow S, et al. Stereotactic ablative radiotherapy for the comprehensive treatment of oligometastatic cancers: long term results of the SABR-COMET phase II randomized trial. J Clin Oncol 2020; 38: 2830–8.

11 Chang DT, Swaminath A, Kozak M, et al. Stereotactic body radiotherapy for colorectal liver metastases: a pooled analysis. Cancer 2011; 117: 4060–9.

Further reading

- UK SABR Consortium (2019). Stereotactic ablative radiotherapy (SABR): a resource. Version 6.1. Available from: www.sabr.org.uk/wp-content/uploads/2019/04/SABRconsortium-guidelines-2019-v6.1.0.pdf (accessed 15 March 2022).

04 Peripheral lung metastasis on a background of bladder cancer

Ben Fulton, Adam Peters

Case history

A 69-year-old man presented to his GP with a lower respiratory tract infection. On chest X-ray he was found to have a right middle lobe lesion. Two years earlier he had received neoadjuvant chemotherapy with cisplatin and gemcitabine, followed by a radical cysto-prostatectomy, for a ypT3ypN1M0 transitional carcinoma of the bladder. The patient denied having any other local or systemic symptoms.

Staging investigations included a CT scan of the chest, abdomen and pelvis followed by FDG PET-CT scan. The results confirmed a solitary 2.8 cm lesion in the inferior aspect of the right upper lobe abutting the parietal pleura but no definite chest wall invasion. Lung function tests confirmed a forced expiratory volume of 1.4 l (62% predicted), forced vital capacity of 2.1 l (71% predicted) and a transfer factor of 55% when corrected for lung volumes.

The patient underwent CT-guided percutaneous biopsy of the lung lesion; pathology confirmed transitional cell carcinoma in keeping with metastasis from his previous bladder cancer. His ECOG performance status remained 1. The case was discussed at the regional uro-oncology and oligometastatic multidisciplinary team (MDT) meetings. The patient was referred to an experienced thoracic surgeon who felt the lesion would require lobectomy in order to achieve surgical resection. Having discussed the risks and benefits, the patient declined surgery and opted to explore non-surgical approaches.

The patient had a consultation with his uro-oncologist to discuss systemic anticancer therapy, following which he elected to proceed with oligometastatic local ablative therapy, with the aim of deferring systemic anticancer therapy until further cancer disease progression. The patient's case was discussed at the regional oligometastatic MDT meeting and he was deemed suitable for stereotactic body radiotherapy (SBRT). After giving informed consent, the patient attended the radiotherapy department for fitting of a beam directional shell and subsequently underwent a respiratory-correlated four-dimensional CT scan in the supine position with arms adducted.

The tumour was outlined according to the UK SABR Consortium guidelines.[1] The lesion was adjacent but not invading or abutting the chest wall and was located peripherally using International Association for the Study of Lung Cancer criteria.[2] The prescribed dose was 55 Gy in five fractions delivered on alternate days, in accordance with Royal College of Radiologists' radiotherapy dose fractionation guidelines for peripheral tumours.[3]

Thoracic SBRT was delivered as scheduled; daily online verification imaging met department tolerance protocols. The patient reported the following grade 1 side effects (defined by the Common Terminology Criteria for Adverse Events): lethargy, cough and chest wall discomfort throughout radiotherapy, which was controlled with regular co-codamol.

Which factors influence patient selection for thoracic SBRT?

What common toxicities are seen when treating a peripheral lung metastasis with SBRT?

What are the common SBRT dose and fractionation schedules for peripherally located lung metastases?

Which factors influence patient selection for thoracic SBRT?

Historically, alternatives to surgery for thoracic tumours have proven unsatisfactory. People with primary lung cancers who were not candidates for surgery were treated with conventional fractionated radiotherapy. In some series this was associated with high rates of local recurrence of 30–40%.[4] SBRT is an alternative strategy to deliver ablative doses of radiotherapy to small tumours in appropriate anatomical locations in the thorax. SBRT has been associated with high rates of local control in primary lung cancers, with 3 year local control rates of up to 90% in some series.[5] One major advantage of thoracic SBRT is that, in appropriately selected patients, the toxicity profile is favourable even in those with significant medical comorbidity. The Radiation Therapy Oncology Group (RTOG) 0236 phase II study of SBRT for early-stage lung tumours (ClinicalTrials.gov NCT00087438) demonstrated risk of grade 3 and 4 toxicities of 13% and 4%, respectively. There were no grade 5 toxicities.[6]

For peripherally located tumours, pulmonary parenchymal tissue is the most relevant critical organ at risk and demonstrates parallel organ radiobiological behaviour.[7] The function of parallel organs is not severely compromised if only a small sub-volume is exposed to high doses of radiation. Tumour size is therefore an important consideration for SBRT. In the initial phase II RTOG study published in 2006,[8] eligibility criteria included T1 or T2 tumours ≤7 cm, staged according to the criteria of the American Joint Committee on Cancer.[9] These have largely been adopted across contemporary thoracic SBRT studies.

Patients with primary or metastatic lung tumours and coexisting interstitial lung disease (ILD) represent a high-risk group for development of treatment-related toxicities with SBRT. Despite the favourable toxicity profile with SBRT in most patients, emerging data indicate that individuals with ILD are at particularly high risk of toxicity after SBRT. A recent meta-analysis found that the use of SBRT for early-stage lung cancer in people with ILD was associated with a 25% risk of grade 3 or higher radiation pneumonitis and a 15% risk of treatment-related death. The latter could be as high as 33% in individuals with idiopathic pulmonary fibrosis.[10] The natural history of ILD is, however, very variable, which makes it difficult to predict outcomes of SBRT in individual patients. The current ASPIRE-ILD (ClinicalTrials.gov NCT03485378) phase II study aims to determine oncological efficacy and toxicity outcomes after lung SBRT in patients with coexistent ILD. Patients will be stratified based on their ILD gender-age-physiology index. While we await publication of the results of this study, it is important in the intervening period to have comprehensive discussions about the merits of SBRT in individuals with ILD, given the significant risks of morbidity and mortality.

What common toxicities are seen when treating a peripheral lung metastasis with SBRT?

The toxicity profile for peripheral lung SBRT is well established in series treating early-stage primary lung cancers. Grade 1–2 toxicities including fatigue are common but generally self-limiting. In 30 studies reporting toxicity outcomes, grade 3–4 toxicities (including pneumonitis, dyspnoea, chest pain and pneumonia) occurred in 2.7–27% of patients.[5] Treatment-related grade 5 toxicities are very rare in peripherally located tumours. The safety and outcomes of SBRT in individuals with chronic obstructive pulmonary disease have been well established. The RTOG 0236 study showed that baseline pulmonary function tests were not predictive of pulmonary toxicity and that poor baseline pulmonary function did not predict decreased overall survival (OS).[11]

Chest wall toxicity from SBRT can include rib fractures or pain due to chest wall necrosis. This has been reported in around 10% of patients, with grade 3 toxicity in 2%. Chest wall toxicity has a median time to onset of 6 months after SBRT. Increased chest wall dose and treatment volume have been the most consistently demonstrated factors associated with toxicity.[12]

What are the common SBRT dose and fractionation schedules for peripherally located lung metastases?

The dose and fractionation regimens for oligometastatic SBRT in the chest are adopted from experiences treating early-stage primary lung cancers. The 2003 Timmerman et al.[13] phase I dose escalation study demonstrated the safety of 3×20 Gy fractions for T1 and T2 peripheral lung tumours. Local failures were seen below a median dose of 3×12 Gy. The subsequent RTOG 0236 phase II study of SBRT in patients with tumours >2 cm from proximal bronchial tree evaluated 55 patients who received 3×18 Gy and reported 5 year disease-free survival and OS rates of 26% and 40%, respectively.[6]

The evidence base for the use of SBRT in early-stage peripherally located lung tumours has steadily grown. The data were reviewed by Murray et al.,[5] which despite the studies' heterogeneous designs and different radiotherapy schedules included outcomes of 4570 patients treated with SBRT. Their report highlighted the importance of the biologically effective dose (BED) on OS in primary lung cancers.[5] The Stahl et al.[14] series also demonstrated that BED_{10} >105 Gy vs <105 Gy remained significantly associated with improved OS. Patients receiving BED_{10} ≥105 Gy had a median survival of 28 months compared with 22 months in those receiving SBRT with BED_{10} <105 Gy (HR 0.78; 95% CI 0.62, 0.98; $p=0.03$). There remains a paucity of data regarding whether the correlation between BED estimations and disease control are homogeneous across different metastatic tumour histologies. This question would be best addressed in well-designed prospective SBRT trials including both agnostic and individual tumour histologies.

The SABR-COMET trial (ClinicalTrials.gov NCT01446744) was conducted among an agnostic oligometastatic patient group.[15] Patients with lung tumours <3 cm surrounded by lung parenchyma were treated with 54 Gy in three fractions on alternate days; patients with tumours abutting the chest wall, but still peripherally situated, were treated with 55 Gy in five fractions on alternate days; patients whose tumour was located within 2 cm of the mediastinum or brachial plexus were treated with 60 Gy in eight fractions on alternate days. In the SBRT arm, 43% of treated lesions had lung metastases vs 51% receiving local control.

Conclusion and learning points

- There is a paucity of data around the role of SBRT for oligometastatic lung lesions and it remains an area demanding high-quality research. The largest volume of data demonstrating efficacy and tolerability of thoracic SBRT comes from treatment of early-stage primary lung cancer.

- There is a clear need to identify and define the population of patients who might benefit from SBRT, addressing multivariate factors such as tumour size, location and comorbidities including ILD among others.

- There remain challenges around patient selection for different thoracic ablative modalities including surgery and SBRT. Thoracic SBRT for peripheral oligometastatic lesions may be considered an appropriate therapeutic modality in medically inoperable individuals or in those who decline surgery. It should ideally be delivered within the framework of well-designed clinical trials.

References

1 UK SABR Consortium (2019). Stereotactic ablative radiotherapy (SABR): a resource. Version 6.1. Available from: www.sabr.org.uk/wp-content/uploads/2019/04/SABRconsortium-guidelines-2019-v6.1.0.pdf (accessed 1 March 2022).

2 Chang JY, Li QQ, Xu QY, et al. Stereotactic ablative radiation therapy for centrally located early stage or isolated parenchymal recurrences of non-small cell lung cancer: how to fly in a 'no fly zone'. Int J Radiat Oncol Biol Phys 2014; 88: 1120–8.

3 The Royal College of Radiologists (2019). Radiotherapy dose fractionation. 3rd. ed. Available from: www.rcr.ac.uk/system/files/publication/field_publication_files/brfo193_radiotherapy_dose_fractionation_third-edition.pdf (accessed 1 March 2022).

4 Wisnivesky JP, Bonomi M, Henschke C, et al. Radiation therapy for the treatment of unresected stage I–II non-small cell lung cancer. Lung Cancer 2003; 41: 1–11

5 Murray P, Franks K, Hanna GG. A systematic review of outcomes following stereotactic ablative radiotherapy in the treatment of early-stage primary lung cancer. Br J Radiol 2017; 90: 20160732.

6 Timmerman RD, Hu H, Michalski J, et al. Long-term results of RTOG 0236: a phase II trial of stereotactic body radiation therapy (SBRT) in the treatment of patients with medically inoperable stage I non-small cell lung cancer. Int J Radiat Oncol 2014; 90 (suppl): S30.

7 Harder EM, Park HS, Chen ZJ, et al. Pulmonary dose-volume predictors of radiation pneumonitis following stereotactic body radiation therapy. Pract Radiat Oncol 2016; 6: e353–9.

8 Timmerman R, McGarry R, Yiannoutsos C, et al. Excessive toxicity when treating central tumors in a phase II study of stereotactic body radiation therapy for medically inoperable early-stage lung cancer. J Clin Oncol 2006; 24: 4833–9.

9 American Joint Committee on Cancer. Lung. In: Amin MB, Edge SB, Greene FL, et al., eds. AJCC cancer staging manual. 8th ed. New York: Springer, 2017; 167–77.

10 Chen H, Senan S, Nossent EJ, et al. Treatment-related toxicity in patients with early-stage non-small cell lung cancer and coexisting interstitial lung disease: a systematic review. Int J Radiat Oncol Biol Phys 2017; 98: 622–31.

11 Stanic S, Paulus R, Timmerman RD. No clinically significant changes in pulmonary function following stereotactic body radiation therapy for early-stage peripheral non-small cell lung cancer: an analysis of RTOG 0236. Int J Radiat Oncol Biol Phys 2014; 88: 1092–9.

12 Shaikh T, Turaka A. Predictors and management of chest wall toxicity after lung stereotactic body radiotherapy. Cancer Treat Rev 2014; 40: 1215–20.

13 Timmerman R, Papiez L, McGarry R, et al. Extracranial stereotactic radioablation: results of a phase I study in medically inoperable stage I non-small cell lung cancer. Chest 2003; 124: 1946–55.

14 Stahl JM, Ross R, Harder EM, et al. The effect of biologically effective dose and radiation treatment schedule on overall survival in stage I non-small cell lung cancer patients treated with stereotactic body radiation therapy. Int J Radiat Oncol Biol Phys 2016; 96: 1011–20.

15 Palma DA, Olson R, Harrow S, et al. Stereotactic ablative radiotherapy for the comprehensive treatment of oligometastatic cancers: long-term results of the SABR-COMET phase II randomized trial. J Clin Oncol 2020; 38: 2830–8.

05 Central lung metastasis on a background of colon cancer

Ben Fulton, Adam Peters

Case history

A 66-year-old woman was found to have a solitary lung metastasis near the right hilum on a surveillance CT scan. She had previously had stage II colorectal cancer, detected after a change in bowel habit and rectal bleeding. Apart from a medical history of stable angina and osteoarthritis affecting both knees, she was otherwise fit and well. Her ECOG performance status was 1.

The patient's previous tumour was an adenocarcinoma of the ascending colon (stage II, Dukes' C, T2N1M0, according to the criteria of the American Joint Committee on Cancer).[1] The tumour was removed with a right hemicolectomy and an R0 resection was achieved. Lymphadenectomy revealed 2/15 positive lymph nodes. The tumour had invaded the submucosa and the muscularis propria but had not penetrated the bowel wall.

Owing to the higher risk of tumour recurrence, the oncology team discussed adjuvant systemic chemotherapy with the patient. She went on to receive 3 months of adjuvant fluorouracil, folinic acid and oxaliplatin (FOLFOX) chemotherapy every 2 weeks. Adjuvant treatment was completed with modest toxicities including Common Terminology Criteria for Adverse Events grade 2 sensory peripheral neuropathy and an isolated episode of febrile neutropenia. The patient had recovered a few weeks after her last cycle, and she returned to her functional baseline after therapy.

CT cross-sectional imaging of the chest, abdomen and pelvis 6 months after completing adjuvant treatment was carried out as part of follow-up. It unfortunately showed a solitary lesion in the right lung near the right hilum. A PET-CT scan characterized it as a small solitary area of intense FDG avidity, roughly 2 cm in diameter. The multidisciplinary team (MDT) thought it likely represented a metachronous lung metastasis from the colorectal cancer.

The patient's case was discussed at an oligometastatic MDT meeting and she was referred to an experienced thoracic surgeon and a clinical oncologist specializing in thoracic stereotactic body radiotherapy (SBRT). A CT-guided biopsy confirmed metastasis from the adenocarcinoma of the colon; pulmonary function testing demonstrated normal spirometry as well as static/dynamic lung function and gas transfer.

The patient declined metastasectomy and elected to proceed with SBRT. A five-point beam directional shell was made and the patient subsequently underwent a contrast-enhanced four-dimensional CT scan in the supine position with arms adducted. The tumour was outlined using UK SABR Consortium guidelines.[2] Because the lesion was close to mediastinal structures and was deemed to be centrally located as it was within the 2 cm margin around the proximal bronchial tree, there were implications with regard to dose fractionation. The prescribed dose was 60 Gy in eight fractions on alternate days as recommended for the treatment of central lung tumours in the Royal College of Radiologists' radiotherapy dose fractionation guidelines.[3]

SBRT to the right lung was delivered with no set-up errors and daily cone-beam CT was carried out with online soft tissue correction. The patient tolerated treatment, the only toxicities being a grade 1 mild skin reaction, grade 1 fatigue and grade 2 oesophagitis, which was managed with oxetacaine/antacid. These had all settled within a matter of weeks and there was no clinical or radiological evidence on post-treatment chest X-ray to suggest pneumonitis.

What are the best practice guidelines for SBRT to the lung in the setting of oligometastatic disease?

What is the definition of central and ultracentral lung tumours?

How does tumour position influence dose fractionation and patient outcomes?

What common toxicities are seen when treating a central lung tumour with SBRT?

What are the best practice guidelines for SBRT to the lung in the setting of oligometastatic disease?

The use of SBRT to both primary and metastatic lung lesions has evolved in the past decade owing to the need to deliver high doses to provide local tumour control. According to the UK SABR Consortium guidelines, dose and fractionation regimens delivering a biologically effective dose (BED) >100 Gy are recommended to give good local control of lung tumours.[2] This dose would carry unacceptable toxicity if given via a conventional fractionation regimen.

In terms of tumour delineation, the UK SABR Consortium guidelines advocate use of a respiratory-correlated four-dimensional CT scan to contour the target volume of the tumour.[2] There are multiple techniques that may be employed to achieve respiratory motion management in localization imaging acquisition. Target volume contouring should be carried out in conjunction with evaluation of all staging investigations and imaging. Gross tumour volume delineation should be done using lung window settings. Mediastinal windowing may aid delineation of lesions situated close to the chest wall or mediastinal structures.

No additional margin is required for the clinical target volume. The internal target volume encompasses either the gross tumour volume at maximum inhale and maximal exhale, generated by registering individual gross tumour volume from the four-dimensional CT dataset as well as additional tumour seen on cine loop, or the full tumour extent on maximum intensity projection. The planning target volume margin is dependent on technique and should be decided by local protocols following internal audit of immobilization device, motion management and delivery technique. Typical internal and planning target volume margins in the lung are 3–5 mm.

There remains controversy around the use of SBRT for ultracentral lung lesions. Several studies of SBRT in primary lung cancers demonstrated significant toxicity and even mortality in SBRT for ultracentral tumours. Contemporary studies, including the UK HALT clinical trial (ClinicalTrials. gov NCT03256981), are exploring the safety of dose-adapted radiotherapy for mediastinal lymph nodes using a prescribed dose of 40–52 Gy in eight fractions, respecting critical organ-at-risk constraints to the proximal bronchial tree and central mediastinal structures.[4]

What is the definition of central and ultracentral lung tumours?

Improvements in radiation technology have led to the advent of hypofractionated radiotherapy schedules for primary and metastatic tumours in the thorax. In 2003, Timmerman et al. published a phase I dose escalation study demonstrating the safety and efficacy of 3×20 Gy fractions of radiotherapy for T1 and T2 peripheral lung tumours.[5] Their subsequent phase II study was the first to report high toxicity after SBRT for centrally located lesions at doses of 60–66 Gy in three fractions without heterogeneity correction.[6] Analysis of peripheral vs central tumour location demonstrated a 2 year incidence of grade ≥3 toxicity of 17% and 46%, respectively. The risk of grades 3–5 toxicities was 11-fold higher in patients with central tumours.

Another high-profile paper published reports in 2012 of fatal airway necrosis 8 months after SBRT (50 Gy in five fractions) for a centrally treated lung lesion.[7] Such reports highlighted the importance of tumour location and associated toxicity with lung SBRT.

The Timmerman et al. phase II study published the initial guidance defining 'central' vs 'peripheral' tumour location, taking into account the proximal bronchial tree (carina, main bronchi, upper/lower lobe bronchi, lingular bronchus and lower lobe branches).[6] Contemporary studies have identified the importance of additional centrally placed organs at risk, including the oesophagus, great vessels and heart. This broader definition of centrality was supported by the study protocol of the RTOG 0813 trial (ClinicalTrials.gov NCT00750269), suggesting that appreciation of other centrally located organs at risk (oesophagus, great vessels, heart) was required.[8] The guidelines on SBRT of the International Association for the Study of Lung Cancer reflect the evolving definition of 'central' tumours, including all lesions within 2 cm of the proximal bronchial tree, mediastinal/pericardial pleura and brachial plexus.[9]

There remain different definitions in the literature of 'ultracentral' tumours. The HILUS trial highlighted the difficulties in treating ultracentral tumours with SBRT. The study definition of ultracentrality was any gross tumour volume ≤1 cm from the proximal bronchial tree, overlapping the trachea or main bronchi.[10] The trial evaluated the use of SBRT at a dose of 56 Gy in eight fractions for ultracentral tumours. Owing to the increase in severe toxicities in ultracentral tumours compared with other tumour locations, the trial results did not support the use of SBRT for ultracentral locations. An equivalent dose of 70–80 Gy in two fractions was found to be an acceptable maximum dose to the trachea and main bronchi.

The phase I dose escalation SUNSET study (ClinicalTrials.gov NCT03306680) is currently assessing the safety and efficacy of SBRT for ultracentral tumours. The trial eligibility criteria for tumour location are any tumour whose planning target volume is expected to touch or overlap the central bronchial tree, oesophagus, pulmonary vein or pulmonary artery.[11] The results of this study are keenly awaited.

How does tumour position influence dose fractionation and patient outcomes?

Tumour location and dose are two important considerations when assessing patient suitability for lung SBRT. Centrality and ultracentrality reflect the tumour location in the thorax and the relationship with important organs at risk. If tumours are located too closely to critical structures, the ability to deliver a high BED to achieve good local control or even cure is often compromised in order to prevent unacceptable toxicity.

Central tumours can still be treated with SBRT with appropriate dose modification to respect tolerance of an organ at risk. The prescribed dosages for central tumours with homogeneity correction are typically 60 Gy in eight fractions over 10–20 days or 50 Gy in five fractions over 12 days.[3] Other dosage regimens may be considered depending on the institution's preference.

There remains controversy about the role of SBRT for ultracentral tumours outside a clinical trial. SUNSET is a multicentre phase I trial investigating the safety and efficacy of delivering treatment in three different doses to ultracentral tumour locations: 60 Gy in eight, 10 and 15 fractions.[11] The UK HALT study includes treatment of mediastinal nodes in an ultracentral tumour location, with appropriate dose mitigation for critical organ-at-risk constraints.[4] There remains a lack of robust clinical outcomes of SBRT for ultracentral tumour locations. The results of prospective clinical trials in this area are awaited.

Other anatomical locations requiring dose adaptations include apical lung tumours because of their proximity to the chest wall and brachial plexus. The updated definition of centrality in the International Association for the Study of Lung Cancer guidelines makes reference to areas such as the lung apex requiring the same dose adaptations as a central lung tumour.[9]

What common toxicities are seen when treating a central lung tumour with SBRT?

Potential toxicities relate to organs at risk adjacent to the treated volume. For central tumours, the main organs at risk include the proximal bronchial tree, oesophagus, great vessels, brachial plexus, chest wall and heart. The UK SABR Consortium outlines current consensus recommendations for organ tolerances that can be applied to SBRT in the thorax.[2]

Acute toxicities of SBRT for central tumours may include dyspnoea, cough, haemoptysis, pericarditis, dermatitis, chest wall pain and oesophagitis as well as constitutional symptoms of lethargy and anorexia. There are reported cases of fatalities due to dyspnoea, upper gastrointestinal perforation/fistulation and haemoptysis. It is of paramount importance that risks are weighed against the benefits of treatment, with informed discussion and decision shared with the patient.

Potential late toxicities of thoracic SBRT include radiation-induced lung fibrosis, necrosis of the bronchus and great vessels, chest wall necrosis/fractures, increased risk of cardiovascular disease, aneurysm formation and brachial plexopathy. These toxicities can adversely influence an individual's quality of life after treatment with SBRT.

Conclusion and learning points

- SBRT to oligometastatic central tumours in the thorax can provide high rates of local tumour control.
- Tumour location within the thorax is of paramount importance, influencing treatment dose, planning and delivery. The location should be assessed on an individual basis by an experienced MDT.
- Consensus guidelines have been published defining centrality and ultracentrality for thoracic tumours and have been serially refined to reflect increasing awareness of the critical importance of central organ-at-risk considerations.
- Recommended dose and fractionation regimens, along with appropriate dose constraints, are available in the UK SABR Consortium and Royal College of Radiologists' guidelines.[2,3]

- Trials to assess the safety and efficacy of SBRT in ultracentral tumour locations are underway and will influence its role in future clinical practice.

References

1   American Joint Committee on Cancer. Lung. In: Amin MB, Edge SB, Greene FL, et al., eds. AJCC cancer staging manual. 8th ed. New York: Springer, 2017; 167–77.

2   UK SABR Consortium (2019). Stereotactic ablative radiotherapy (SABR): a resource. Version 6.1. Available from: www.sabr.org.uk/wp-content/uploads/2019/04/SABRconsortium-guidelines-2019-v6.1.0.pdf (accessed 1 March 2022).

3   Royal College of Radiologists (2019). Radiotherapy dose fractionation. 3rd. ed. Available from: www.rcr.ac.uk/system/files/publication/field_publication_files/brfo193_radiotherapy_dose_fractionation_third-edition.pdf (accessed 1 March 2022).

4   McDonald F, Gukenberger M, Popat S, et al. HALT: targeted therapy beyond progression with or without dose-intensified radiotherapy in oligo-progressive disease in oncogene addicted lung tumours. Lung Cancer 2017; 103 (suppl): S57.

5   Timmerman R, Papiez L, McGarry R, et al. Extracranial stereotactic radioablation: results of a phase I study in medically inoperable stage I non-small cell lung cancer. Chest 2003; 124: 1946–55.

6   Timmerman R, McGarry R, Yiannoutsos C, et al. Excessive toxicity when treating central tumors in a phase II study of stereotactic body radiation therapy for medically inoperable early-stage lung cancer. J Clin Oncol 2006; 24: 4833–9.

7   Corradetti MN, Haas AR, Rengan R. Central-airway necrosis after stereotactic body-radiation therapy. N Engl J Med 2012; 366: 2327–9.

8   Bezjak A, Paulus R, Gaspar LE, et al. Safety and efficacy of a five-fraction stereotactic body radiotherapy schedule for centrally located non-small-cell lung cancer: NRG Oncology/RTOG 0813 trial. J Clin Oncol 2019; 37: 1316–25.

9   Chang JY, Li QQ, Xu QY, et al. Stereotactic ablative radiation therapy for centrally located early stage or isolated parenchymal recurrences of non-small cell lung cancer: how to fly in a 'no fly zone'. Int J Radiat Oncol Biol Phys 2014; 88: 1120–8.

10 Lindberg K, Grozman V, Karlsson K, et al. The HILUS trial – a prospective Nordic multicenter phase 2 study of ultracentral lung tumors treated with stereotactic body radiotherapy. J Thorac Oncol 2021; 16: 1200–10.

11 Giuliani M, Mathew AS, Bahig H, et al. SUNSET: Stereotactic Radiation for Ultracentral Non-Small-Cell Lung Cancer – A Safety and Efficacy Trial. Clin Lung Cancer 2018; 19: e529–32.

06 Colorectal cancer and a solitary tibial metastasis

Rebecca Muirhead

Case history

A 52-year-old woman underwent a high anterior resection for a sigmoid adenocarcinoma. The pathology was pT2pN0, Ras/*BRAF* wild-type, mismatch repair-proficient. Owing to the early stage, negative nodal status and good prognosis, there was no indication for adjuvant treatment, and she commenced routine surgical follow-up.

Two months later, she presented to the orthopaedic team with pain in her right shin. An X-ray revealed a 2 cm lucent lesion in the mid-tibia (Figure 6.1). She had a biopsy, as initially it was thought to be a primary bone lesion. The biopsy unexpectedly revealed a metastatic adenocarcinoma. The pathology was reviewed and was identical both morphologically and immunohistochemically to her previous sigmoid adenocarcinoma. She underwent whole body CT and PET-CT scans, which confirmed the tumour was a solitary lesion breaching the cortex of the tibia.

Over a short period of time oncologists and orthopaedic surgeons discussed with her the different treatment options, during which the lesion was visibly increasing in size beneath the skin. In addition, mobilizing was becoming difficult because of rapidly increasing pain.

What different concerns should be considered in this case?

What treatment options were available?

What are the risks and benefits of stereotactic body radiotherapy (SBRT)?

What is the delivery technique for SBRT?

What is the appropriate follow-up schedule after SBRT?

What different concerns should be considered in this case?

Pain

When the patient was seen by the oncologists, pain was a major issue. As the lesion grew it was becoming more painful and mobilization was becoming more difficult. The first step was to instigate appropriate analgesics and support. Because of the rapid escalation in pain it was important to tailor treatment to provide an early, more definitive treatment for her local symptoms.

Fracture risk

Malignant bony lesions carry a risk of fracture. The Mirels' score was used to calculate the percentage risk based on the site and size of the metastasis, the nature of the metastasis (lytic or

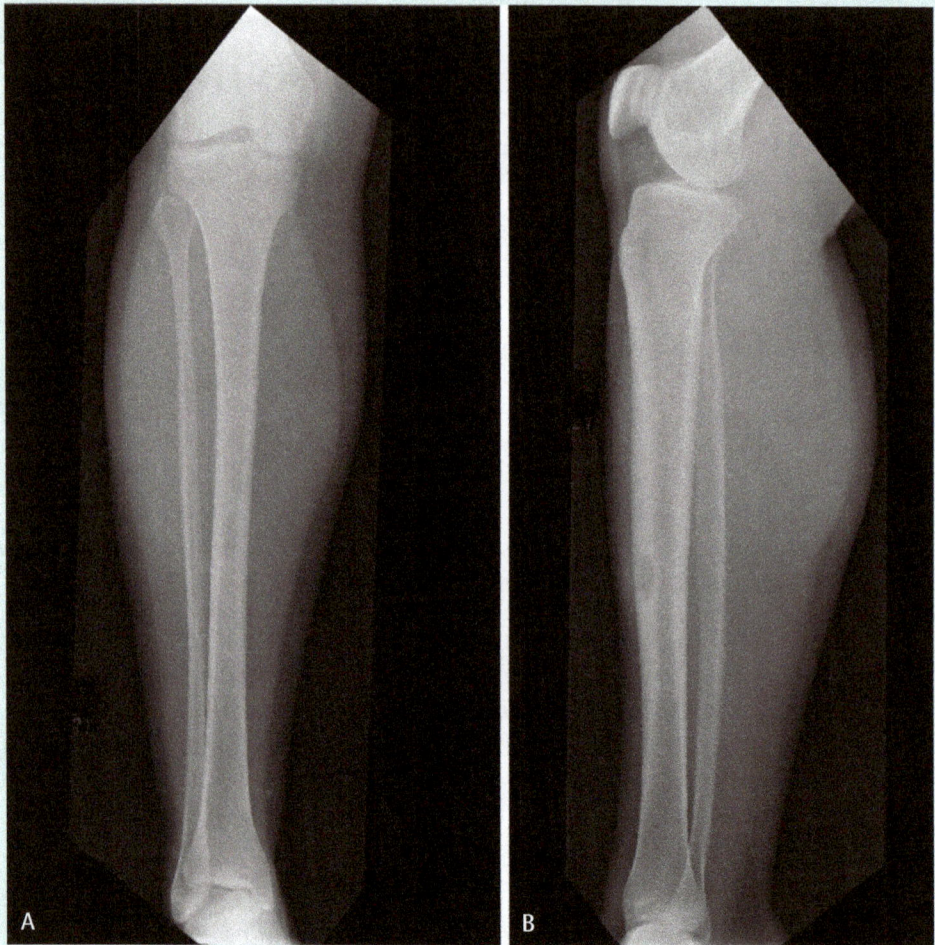

Figure 6.1 X-ray image of the right lower leg, demonstrating a radiolucent area in the mid-tibia. (A) Anterior posterior view; (B) sagittal view.

sclerotic) and the degree of pain.[1] The risk of fracture was calculated to be >33% at 3 months post-irradiation. At this level of risk, fixation should be considered.

Systemic disease risk

The length of the disease-free interval from primary surgery to the development of further disease is an excellent indicator of overall survival (OS).[2] The shorter the interval, the more likely there are to be systemic micrometastases and worsening biology. As such, radical treatment of oligometastatic disease is usually undertaken when there is a minimum disease-free interval of 6 months; however, this patient had had a very short disease-free interval. In deciding on treatment it was important to fully discuss the likely poor oncological outcome and make management decisions with that in mind.

What treatment options were available?

Palliative treatment: single fraction of radiotherapy +/– systemic therapy in due course

Because of the short disease-free interval it would have been appropriate to consider this a pallia-tive situation. A single fraction of 8 Gy to the tibia would have offered excellent pain relief. Sys-temic therapy could have been started thereafter or, more likely, when further disease developed and a response to chemotherapy could be meaningfully measured.

Radical option 1: radical surgery +/– neoadjuvant or adjuvant chemotherapy

The orthopaedic team felt that radical surgery to remove and replace the bone would carry significant morbidity and mortality. In view of the short disease-free interval and likely poor on-cological outcome they did not feel that radical surgery was appropriate. Neoadjuvant chemo-therapy was considered as a test of biology, to ascertain whether the disease remained localized, before embarking on significant surgery; however, this course of action was dismissed because chemotherapy would have little impact on the patient's pain, which was significantly impacting her quality of life.

Radical option 2: SBRT +/– adjuvant chemotherapy

SBRT is the delivery of a very high ablative dose of radiation concentrated on a tumour, while limiting the dose to the surrounding organs. This would have the potential of eradicating the tibial disease, requiring five outpatient visits and with minimal toxicity. In a setting with a likely poor oncological outcome, it was considered of paramount importance to maximize quality of life.

What are the risks and benefits of SBRT?

There were a number of benefits of SBRT for this patient. In colorectal cancer, SBRT has local control rates at 1 and 2 years of 81% and 62%, respectively.[3] A significant pain response was re-ported in the phase II VERTICAL study (ClinicalTrials.gov NCT02364115) in 96% of patients within 3 months of receiving SBRT.[4] Cohort studies and retrospective series of ablative treatments in oligometastatic disease have demonstrated consistently better outcomes than are seen in trials of systemic therapy.[5-7] However, without randomized evidence, it is possible these outcomes re-flect patient selection. The SABR-COMET trial (ClinicalTrials.gov NCT01446744) provides ran-domized prospective evidence of an OS benefit using SABR as the directed therapy.[8]

Additionally, SBRT is convenient and low cost and it has low toxicity. Delivery requires between three and five outpatient visits to the radiotherapy department. The patient gave informed consent for the acute toxicities of a potential 1–2 week pain flare, skin redness and itch and mild fatigue. Because of the low risk of morbidity she would be fit for systemic therapy immediately after com-pleting her treatment if it was deemed appropriate. The potentially serious late toxicities were a <5% risk of grade 3 skin ulceration and a significant continued risk of fracture.

What is the delivery technique for SBRT?

SBRT is entirely reliant on optimal immobilization. One must also avoid using the other leg where possible. The patient was therefore immobilized supine, with her left leg bent and her right leg on a knee rest and a thermoplastic shell was fitted around her right foot to keep it immobile (Figure 6.2). The target volume (gross tumour volume) was outlined with an additional margin for set-up errors to create a planning target volume. The primary organs at risk for consideration in this case were the skin and fibula. The radiation was delivered in two arcs, a clockwise and

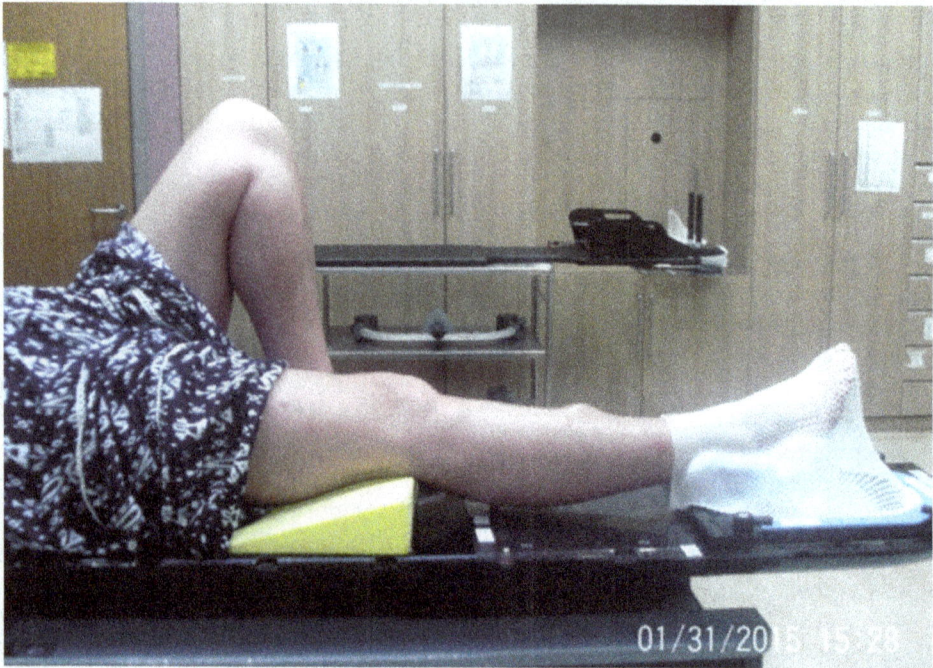

Figure 6.2 Position of the patient on the radiotherapy bed with her left knee bent, her right knee resting and an individualized foot mask fitted around her right foot. The mid-tibial lesion can be seen protruding from the skin.

an anticlockwise arc, with two further static anterior oblique beams in order to minimize the dose to the posterior leg and fibula (Figure 6.3). The dose delivered was 40 Gy in five fractions with a peak dose within the gross tumour volume of 112.5% (Figure 6.4).

What is the appropriate follow-up schedule after SBRT?

In this case, whether to deliver adjuvant chemotherapy following SBRT was a challenging decision. There is increasing phase III evidence reporting no OS benefit of either neoadjuvant or adjuvant chemotherapy following treatment of oligometastatic disease.[9] However, in these studies there had been a minimum of 6 months between primary surgery and oligometastatic treatment, and many of the study patients had undergone a course of adjuvant systemic therapy after primary surgery. As our patient had had a 2 month disease-free interval and had not received any adjuvant systemic therapy, the chance of her having micrometastasis that may be amenable to adjuvant therapy was deemed significant. She therefore received 6 months of adjuvant capecitabine and oxaliplatin (CAPOX), which was the standard of care at the time.

Imaging follow-up after SBRT was challenging. SABR-COMET showed that patients who received SBRT often required, and benefited from, further intervention with SBRT.[10] The residual necrotic mass may be mistaken for residual disease, particularly as it can remain FDG-avid for several years. Patients should have baseline imaging 3 months after SBRT, and recurrence should be considered in lesions that demonstrate consistent growth from that baseline. In this case, the

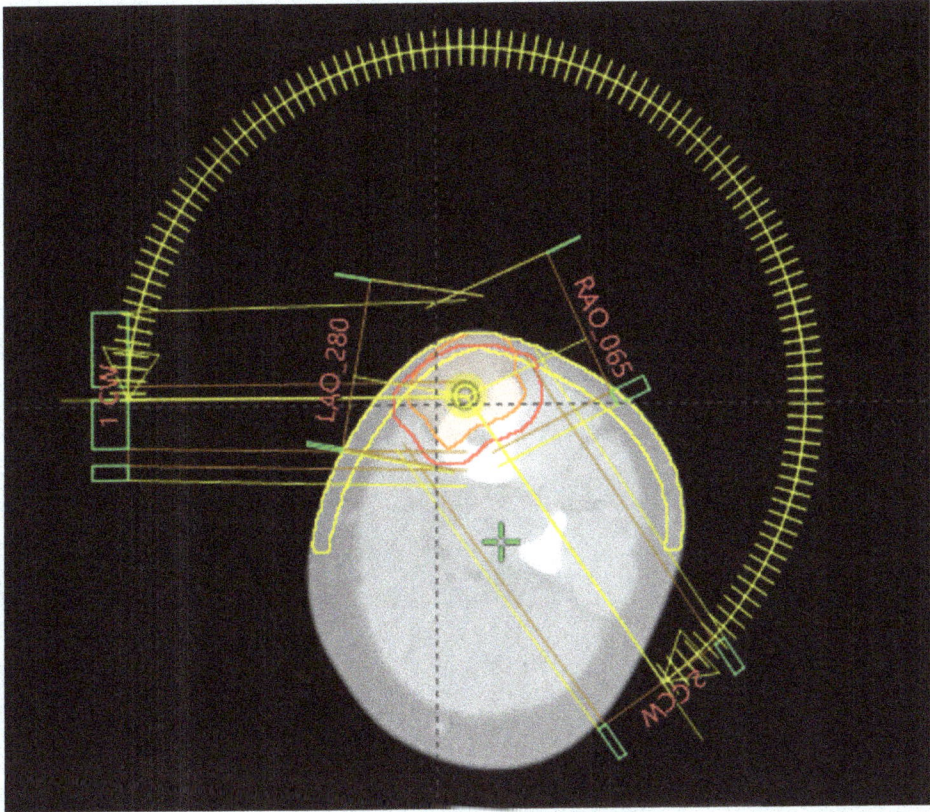

Figure 6.3 CT planning scan image of the right tibia showing the gross tumour volume (orange), planning target volume (red) and organ at risk (skin, yellow). The beams show two arcs with two anterior oblique fields.

patient was referred back to the primary oncology centre for local follow-up and the SBRT team were not consulted regarding further imaging. The residual mass remained FDG-avid. Following communication with the orthopaedic and sarcoma teams, the view was this represented residual disease, and the orthopaedic team undertook surgical replacement of her right tibia, 13 months after her SBRT. The pathology revealed a pathological complete response. Unfortunately, the patient has required two further surgical procedures and a number of inpatient stays for infection and morbidity relating to the surgery. Three years since her SBRT, she remains free of disease.

Conclusion and learning points

- SBRT is one of the multiple local treatments available for oligometastatic disease in colorectal cancer.
- SBRT requires between three and five outpatient visits and causes minimal toxicity. It can be used to target most metastatic sites such as bones, lymph nodes, lung, liver, peritoneal deposits and local recurrences.

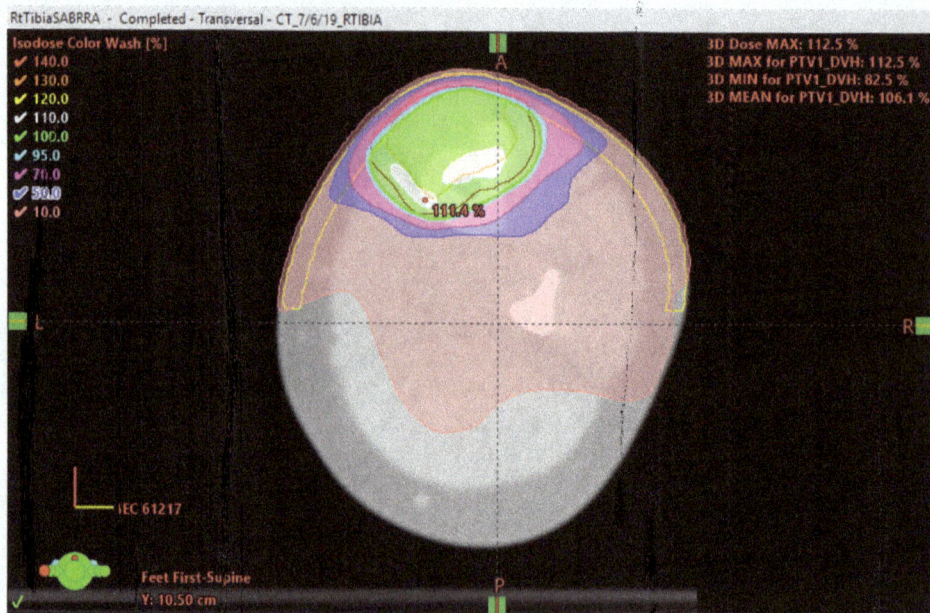

Figure 6.4 CT planning scan image of the right tibia showing the dose distribution. Isodose lines of 10%, 50%, 70%, 100% and 110% are shown in pink, blue, magenta, green and white, respectively.

- Prospective trial data demonstrate efficacy of SBRT as regards local control, pain control and OS.

- SBRT, like all targeted therapies, is usually reserved for patients demonstrating good biology with three or fewer lesions and a minimum disease-free interval of 6 months. The present case, however, highlights that in selected clinical circumstances, it may be appropriate therapy notwithstanding these stringent criteria.

References

1   Mirels H. Metastatic disease in long bones: a proposed scoring system for diagnosing impending pathologic fractures. Clin Orthop Relat Res 1989; 249: 256–64.

2   Sargent DJ, Wieand HS, Haller DG, et al. Disease-free survival versus overall survival as a primary end point for adjuvant colon cancer studies: individual patient data from 20,898 patients on 18 randomized trials. J Clin Oncol 2005; 23: 8664–70.

3   Chalkidou A, Macmillan T, Grzeda MT, et al. Stereotactic ablative body radiotherapy in patients with oligometastatic cancers: a prospective, registry-based, single-arm, observational, evaluation study. Lancet Oncol 2021; 22: 98–101.

4   Pielkenrood BJ, van der Velden JM, van der Linden YM, et al. Pain response after stereotactic body radiation therapy versus conventional radiation therapy in patients with bone metastases – a phase 2 randomized controlled trial within a prospective cohort. Int J Radiat Oncol Biol Phys 2021; 110: 358–67.

5   Ashworth A, Rodrigues G, Boldt G, Palma D. Is there an oligometastatic state in nonsmall
    cell lung cancer? A systematic review of the literature. Lung Cancer 2013; 82: 197–203.

6   Utley M, Treasure T, Linklater K, Moller H. Better out than in? The resection of pulmonary
    metastases from colorectal tumours. Presented at: 33rd International Conference on
    Operational Research Applied to Health Services, Saint-Étienne, France, 15–20 July 2007;
    493–500.

7   Palma DA, Salama JK, Lo SS, et al. The oligometastatic state – separating truth from wishful
    thinking. Nat Rev Clin Oncol 2014; 11: 549–57.

8   Palma DA, Olson R, Harrow S, et al. Stereotactic ablative radiotherapy versus standard
    of care palliative treatment in patients with oligometastatic cancers (SABR-COMET): a
    randomised, phase 2, open-label trial. Lancet 2019; 393: 2051–8.

9   Booth C, Berry S. Perioperative chemotherapy for resectable liver metastases in colorectal
    cancer: do we have a blind spot? J Clin Oncol 2021; 39: 3767–9.

10 Palma DA, Olson R, Harrow S, et al. Stereotactic ablative radiotherapy for the comprehensive
    treatment of oligometastatic cancers: long-term results of the SABR-COMET phase II
    randomized trial. J Clin Oncol 2020; 38: 2830–8.

07 Prostate cancer and an isolated spinal metastasis

Sara Walker, Séan M. O'Cathail

Case history

A 69-year-old man presented with a 6 week history of mild back pain. His medical history included a diagnosis of adenocarcinoma of the prostate (Gleason score 4+3=7, T3bN0M0) 4 years earlier. He was treated with neoadjuvant androgen deprivation therapy followed by radical, moderately hypofractionated external beam radiotherapy 60 Gy in 20 fractions. He tolerated his radiotherapy well and his prostate-specific antigen (PSA) level reached a nadir of <0.01 ng/ml 6 months after completing treatment. He had no other medical history of note and did not take any regular medications.

He had been well until he began noticing a pain in the mid-lower thoracic region of his spine, particularly at night and during periods of exertion, but he was not taking any regular analgesia. A blood test arranged by his GP revealed an elevated PSA level of 8.2 ng/ml. He was referred back to his treating oncologist. A bone scan showed an area of increased uptake in the T9 region that suggested a metastatic deposit. No other concerning skeletal deposits were noted. A CT scan of the thorax, abdomen and pelvis confirmed an osteosclerotic metastasis in the T9 region and no areas of visceral or nodal metastases.

The patient's case was discussed by the uro-oncology multidisciplinary team and the prospect of spinal stereotactic body radiotherapy (SBRT) was raised. A subsequent MRI scan showed that his disease was limited to the vertebral body, there was no evidence of spinal canal compromise or body collapse, there was normal alignment and there were no other spinal metastases. His clinical oncologist calculated a low spinal instability neoplastic score of 6/18, indicating a stable spine.[1] He was referred to his local SBRT team for consideration of treatment to his T9 vertebra.

Was SBRT a legitimate treatment option in this case?

What would be the benefits of SBRT in this patient?

What is the evidence base for his treatment options?

What are the likely acute and long-term complications?

What role does SBRT play in his future management?

Was SBRT a legitimate treatment option in this case?

Since prostate cancer is regarded as a relatively radiosensitive cancer, either conventional external beam radiotherapy (EBRT) or SBRT were felt to be reasonable treatment options. Breast, ovarian

Measurement	SBRT	EBRT
Aim of treatment	Local control and not an emergency (e.g. spinal cord compression)	Symptom control (e.g. pain) or an emergency (e.g. spinal cord compression)
Performance status	ECOG 0–1 KPS ≥80%	ECOG ≥2 KPS <80%
Neurological symptoms	Asymptomatic or mild symptoms without rapid progression	Severe or rapidly progressing neurological symptoms
No. of spinal metastases	≤3 contiguous vertebral bodies and no cord compression	>3 contiguous vertebral bodies, non-contiguous vertebral body involvement or evidence of spinal cord compression
Extent of metastatic disease	≤5 metastatic sites	>5 metastatic sites
Response to SACT	Partial response or stable disease	Progressive disease

Table 7.1 Clinical factors to aid initial treatment decision: SBRT vs EBRT (adapted from Singh et al.[5]).

KPS, Karnofsky performance scale score; SACT, Systemic anticancer therapy.

and neuroendocrine cancers are included in this category. Radioresistant tumour types include renal, thyroid and hepatocellular, as well as non-small-cell lung carcinoma, sarcoma and melanoma, and it is felt that these tumours require SBRT to better achieve local control.[2] Lymphoma, seminoma and myeloma are globally recognized as radiosensitive histologies; therefore, irrespective of neurological compromise, EBRT should be used instead of SBRT or spinal surgery for metastatic spinal disease, even in the clinical setting of cord compression.[2]

A consensus document from the European Society for Radiotherapy and Oncology (ESTRO) and the American Society for Radiation Oncology (ASTRO) defines oligometastatic disease as involving up to five metastatic lesions. All metastatic sites can be safely treated and the primary tumour controlled.[3] The treatment of oligometastatic disease is a relatively new and emerging area of interest and research in oncology. Further work is required to determine, ideally in a prospective series, which patients are best suited to treatment with metastasis-directed therapy.[4]

Nevertheless, the use of metastasis-directed therapy is increasing, meaning that there are now multiple ways to treat metastatic prostatic spinal disease with radiotherapy. Options include EBRT, fractionated SBRT or single fraction SBRT. Table 7.1 summarizes a number of clinical factors to aid the initial treatment decision between SBRT and EBRT for metastatic spinal disease.[5]

Our patient had a good ECOG performance status of 1 (Karnofsky performance scale score ≥80%). He had fewer than five sites of metastatic disease and no neurological compromise or spinal cord compression, and his underlying primary tumour was associated with a good prognosis. As the aim of treatment in this man was therefore both local control and alleviation of symptoms, SBRT was seen as a legitimate choice.

What would be the benefits of SBRT in this patient?

Because of the more favourable risk factors associated with our patient's presentation, the aim of treatment was to improve his symptom burden and local control as well as his overall survival (OS). Mounting evidence suggests that SBRT treatment of oligometastatic prostate cancer is associated with better local control outcomes and androgen deprivation therapy-free survival.[4,6-8] SBRT is also delivered in fewer outpatient visits compared with EBRT.

What is the evidence base for his treatment options?

The STOMP trial (ClinicalTrials.gov NCT01558427) investigated whether metastasis-directed therapy for oligometastatic prostate cancer improved progression-free survival (PFS) (androgen deprivation therapy-free).[7,8] Participants comprised 62 men with asymptomatic biochemical recurrence of prostate cancer following primary treatment with curative intent, with up to three metastases and serum testosterone levels >50 ng/ml (>173.35 nmol/l). Between August 2012 and August 2015, participants were randomly assigned 1:1 to either surveillance or metastasis-directed therapy. Androgen deprivation therapy was commenced at symptomatic progression if more than three metastases developed or if there was local progression of known metastases. At both 3 and 5 year follow-up androgen deprivation therapy-free survival was found to be longer with metastasis-directed therapy than with surveillance alone for oligorecurrent prostate cancer: 8% for the surveillance group vs 34% for the metastasis-directed therapy group (HR 0.57; 80% CI 0.38%, 0.84%; p=0.06). The safety of metastasis-directed therapy was very good, with 17% grade 1 toxicity and no grade 2 or higher toxicity reported. The 5 year castrate-resistant prostate cancer-free survival, a secondary endpoint, was 53% for the surveillance group and 76% for the metastasis-directed therapy group (HR 0.62; 80% CI 0.35%, 1.09%; p=0.27). It is recommended to test metastasis-directed therapy in larger phase III trials.

A multicentre phase III study by the Radiation Therapy Oncology Group (RTOG 0631; ClinicalTrials.gov NCT00922974) randomized 339 eligible individuals with up to three spinal metastases to pain relief with SBRT or EBRT.[9] Participants were randomly assigned to receive SBRT at a dose of 16 or 18 Gy in one fraction to the involved spinal segment or to receive EBRT at a dose of 8 Gy in one fraction to the involved vertebrae plus the vertebrae above and below. The primary outcome was pain control, which was identified as a three point improvement on the numerical rating pain scale at the treated spinal segment, 3 months post-treatment. The investigators concluded that there was no significant difference in pain control achieved at 3 months post-treatment between the two groups (40.3% vs 57.9%; one-sided p=0.99).

The CCTG SC.24/TROG 17.06 trial (ClinicalTrials.gov NCT02512965) comprised 229 individuals with new, painful spinal metastases (brief pain inventory score ≥2) and ECOG performance status 0-2.[10] Participants were randomized 1:1 to receive SBRT at a dose of 24 Gy in two fractions or EBRT at a dose of 20 Gy in five fractions to painful spinal metastases. Three months post-radiation, 14% in the EBRT group reported a complete response to pain vs 36% in the SBRT group. Significance was retained in multivariable analyses (risk ratio 1.33; 95% CI 1.14, 1.55; p<0.001) in support of SBRT. At 6 months, 16% in the EBRT group vs 32% in the SBRT group reported a complete pain response (p=0.0036). The 3 month PFS was 86% for EBRT vs 92% for SBRT (p=0.18) and at 6 months it was 69% for EBRT vs 75% for SBRT (p=0.34). The investigators concluded that SBRT was superior to EBRT in delivering pain relief associated with spinal metastases.

What are the likely acute and long-term complications?

SBRT to spinal metastases may be complicated by acute pain flare, which is ameliorated effectively with the use of high-dose steroid cover.[11] It is recommended that all individuals receiving spinal SBRT should be prescribed concurrent high-dose steroid cover (8 mg oral dexamethasone, twice daily).

Another recognized acute complication secondary to spinal SBRT is the risk of vertebral compression fracture (VCF).[12] As VCF is substantially higher in association with SBRT (11–39%) than with EBRT (<5%), patients offered spinal SBRT should be assessed using the spinal instability neoplastic score.[1] As the thoracic spine was the area receiving SBRT in our patient, specific acute complications would potentially include oesophagitis, nausea, chest pain or rib fracture as well as a small long-term risk of tracheo-oesophageal fistula or stricture formation.[11]

Late complications of spinal SBRT are poorly understood, mainly because this patient group has a poor prognosis and follow-up data are scarce, but increasing length of survival brings a longer term risk of complications. Radiation-induced myelopathy is a concern; however, the risk of radiation-induced myelopathy was reported to be ≤5% when limiting the thecal sac point maximum volume doses to 12.4 Gy in one fraction, 17 Gy in two fractions, 20.3 Gy in three fractions, 23 Gy in four fractions and 25.3 Gy in five fractions.[13] Close monitoring, long-term follow-up and measurement of patient-reported outcomes, particularly in the context of clinical trials, are crucial in this patient group to better evaluate the longer term risk of complications associated with spinal SBRT.

What role does SBRT play in his future management?

A retrospective study was carried out at the Royal Marsden hospital, London, using the ESTRO/European Organisation for Research and Treatment of Cancer classification to predict progression in individuals treated for bone-only oligometastatic prostate cancer.[4] The study recruited 105 men (119 separate treatments) and reported a 3 year metastatic PFS of 23% (95% CI 13%, 32%) and a 3 year OS of 88% (95% CI 80%, 96%). Patients may benefit from further metastasis-directed therapy in the future, as seen in the SABR-COMET trial (ClinicalTrials.gov NCT01446744).[14]

Future considerations following spinal SBRT treatment should include the management of vertebral fracture risk. The risk of VCF associated with spinal SBRT treatment is far higher (28.5% 1 year after SBRT [or generally recognized as 11–39%]) than that associated with EBRT (~5%). The mechanism of action of SBRT-related VCF is thought to be osteoradionecrosis. Other risk factors associated with a higher VCF rate include pre-existing VCF and osteolytic disease.[11,12,15]

One-third of post-SBRT VCFs require intervention: percutaneous, minimally invasive or open spinal surgery. There is therefore a suggestion, though debated, that if pre-existing VCF and/or osteolytic disease is present, then early preventative vertebroplasty should be considered for high-risk vertebral segments.[12,15] Another method proposed to try to reduce the potential VCF risk associated with spinal SBRT is to deliver treatment over multiple fractions rather than in a single fraction, mainly to minimize the degree of osteoradionecrosis caused.[16]

A more holistic approach to VCF risk management is to prevent and treat for osteoporosis: encouraging patients to stop smoking and minimize alcohol consumption, recommending weight-bearing and muscle-strengthening exercises and assessing the patient's risk of falls will all help to prevent the occurrence of VCF.[17]

Conclusion and learning points

- There are now multiple radiotherapy treatment options for metastatic spinal disease. The individual's clinical factors determine which modality of radiotherapy may be best to use. Tools such as that given in Table 7.1, the neurologic, oncologic, mechanical and systemic decision framework[2] and the ESTRO-ASTRO oligometastatic classification system[3] can aid treatment modality decisions, but research on how to improve patient selection is still required.

- More prospective trial data are required to better evidence the improved local control and symptomatic outcomes associated with SBRT to spinal metastases, the results of which are so far encouraging.

- Spinal SBRT treatment is generally well tolerated and few severe-grade toxicities have been reported.

- Close clinical follow-up to better determine the longer term complications associated with spinal SBRT treatment is needed because it will aid optimization of survivorship in this patient population.

References

1 Fisher CG, DiPaola CP, Ryken TC, et al. A novel classification system for spinal instability in neoplastic disease: an evidence-based approach and expert consensus from the Spine Oncology Study Group. Spine 2010; 35: E1221.

2 Laufer I, Rubin DG, Lis E, et al. The NOMS framework: approach to the treatment of spinal metastatic tumors. Oncologist 2013; 18: 744–51.

3 Lievens Y, Guckenberger M, Gomez D, et al. Defining oligometastatic disease from a radiation oncology perspective: an ESTRO-ASTRO consensus document. Radiother Oncol 2020; 148: 157–66.

4 Nicholls L, Chapman E, Khoo V, et al. Metastasis-directed therapy in prostate cancer: prognostic significance of the ESTRO/EORTC classification in oligometastatic bone disease. Clin Oncol (R Coll Radiol) 2022; 34: 63–9.

5 Singh R, Lehrer EJ, Dahshan B, et al. Single fraction radiosurgery, fractionated radiosurgery, and conventional radiotherapy for spinal oligometastasis (SAFFRON): a systematic review and meta-analysis. Radiother Oncol 2020; 146: 76–89.

6 Phillips R, Shi WY, Deek M, et al. Outcomes of observation vs stereotactic ablative radiation for oligometastatic prostate cancer: the ORIOLE phase 2 randomized clinical trial. JAMA Oncol 2020; 6: 650.

7 Ost P, Reynders D, Decaestecker K, et al. Surveillance or metastasis-directed therapy for oligometastatic prostate cancer recurrence (STOMP): five-year results of a randomized phase II trial. J Clin Oncol 2020; 38 (6 suppl): 10.

8 Ost P, Reynders D, Decaestecker K, et al. Surveillance or metastasis-directed therapy for oligometastatic prostate cancer recurrence: a prospective, randomized, multicenter phase II trial. J Clin Oncol 2018; 36: 446–53.

9 Ryu S, Deshmukh S, Timmerman RD, et al. Radiosurgery compared to external beam radiotherapy for localized spine metastasis: phase III results of NRG Oncology/RTOG 0631. Int J Radiat Oncol Biol Phys 2019; 105 (suppl): S2–3.

10 Sahgal A, Myrehaug SD, Siva S, et al. Stereotactic body radiotherapy versus conventional external beam radiotherapy in patients with painful spinal metastases: an open-label, multicentre, randomised, controlled, phase 2/3 trial. Lancet Oncol 2021; 22: 1023–33.

11 UK SABR Consortium (2019). Stereotactic ablative radiotherapy (SABR): a resource. Version 6.1. Available from: www.sabr.org.uk/wp-content/uploads/2019/04/SABRconsortium-guidelines-2019-v6.1.0.pdf (accessed 12 March 2022).

12 Sahgal A, Whyne CM, Ma L, et al. Vertebral compression fracture after stereotactic body radiotherapy for spinal metastases. Lancet Oncol 2013; 14: e310–20.

13 Sahgal A, Weinberg V, Ma L, et al. Probabilities of radiation myelopathy specific to stereotactic body radiation therapy to guide safe practice. Int J Radiat Oncol Biol Phys 2013; 85: 341–7.

14 Palma DA, Olson R, Harrow S, et al. Stereotactic ablative radiotherapy versus standard of care palliative treatment in patients with oligometastatic cancers (SABR-COMET): a randomised, phase 2, open-label trial. Lancet 2019; 393: 2051–8.

15 Yoo GS, Park HC, Yu JI, et al. Stereotactic ablative body radiotherapy for spinal metastasis from hepatocellular carcinoma: its oncologic outcomes and risk of vertebral compression fracture. Oncotarget 2017; 8: 72860–71.

16 Mehta N, Zavitsanos PJ, Moldovan K, et al. Local failure and vertebral body fracture risk using multifraction stereotactic body radiation therapy for spine metastases. Adv Radiat Oncol 2018; 3: 245–51.

17 Cosman F, de Beur SJ, LeBoff MS, et al. Clinician's guide to prevention and treatment of osteoporosis. Osteoporos Int 2014; 25: 2359–81.

08 Lung metastases from colorectal cancer

Fergus Macbeth, Tom Treasure

Case history

A 65-year-old man was being followed up by his GP after surgery and adjuvant chemotherapy with 6 months of fluorouracil, folinic acid and oxaliplatin (FOLFOX) for stage III (T2N1M0) colon cancer 3 years previously.

A chest X-ray taken following an acute chest infection had shown possible metastases; CT confirmed that there were two small metastases (<1 cm in diameter), one peripherally in the left upper lobe and the other more central in the middle lobe. Fine needle aspiration of the more peripheral metastasis confirmed a diagnosis of metastatic adenocarcinoma consistent with an origin in the colon. A subsequent PET-CT scan showed no other metastases or signs of local recurrence.

The man was asymptomatic apart from mild dyspnoea on exertion. He had been a heavy smoker in the past but had given up 5 years previously. His lung function tests were consistent with mild emphysema. He was otherwise fit and well with no recent weight loss, normal liver function tests and a carcinoembryonic antigen (CEA) level of 6 μg/l.

What are the treatment options?

What is the evidence on how best to manage lung 'oligometastases' from colorectal cancer?

What are the risks and benefits of the different treatment options?

What should this man be told?

Should he have been followed up more closely with regular CT scans and CEA measurements?

What are the treatment options?

There are four main treatment options:

- observation and no further therapy until there is obvious symptomatic progression;
- surgery to remove the metastases;
- ablation of the metastases by either stereotactic radiotherapy (SBRT) or radiofrequency ablation;
- systemic treatment with chemotherapy and/or immunotherapy depending on molecular testing.

What is the evidence on how best to manage lung 'oligometastases' from colorectal cancer?

It should be noted that we question the existence of 'oligometastasis' as an entity rather than just the tail end of a distribution for whom the fewness of their discoverable metastases at that point in time makes them amenable to local treatments.[1]

Surgical removal and ablation of colorectal cancer lung metastases have been carried out for many years. The wide belief in their usefulness is based on many retrospective observational studies which have claimed to show that the intervention improves overall survival (OS). These studies may show the safety and technical efficacy of the interventions but as they were not randomized and lacked controls they do not provide evidence of effectiveness.

There have been a few randomized controlled trials (RCTs) investigating the removal or ablation of so-called 'oligometastases', but only the PulMiCC study (ClinicalTrials.gov NCT01106261) directly investigated whether removal of lung metastases benefits people with colorectal cancer. An RCT (N=93) was nested within a large, careful observational study (N=512). The participants selected for metastasectomy (n=263) had longer OS (median 4.4 years) than those not selected for surgery (n=128) (median 2.8 years) but also much more favourable prognostic factors (Figure 8.1, upper panel).[2] Those entered into the RCT were well balanced for known prognostic factors and there was no significant difference in OS between the two arms. Median survival was in fact longer (3.8 vs 3.5 years) for controls (Figure 8.1, lower panel).[3] These results cannot exclude a small difference in survival attributable to intervention, but if it does exist it must be much smaller than widely believed.

The SABR-COMET trial (ClinicalTrials.gov NCT01446744) was a small (N=99) phase II RCT that included participants with lung metastases from six or more primary cancer types of which only 18 were colorectal. The trial compared SBRT plus standard care with standard care alone, randomized 2:1.[4] Since other ablative therapy such as radiofrequency ablation and surgery were not allowed for participants randomized to the standard care arm, these individuals were assumed to receive either chemotherapy or observation. SABR-COMET was imbalanced: there were more participants with a single metastasis and more with better prognosis breast and prostate cancer in the SBRT arm. Although the survival advantage appeared good (HR 0.57), the significance of the results should be considered in the context of how the trial was powered.

In summary, there is no substantial RCT evidence that local intervention to lung metastases improves survival, but there is clear evidence that it is associated with adverse events. It should also be noted just how selective was the practice upon which clinical impressions were based. Between 2005 and 2013 in the English NHS 173,354 individuals had a colorectal cancer resection of whom 3434 (2%) had a lung operation within 3 years.[5] Not only is there a very high level of expert selection but that selection can be refined during a period of observation and reinvestigation allowing guarantee time bias.[6]

What are the risks and benefits of the different treatment options?

The man was well and asymptomatic with mild dyspnoea, consistent with his history of smoking and diagnosis of emphysema. The finding of lung metastases was incidental, and the normal CEA and 3 year disease-free interval meant that his prognosis was relatively good. As well as anaesthetic risks, surgical intervention in the lung, even by minimal access, carries a real risk of harm such as pneumothorax, haemothorax and empyema. In a study of 566 patients, radiofrequency ablation was associated with a pneumothorax rate of 67% and 39% of patients had a chest tube inserted.[7] SBRT can also result in adverse events (29% grade 2 or worse in one study)

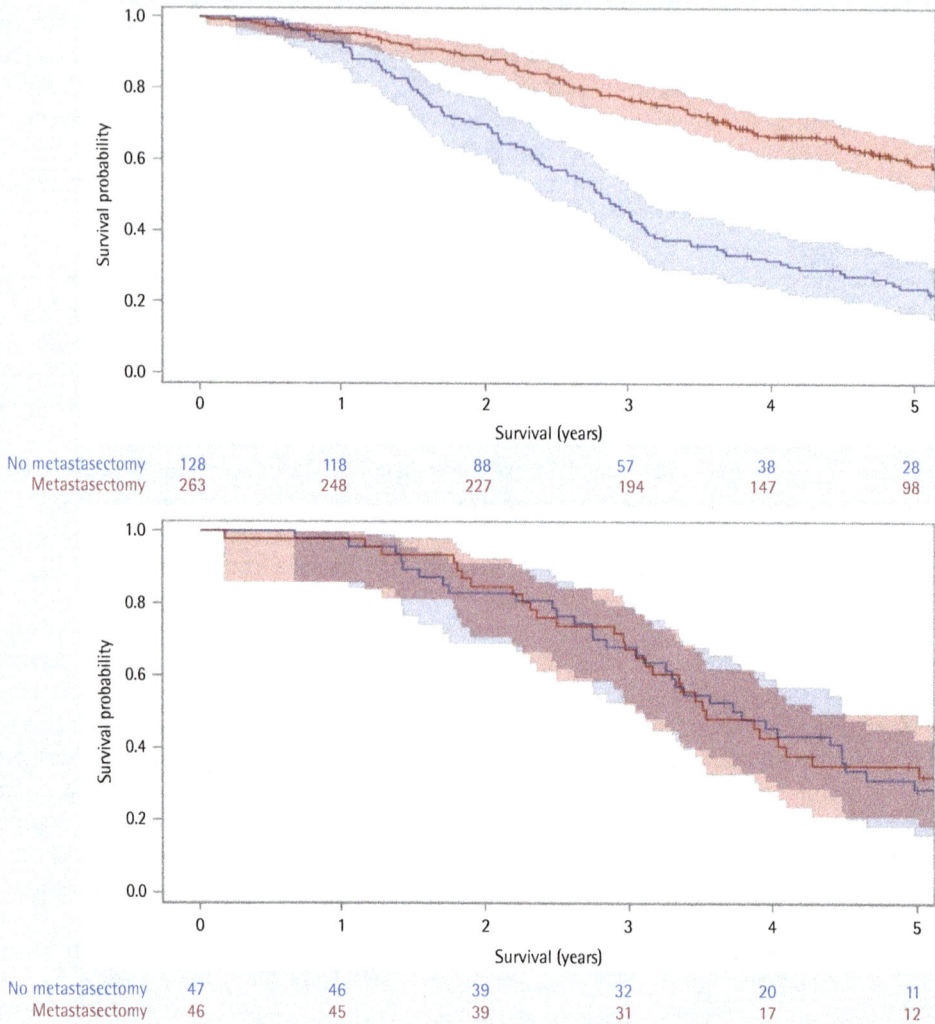

Figure 8.1 Kaplan–Meier curves from the PulMiCC study showing estimated probability of survival (with 95% CIs) for participants treated electively (upper panel; adapted from Treasure et al.[3]) or randomly assigned to metastasectomy (red) or no metastasectomy (blue) (lower panel; adapted from Milosevic et al.[2]).

and even occasional deaths.[4] The possible benefit for this man for whom the risks of intervention might have been higher is very uncertain.

The man would almost certainly be offered systemic therapy at some time, as most individuals like him eventually develop progressive disease. This is likely to entail significant toxicity, possibly severe. There is little evidence that in a person with colorectal cancer, minimal metastatic disease and no symptoms, early systemic therapy is more effective than waiting until disease clearly progresses and symptoms develop. Provided he is fully informed and accepts that intervention is associated with real risks and uncertain benefits, a reasonable option is observation alone with regular follow-up. His disease can easily be monitored with chest X-rays to assess the pace of progression.

What should this man be told?

The man should be told about the metastases and advised that any intervention at this stage would be associated with some risk of unpleasant adverse events and that the evidence that intervention would either cure him or improve his chances of living longer is uncertain. He could be reassured, however, that although his condition is almost certainly incurable his very low CEA level and relatively long disease-free interval indicate a relatively good prognosis. He has perhaps a 50% chance of living for 5 years without local intervention, and the lung metastases are very unlikely to cause symptomatic problems. In the very unlikely event that they do cause symptoms, they can still be effectively treated. All the treatment options and their possible risks and benefits should be openly discussed and he should share in the decision making.

Should he have been followed up more closely with regular CT scans and CEA measurements?

Current practice is to follow all individuals after potentially curative treatment for colorectal cancer with regular CT scans and CEA measurements, to find locally recurrent or metastatic disease as soon as possible. Two systematic reviews and meta-analyses of RCTs of various strategies of increased follow-up have shown that although the diagnosis of metastatic disease was brought forward by an average of 10 months, OS was not significantly improved. These follow-up strategies generate significant costs and are very unlikely to be cost-effective. Intensive follow-up does not seem to be worthwhile and any reassurance provided by it may be misleading and contribute to anxiety and distress with no advantage to the individual.[8,9]

Conclusion and learning points

- It is uncertain what is the optimal treatment of people with colorectal cancer and a few lung metastases.
- If the person is asymptomatic, observation without treatment is a valid option.
- There is no strong evidence that removing or ablating lung metastases is associated with cure or an improvement in OS.
- Intervention is associated with a risk of adverse events especially in those with underlying lung disease.
- People should be fully and impartially informed of the possible risks and uncertain benefits of any intervention and allowed to share in decision making.

References

1 Treasure T. Oligometastatic cancer: an entity, a useful concept, or a therapeutic opportunity? J R Soc Med 2012; 105: 242–6.

2 Milosevic M, Edwards J, Tsang D, et al. Pulmonary metastasectomy in colorectal cancer: updated analysis of 93 randomized patients – control survival is much better than previously assumed. Colorectal Dis 2020; 22: 1314–24.

3 Treasure T, Farewell V, Macbeth F, et al. The Pulmonary Metastasectomy in Colorectal Cancer cohort study: analysis of case selection, risk factors and survival in a prospective observational study of 512 patients. Colorectal Dis 2021; 23: 1793–803.

4 Palma DA, Olson R, Harrow S, et al. Stereotactic ablative radiotherapy versus standard of care palliative treatment in patients with oligometastatic cancers (SABR-COMET): a randomised, phase 2, open-label trial. Lancet 2019; 393: 2051–8.

5 Fenton HM, Finan PJ, Milton R, et al. National variation in pulmonary metastasectomy for colorectal cancer. Colorectal Dis 2021; 23: 1306–16.

6 Giobbie-Hurder A, Gelber RD, Regan MM. Challenges of guarantee-time bias. J Clin Oncol 2013; 31: 2963–9.

7 de Baere T, Auperin A, Deschamps F, et al. Radiofrequency ablation is a valid treatment option for lung metastases: experience in 566 patients with 1037 metastases. Ann Oncol 2015; 26: 987–91.

8 Mokhles S, Macbeth F, Farewell V, et al. Meta-analysis of colorectal cancer follow-up after potentially curative resection. Br J Surg 2016; 103: 1259–68.

9 Jeffery M, Hickey BE, Hider PN, et al. Follow-up strategies for patients treated for non-metastatic colorectal cancer. Cochrane Database Syst Rev 2016; 11: CD002200.

09 A novel, non-invasive treatment for liver tumours using focused ultrasound

Claire Ryan, Dhakshinamoorthy Vijayanand, Adel Samson, Ian Rowe, Tze Min Wah

Case history

A 68-year-old woman, under imaging surveillance for alcohol-related cirrhosis, was found to have a 2.2 cm lesion in the left lobe of her liver on an ultrasound scan. Her medical history included urticarial vasculitis (treated with long-term steroids), hypertension and type 2 diabetes mellitus. She had an ECOG performance status of 1.

A fast-track MRI scan performed locally found two other subcentimetre lesions in segment VIII. All three lesions had malignant features. No extrahepatic disease was present on staging CT; her case was referred to the regional liver multidisciplinary team (MDT).

Radiological findings supported hepatocellular carcinoma (HCC) (T2N0M0; Liver Reporting and Data System category 5) (Figure 9.1). Her liver cirrhosis was classified as Child–Pugh class A. She had abstained from alcohol for 18 months. The lesions were considered amenable to ablation, and an interventional oncologist saw the patient for consideration of ablative techniques.

Once the largest lesion was confirmed to be readily identifiable on ultrasound, she chose to enrol in the experimental #Hope4Liver trial (ClinicalTrials.gov NCT04573881), which uses histotripsy to treat primary and metastatic liver tumours; as the segment VIII lesions were sonographically invisible, treatment was offered with conventional thermal ablation. Histotripsy uses a non-thermal, focused ultrasound technique requiring no needles or ionizing radiation. The segment II/III HCC was treated using a HistoSonics prototype under ultrasound guidance with the patient under general anaesthesia. The treatment time was just 36 min.

The patient was discharged home the following day. She was delighted with the rapid non-invasive therapy and gave excellent feedback (see Further reading). Her post-treatment MRI scan showed good treatment coverage on day 1, with no viable tumour. The smaller, untreated segment VIII lesions were stable.

She complained of symptoms of fatigue in the week following the procedure and was admitted after 8 days for a 2 U red blood cell transfusion (haemoglobin pre-procedure 86 g/l and pre-transfusion 70 g/l). Her haemoglobin level then remained in the normal range without further intervention. Three months later, she underwent conventional image-guided (microwave) ablation to both smaller lesions using one 15G PR XT NeuWave probe to each at 65 W for 10 min.

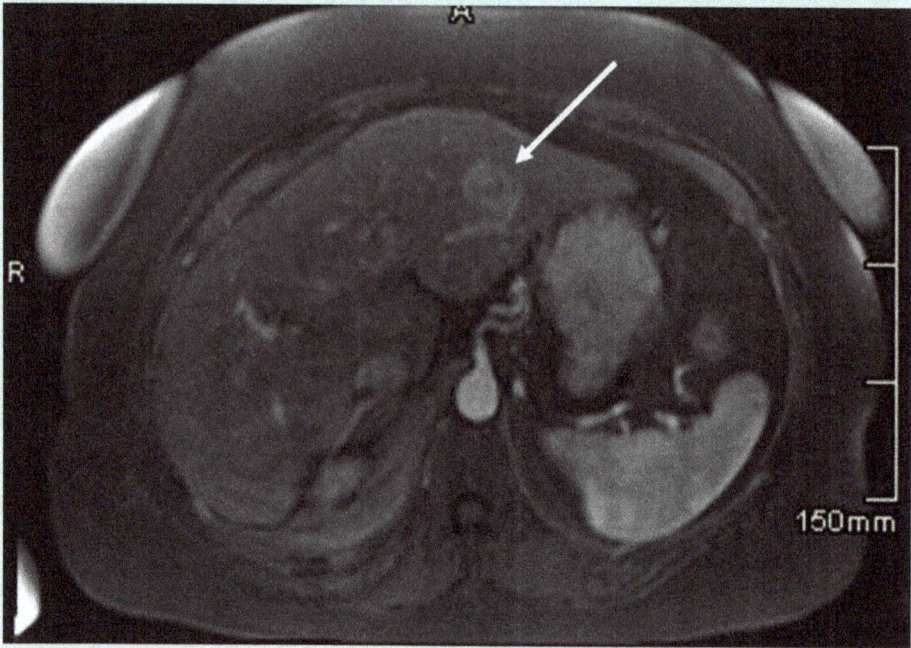

Figure 9.1 Pretreatment contrast-enhanced MRI appearance of the largest lesion located in the left lobe of the liver.

This time her recovery time was protracted: she had a severe post-ablation syndrome, a 1 week hospital stay and pain for several weeks after discharge. Six months after treatment, however, she was well and her 6 month post-histotripsy MRI showed no evidence of a viable tumour.

What were the patient's treatment options for these lesions?

What is the #Hope4Liver trial?

What is the current evidence around histotripsy?

What is the procedure for histotripsy using HistoSonics?

What are the considerations when inviting a patient for trial treatments?

What might the patient's perspectives be?

What were the patient's treatment options for these lesions?

A summary of the primary treatment modalities is explored below:

- A minority of patients with chronic liver disease are anatomically and clinically suitable for surgical treatment of HCC:
  - Transplant in endstage cirrhosis and early-stage HCC is curative for malignancy and underlying liver disease.

- Anatomical or non-anatomical liver resection is the first line of definitive treatment for HCC in a non-cirrhotic liver. The risk of liver decompensation and mortality should be considered in patients with cirrhosis and portal hypertension.
- Stereotactic body radiotherapy is a precisely targeted high-dose radiotherapy option in early-stage HCC. It has been shown to have comparable outcomes to those with ablative therapy and favourable results with respect to transarterial chemoembolization (TACE) in terms of toxicity, retreatment and hospitalization rates.[1]
- Image-guided techniques:
  - Ablative techniques comprise thermal (radiofrequency ablation, microwave ablation and cryoablation) and non-thermal ablation. Irreversible electroporation is a non-thermal ablative therapy that has become available in the last decade.
  - HCCs predominantly receive supply from hepatic arteries. With selective microcatheter placement, chemotherapy (commonly doxorubicin) is either directly injected or loaded on to drug-eluting beads, emitting the agent for minutes to hours.
  - Selective internal radiation therapy comprises the injection of yttrium-90-labelled microspheres via a selective microcatheter, similar to the procedure for TACE.
- Systemic anticancer therapy:
  - For patients with more advanced HCC, combination conventional chemotherapy (doxorubicin, platinum-based drugs, anthracyclines), tyrosine kinase inhibitors (sorafenib) and immunotherapy are options. Combination with local therapies may enhance (or mitigate) the effects on HCC; MDT input is crucial.

The 2022 update to the Barcelona Clinic Liver Cancer staging system outlines the rationale for treatment selection, considering clinical (performance status, liver function) and oncological (staging, size and number of tumours) factors.[2] The potential for a place for histotripsy in future iterations is an exciting prospect.

What is the #Hope4Liver trial?

HistoSonics is a private medical devices company based in Michigan. The #Hope4Liver trial (The HistoSonics System for Treatment of Primary and Metastatic Liver Tumors Using Histotripsy) is a non-randomized prospective study with recruitment from the USA and Europe. Leeds Teaching Hospitals NHS Trust is the chief investigator site in the UK; Newcastle upon Tyne Hospitals NHS Foundation Trust is also participating. The trial aims to evaluate the efficacy and safety of the HistoSonics system for treating both primary and metastatic liver tumours. Participants are proposed to undergo treatment, with imaging follow-up within 36 h of treatment completion and 30 day, 6 month and 1 year clinical follow-up.

Technique efficacy is defined as a 'lack of a nodular or mass-like area of enhancement within or along the edge of the treatment volume' on CT or MRI assessment within 36 h of procedure completion. Safety is defined as the avoidance of 'major complications, defined as Common Terminology Criteria for Adverse Events grade 3 or higher toxicities', up to 30 days after the index procedure. The main inclusion criteria are: individual tumours <3 cm, a maximum of three tumours, adult patients (older than 18 years), performance status 0–2 and Child–Pugh A/B disease.

What is the current evidence around histotripsy?

Histotripsy uses the mechanical effects of focused, pulsed ultrasound waves, which lead to the formation, oscillation and collapse of microbubbles. This fractures cells, liquefying tissues and leaving a cavity, which later resorbs to form a scar.[3] Conversely, high-intensity focused ultrasound ablation is based on thermal energy from continuous or long-burst ultrasound waves, inducing coagulation necrosis. However, it has had variable success and has been reported to be time-consuming, susceptible to the heat sink, and often technically challenging to perform in the liver.[4,5]

Although early impressions of histotripsy techniques are optimistic, there are minimal data on the efficacy and safety of histotripsy for treating cancer in humans. Longo et al.[6] investigated the ablative effects of histotripsy on porcine livers (the closest to the human liver in size, although variations in shape and neighbouring anatomy, such as ribs and stomach, impact comparisons). The investigators found that the treatment was effective at destroying the tumour and was safe, i.e. there were no significant complications such as focal bile duct damage (which is of concern in other ablative techniques). However, as the animals were euthanized after treatment, longer term outcomes were not assessed.

Similarly, Knott et al.[7] demonstrated efficacy – again in a porcine animal model – in renal ablation, with minimal injury to neighbouring urothelium. This suggests that collagenous tissues, such as bile ducts and collecting systems, are preserved while highly cellular tissue is destroyed. Another good effect of histotripsy is the abscopal effect observed in non-human trials, whereby treating one tumour produces an immunological response against other tumours.[8] This is an exciting area to consider in future research after completion of the #Hope4Liver trial, focusing on patients with several tumours but only one treated with histotripsy.

What is the procedure for histotripsy using HistoSonics?

Performed under general anaesthesia according to the trial protocol, the procedure takes place in a sterile environment, such as an interventional radiology theatre or a room used for CT-guided interventional procedures, with an interventional radiology (interventional oncology) and anaesthesia team.

The HistoSonics system integrates a planning-phase feature, allowing the operator to select a target using live ultrasound and up-to-date cross-sectional imaging on the same screen. In addition, a region-of-interest facility allows the interventional radiologist accurately to choose the target site and volume.

The technique involves placing a sterile, gasless water bath over the treatment area (which acts as a medium) before positioning the probe over the target. Real-time dynamic ultrasound images are visible to the operator, who can monitor the treatment effect and see the echogenic microbubbles as they arise in the treatment field. The changes in echogenicity in the target are observable in real time. Treatment times are typically 20–30 min for a 2 cm tumour.

What are the considerations when inviting a patient for trial treatments?

HCC is the fifth and seventh most common cancer in the world for men and women, respectively, and a healthcare priority globally.[9] Therefore, safe, effective and non-invasive treatments are crucial, especially in a population comorbid with cirrhosis.

An ethical requirement in undertaking the #Hope4Liver clinical trial is that histotripsy must be expected to be at least as safe and effective as the best available treatments (such as surgery or existing ablative techniques).[10] There is a potential for patients to be exploited during clinical trials, and the competing interests of investigators should be stated, minimized or nullified. Established research protocols exist to protect patients and consider questions including the social and clinical value of the research (how much will it benefit present or future patients); scientific feasibility (is the question answerable and the methodology sound); participant selection (who should be included to answer the question); and is the risk vs benefit ratio favourable? Basic ethical principles such as beneficence, autonomy and confidentiality must be respected. Informed consent is imperative: participants must understand the implications of entering a trial as well as its purpose, risks and benefits; they must appreciate how the practice aligns with their personal clinical needs. They must be allowed to withdraw at any time without justification.

What might the patient's perspectives be?

Entering a trial can be daunting for a patient: their questions and concerns may need answers, either provided by clinicians or through their own research. They are unlikely to have friends or acquaintances who have been through the same or similar treatment. If the treatment is not practical, might they lose the chance to have treatment that is known to be effective? Counselling, offering a range of options (potentially from a range of clinicians) and providing a specialist nurse point of contact are essential in trial scenarios.

Conclusion and learning points

- There are multiple treatment options for HCC, but the choice often depends on clinical and oncological features.
- MDT involvement is vital.
- Histotripsy is a novel, non-thermal ultrasound-based technique that requires no breach of the patient's skin and is performed without radiation. It was pioneered by HistoSonics and invented at the University of Michigan.
- The involvement of patients in clinical trials requires careful ethical considerations and sensitive communication.

References

1   Rhieu BH, Narang AK, Meyer J. Stereotactic ablative radiotherapy (SABR/SBRT) for hepatocellular carcinoma. Curr Hepatol Rep 2018; 17: 392–8.

2   Reig M, Forner A, Rimola J. BCLC strategy for prognosis prediction and treatment recommendation: the 2022 update. J Hepatol 2022; 76: 681–93.

3   Xu Z, Hall TL, Vlaisavljevich E, Lee FT Jr. Histotripsy: the first noninvasive, non-ionizing, non-thermal ablation technique based on ultrasound. Int J Hyperthermia 2021; 38: 561–75.

4   Haar GT, Coussios C. High intensity focused ultrasound: physical principles and devices. Int J Hyperthermia 2007; 23: 89–104.

5   Wijlemans JW, Bartels LW, Deckers R, et al. Magnetic resonance-guided high-intensity focused ultrasound (MR-HIFU) ablation of liver tumours. Cancer Imaging 2012; 12: 387–94.

6   Longo KC, Knott EA, Watson RF, et al. Robotically assisted sonic therapy (RAST) for noninvasive hepatic ablation in a porcine model: mitigation of body wall damage with a modified pulse sequence. Cardiovasc Intervent Radiol 2019; 42: 1016–23.

7   Knott EA, Swietlik JF, Longo KC, et al. Robotically-assisted sonic therapy for renal ablation in a live porcine model: initial preclinical results. J Vasc Interv Radiol 2019; 30: 1293–302.

8   Pahk KJ, Shin CH, Bae IY, et al. Boiling histotripsy-induced partial mechanical ablation modulates tumour microenvironment by promoting immunogenic cell death of cancers. Sci Rep 2019; 9: 9050.

9   American Society of Clinical Oncology (2022). Liver cancer: statistics. Available from: www.cancer.net/cancer-types/liver-cancer/statistics (accessed 5 February 2023).

10 Miller FG, Brody H. A critique of clinical equipoise. Therapeutic misconception in the ethics of clinical trials. Hastings Cent Rep 2003; 33: 19–28.

Further reading

- Cardona K, Maithel SK, eds. Primary and metastatic liver tumors. Cham, Switzerland: Springer, 2018; 37–98.

- Jackson J (2021). First UK patients treated for liver cancer using ultrasound technology. Available from: www.nationalhealthexecutive.com/articles/uk-patients-liver-cancer-NHS-ultrasound-technology.

- Monti A (2022). Tiny exploding bubbles can destroy tumours in as little as seven minutes. Available from: www.dailymail.co.uk/health/article-10612197/Radical-new-therapy-uses-tiny-bubbles-gas-destroy-tumours.html.

- Saheed H (2021). Bradford women [sic] has cancer treated with new treatment. Available from: www.thetelegraphandargus.co.uk/news/19584347.bradford-women-cancer-treated-new-treatment.

10 *De novo* hepatocellular carcinoma treated with navigation–assisted stereotactic irreversible electroporation

Omar Abdel-Hadi, James Lenton, Tze Min Wah

Case history

A 66-year-old man with known cirrhosis was found on surveillance following previous treatment for hepatocellular carcinoma (HCC) to have a new 2.6 cm LR-5 HCC in segment III. His medical history included cirrhosis secondary to genetic haemochromatosis (for which he had been undergoing venesection since 2010), type 2 diabetes, portal hypertension, joint stiffness and hypopituitarism. He had undergone irreversible electroporation (IRE) ablative therapy in 2020 for an 18 mm segment III LR-5 lesion; initial follow-up imaging showed a successful ablation zone with no residual disease. A follow-up CT scan at 18 months, however, revealed a new focus of arterial phase non-rim hyperenhancement with washout, suggesting *de novo* HCC.

The regional tertiary liver multidisciplinary team (MDT) recommended further evaluation with MRI. Imaging confirmed a 2.6 cm segment III LR-5 lesion with arterial enhancement, portal venous washout with an enhancing capsule, diffusion restriction and reduced Primovist concentration.

Blood tests revealed alpha-fetoprotein (AFP) 258 µg/l, platelets 152×10⁹/l, normal clotting profile and Child–Pugh score A-6. The man appeared frail and had a recent history of weight loss and progression in cognitive impairment.

Following MRI, MDT discussions centred upon the therapeutic options for treating the segment III HCC. There were concerns about the suitability of loco-regional treatments given the proximity of the lesion to the traversing gastric pylorus posteriorly. The patient was not felt to be suitable for transplantation or resection, and he had decided against surgical treatment when seen in the clinic. In addition, stereotactic body radiotherapy (SBRT) was unsuitable because of the proximity to the bowel and the high risk of bowel injury.

According to the modified Barcelona Clinic Liver Cancer (BCLC) algorithm, he was referred for image-guided ablation. This algorithm guides treatment for small early-stage HCC when a patient is not a surgical candidate.[1] The interventional oncology team explained that more conventional therapies, such as microwave ablation (first-line treatment for HCC at our institution) or radiofrequency ablation, would be at high risk of complications. A discussion was had with the patient regarding the use of IRE to minimize any potential complications due to bleeding and organ injury.

Moreover, using navigation-assisted probe placement would enable a more concise positioning of probes relative to the target lesion, minimizing the risks of incomplete treatment and injury to surrounding structures.

What was the goal of cancer treatment in this patient?

What is the mechanism of action of IRE?

What are the common image-guided ablative energies used for HCC? What are their mechanisms of action?

What technical considerations are key to deciding whether lesions are amenable to image-guided ablation?

How has the development of navigation-assisted stereotactic ablative techniques changed how the treatment is delivered?

What was the goal of cancer treatment in this patient?

Treatment in this patient was performed with curative intent. The initial lesion appeared to have been successfully treated, but a new HCC had developed in the same lobe. The therapeutic goal should always be balanced against the patient's comorbidities and disease staging as well as quality of life considerations. Given that he had signalled a reluctance for transplant, a cure could only be reliably achieved with image-guided ablation using radiofrequency or microwave ablation. IRE or SBRT, while performed with curative intent, are still evolving treatments.

What is the mechanism of action of IRE?

IRE is a relatively new non-thermal ablative technique in which microsecond to millisecond electrical pulses are delivered to target tissue to produce cell necrosis.[2] Necrosis is achieved by the irreversible formation of nanopores in the cellular membrane and subsequent cellular apoptosis. The main advantage is the preservation of collagen structures (e.g. phospholipid bilayer of bile ducts/vessels) close to the ablation zone.[3,4] This is particularly beneficial in liver HCC as it markedly reduces bleeding risk and biliary injury. In addition, such ablative therapeutic options are now available for individuals deemed at too high risk with use of conventional thermal ablative technology such as radiofrequency or microwave ablation.

What are the common image-guided ablative energies used for HCC? What are their mechanisms of action?

Radiofrequency ablation is based on the generation of an alternating current (370–505 kHz) through an electrode tip inserted into the target tumour, which induces frictional thermal energy to raise temperatures to between 55°C and 90°C, causing tissue necrosis. However, the heat propagates in a centrifugal direction, which decreases the temperature and hence is less effective in lesions >2 cm.

Microwave ablation is a thermal technique that creates an electromagnetic field around a monopolar electrode inducing homogenous heating and necrosis.[5-7] The advantage over radiofrequency ablation is that larger volumes of necrosis are induced, and faster ablation rates can be reached, mitigating the heat sink effect.[8]

Radiofrequency ablation was previously the mainstay of image-guided ablation for liver HCC; however, microwave ablation has emerged in the last decade as an alternative. Poulou et al.[9] suggested similar efficacy and safety between radiofrequency and microwave ablation for early HCC treatment. Although there is early evidence of slight advantages to using microwave over radiofrequency ablation in terms of overall survival, further long-term studies and higher level evidence are required to validate it.[10]

What technical considerations are key to deciding whether lesions are amenable to image–guided ablation?

There are several important considerations when assessing patients' suitability for ablative therapies. The first is a holistic consideration of their expectations, needs, quality of life and comorbidities. Therefore, a clinical review is essential for the interventional oncologist to evaluate these factors in partnership with the patient. Although image-guided ablation is minimally invasive, it is not without risk, and the convention is that ablative therapies are performed with sedation or under general anaesthesia. Therefore, patients should be pre-assessed for their suitability in this regard. It is essential to establish the proximity of the lesion to blood vessels because of the increased risk of severe bleeding and the heat sink effect. Heat sink occurs because blood flow in the surrounding vasculature conducts thermal energy away from the target tissue, reducing the efficacy of the ablative therapy. This is important for lesions near the portal vein and hepatic arteries.

The proximity of the lesion to the bowel, stomach, gallbladder and pleura should be considered in the treatment planning phase. Lesions close to the hollow viscera significantly increase potential bowel injury (ranging from inflammation to perforation) and could substantially increase morbidity post-treatment. Moreover, lesions in the superior aspect of segments VII and VIII are at higher risk of diaphragmatic injury. To prevent such adverse events, hydrodissection, or hydropneumodissection, helps to displace them away from the target by instilling a mixture of contrast, saline and gas within the space between at-risk structures, thereby allowing a greater distance between the ablation zone and at-risk tissues.[11,12]

How has the development of navigation–assisted stereotactic ablative techniques changed how the treatment is delivered?

Using navigational devices as adjuncts has helped to improve the precise targeting of technically challenging-to-reach lesions. These devices have varying levels of sophistication but have developed to allow a safe insertion of probes to a target lesion, adjusting the position of the entry in the skin and the trajectory angle to avoid other vital structures. This is particularly important in IRE, as successful ablation requires placing two or more applicator probes in a parallel distribution with a gap of between 1.5 and 2.0 cm. The placement of multiple parallel needles can be very challenging. Navigation-assisted devices have therefore emerged as a solution to overcome these technical challenges by comprehensively planning needle configurations using three-dimensional image data to support needle placement. This is usually achieved using a camera, fiducial markers, computer software and manoeuvrable probe guides.[13,14] A further advantage is that fusion imaging (e.g. liver MRI) can target lesions that are difficult to see using CT or ultrasound. Multiple studies have demonstrated reduced procedural times and radiation doses as well as greater accuracy and comparatively higher numbers of complete treatments achieved using navigation-assisted stereotactic ablation compared with conventional CT-guided microwave ablation.[13–15]

Conclusion and learning points

- MDT consensus regarding therapeutic options is vital, especially when considering new and evolving modalities.

- Clinical assessment by an interventional oncologist is required to provide patients with all the appropriate information regarding the risks and benefits of undertaking treatment.

- Selecting the appropriate ablation energy and guidance method is vital to achieving successful ablation with a reduced risk of complications.

- Image-guided thermal microwave or radiofrequency ablation is accepted as a standard treatment for very-early-stage and some early-stage HCCs according to the modified BCLC guidelines.

- IRE is an emerging non-thermal technique that may be used where a tumour is close to vital structures, to mitigate the risk of thermal injury.

- Navigation-assisted stereotactic ablation is now increasingly used to facilitate electrode placement, shorten the procedural time and significantly reduce procedural radiation.

References

1   Llovet JM, Fuster J, Bruix J, Barcelona-Clínic Liver Cancer Group. The Barcelona approach: diagnosis, staging, and treatment of hepatocellular carcinoma. Liver Transpl 2004; 10 (2 suppl 1): S115–20.

2   Rubinsky B, Onik G, Mikus P. Irreversible electroporation: a new ablation modality – clinical implications. Technol Cancer Res Treat 2007; 6: 37–48.

3   Lee EW, Loh CT, Kee ST. Imaging guided percutaneous irreversible electroporation: ultrasound and immunohistological correlation. Technol Cancer Res Treat 2007; 6: 287–93.

4   Sánchez-Velázquez P, Castellví Q, Villanueva A, et al. Long-term effectiveness of irreversible electroporation in a murine model of colorectal liver metastasis. Sci Rep 2017; 7: 44821.

5   Giorgio A, Gatti P, Montesarchio L, et al. Microwave ablation in intermediate hepatocellular carcinoma in cirrhosis: an Italian multicenter prospective study. J Clin Transl Hepatol 2018; 6: 251–7.

6   Galle PR, Forner A, Llovet JM, et al. EASL clinical practice guidelines: management of hepatocellular carcinoma. J Hepatol 2018; 69: 182–236.

7   Nault JC, Sutter O, Nahon P, et al. Percutaneous treatment of hepatocellular carcinoma: state of the art and innovations. J Hepatol 2018; 68: 783–97.

8   Lahat E, Eshkenazy R, Zendel A, et al. Complications after percutaneous ablation of liver tumors: a systematic review. Hepatobiliary Surg Nutr 2014; 3: 317–23.

9   Poulou LS, Botsa E, Thanou I, et al. Percutaneous microwave ablation vs radiofrequency ablation in the treatment of hepatocellular carcinoma. World J Hepatol 2015; 7: 1054–63.

10 Ricci AD, Rizzo A, Bonucci C, et al. The (eternal) debate on microwave ablation versus radiofrequency ablation in BCLC-A hepatocellular carcinoma. In vivo 2020; 34: 3421–9.

11 Campbell C, Lubner MG, Hinshaw JL. Contrast media-doped hydrodissection during thermal ablation: optimizing contrast media concentration for improved visibility on CT images. Am J Roentgenol 2012; 199: 677.

12 Lee SJ, Choyke LT, Locklin JK, Wood BJ. Use of hydrodissection to prevent nerve and muscular damage during radiofrequency ablation of kidney tumors. J Vasc Interv Radiol 2006; 17: 1967.

13 Beyer LP, Lürken L, Verloh N, et al. Stereotactically navigated percutaneous microwave ablation (MWA) compared to conventional MWA: a matched pair analysis. Int J Comput Assist Radiol Surg 2018; 13: 1991–7.

14 Beyer LP, Pregler B, Niessen C, et al. Stereotactically-navigated percutaneous irreversible electroporation (IRE) compared to conventional IRE: a prospective trial. PeerJ 2016; 4: e2277.

15 Beyer LP, Pregler B, Michalik K, et al. Evaluation of a robotic system for irreversible electroporation (IRE) of malignant liver tumors: initial results. Int J Comput Assist Radiol Surg 2017; 12: 803–9.

11 Image-guided liver cryoablation for colorectal liver metastases post-hepatectomy

Jack McKenna, Helen Ng, Peter Lodge, Dhakshinamoorthy Vijayanand, Tze Min Wah

Case history

A 65-year-old woman presented with recurrent colorectal liver metastasis from a sigmoid adenocarcinoma. She was initially diagnosed with carcinoma of the sigmoid colon in 2008, following which she had a laparoscopic sigmoid colectomy, adjuvant chemotherapy and multiple surgeries to the liver (right hemihepatectomy in 2011, segment II metastasectomies with resection and reconstruction of the left portal vein in 2015, segment II metastasectomy with left hepatic vein resection in 2018), as well as stereotactic body radiotherapy (SBRT) to locally recurrent disease in the liver remnant. Her medical history included hypertension, Graves' disease, osteoarthritis and depression. In 2021 she presented with a residual disease that had increased in size from 22 mm to 28 mm at the site of previous SBRT treatment. The disease site was near the left portal vein in hepatic segment III (Figure 11.1).

The patient underwent percutaneous image-guided cryoablation of the liver metastasis under general anaesthetic with CT guidance. A total of six IceRod cryoprobes were inserted into the local recurrent disease near the surgical clips. Two complete freezing and thawing cycles were performed during a total treatment time of 33 min (Figure 11.2). No immediate complications were observed.

Unfortunately, on day 1 post-procedure, the patient developed hypovolaemic shock with a haematoma adjacent to the hepatic capsule. Hepatic angiography was performed with the goal of selective hepatic artery embolization. However, the active focus of haemorrhage could not be identified. The bleeding settled with conservative management; concurrent *Escherichia coli* septicaemia was resolved with intravenous antibiotics.

A complication arose 10 days post-cryoablation: a biliary fistula was identified, causing a persistent biliary cutaneous leak (Figure 11.3). The initial plan was for the patient to receive endoscopic retrograde cholangiopancreatography (ERCP) at her local hospital, but the attempt was unsuccessful. More than 1 month later, she was transferred to a tertiary centre to reattempt ERCP or consider percutaneous transhepatic cholangiography (PTC) if unsuccessful. ERCP was completed, and the

Case 11: Image-guided cryoablation
for colorectal liver metastases
post-hepatectomy
91

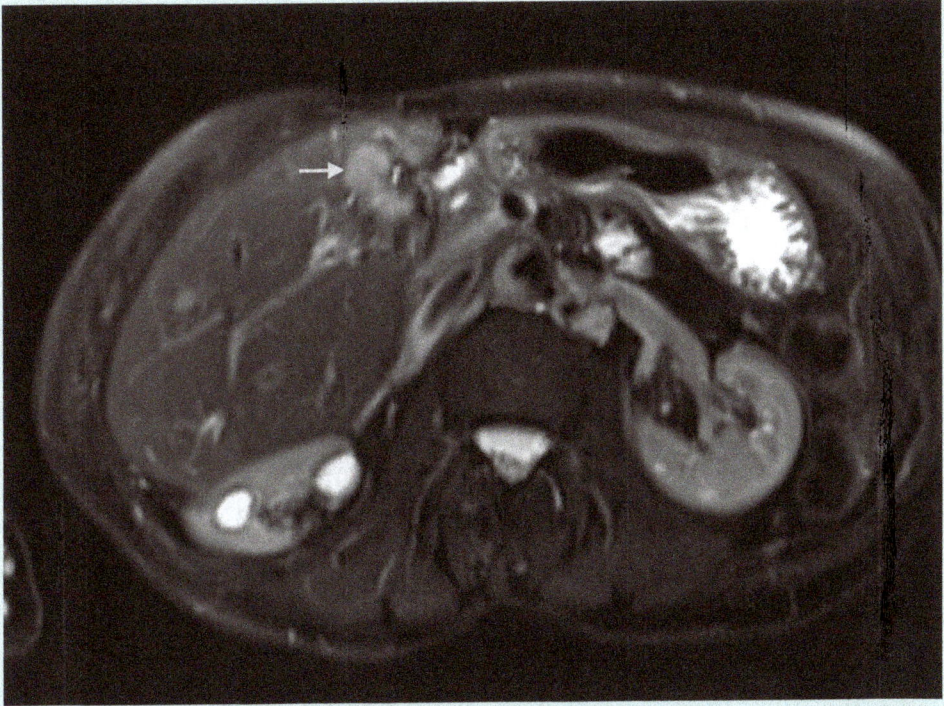

Figure 11.1 Axial T2-weighted HASTE MRI scan demonstrating the T2 hyperintense hepatic lesion (arrow) proximal to the left portal vein in hepatic segment III.

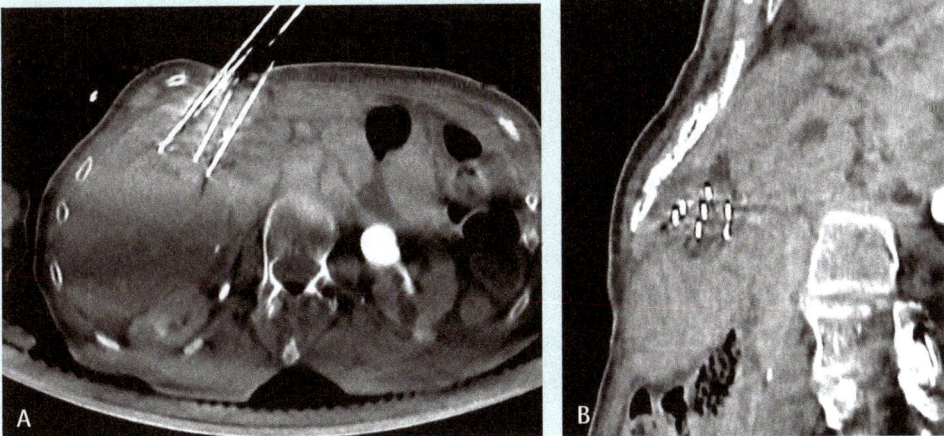

Figure 11.2 (A) Axial CT view and (B) coronal CT view of the placement of the six cryoprobes into the lesions during cryoablative treatment.

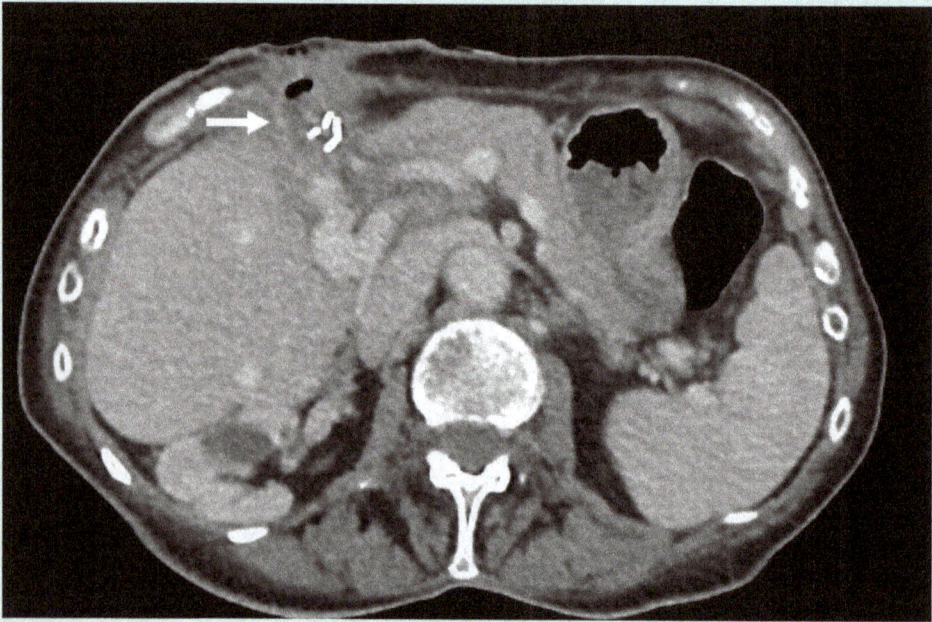

Figure 11.3 Axial CT view showing the biliary fistula (arrow) post-cryoablation: dilated segment II/III ducts with subcutaneous gas locules and a contiguous fluid cavity.

cholangiogram showed a complete blockage of the common bile duct, with no contrast filling the liver because of a combination of distorted biliary anatomy and a possible stricture. A percutaneous approach (PTC) was planned for 1 month later, but the patient showed improvement in her liver function tests. The reassessment scan revealed that the biliary fistula had closed spontaneously and the liver enzymes had normalized; thus, there was no need for further interventions. The patient was discharged to her local oncologist's care. A recent surveillance CT scan of the chest, abdomen and pelvis, almost 6 months after the cryoablation, showed no evidence of residual or recurrent disease.

What was the goal of treatment in this patient?

Why was one treatment modality picked over the others?

What is the evidence base for the treatment decision?

How did her surgical and medical history affect the final treatment outcome?

What complications of image–guided ablation should one be aware of?

What was the goal of treatment in this patient?

On preoperative imaging of patients with colorectal cancer, 30–50% are found to have liver metastases. Curative treatment intended for liver metastases is largely by surgical resection. Alternative treatment options must be considered carefully depending on the patient's fitness for surgery and

Case 11: Image-guided cryoablation
for colorectal liver metastases
post-hepatectomy

93

the size, disease burden and location of the liver metastases. The multidisciplinary team (MDT) decided that a redo liver resection for metastasis excision was a high risk; hence, ablative treatments were considered to control disease recurrence. Percutaneous image-guided ablative techniques were therefore considered with local curative intent. Image-guided ablation with thermal technology includes radiofrequency ablation, microwave ablation and cryoablation. Other emerging non-thermal technologies for tumour ablation use high-voltage electrical pulses through irreversible electroporation (IRE) and electrochemotherapy. IRE induces cell death within a soft tissue lesion by causing membrane disruption. Electrochemotherapy temporarily increases the permeability of a cell membrane, subsequently allowing increased transportation of cytotoxic chemotherapy agents into the cell. Another treatment option is selective internal radiation therapy (SIRT) for unresectable colorectal metastases in the liver. However, surgical resection after SIRT is associated with increased morbidity compared with resections in patients who have not undergone SIRT.[1]

Direct comparisons between surgical resection and image-guided ablation are difficult as there is a lack of prospective studies. Recruitment for randomized controlled trials is challenging for ethical reasons, as patients considered for image-guided ablation are mostly deemed unsuitable for surgery. It is difficult for eligible patients to consent to such trials, as, if ablation fails, patients can resort to surgical resection, which remains the gold standard treatment. In patients unsuitable for surgical resection, image-guided microwave ablation is the preferred thermal technology and has been increasingly considered owing to emerging evidence in its favour.[2] The debate comparing microwave ablation with liver resection is ongoing. Other technologies, such as cryoablation and IRE, are used in problem-solving cases.[3,4]

Why was one treatment modality picked over the others?

A surgical approach was deemed inappropriate as the patient had undergone multiple liver resections and there had been significant vascular involvement on the last two occasions, meaning further surgery would be very high risk. Image-guided ablation, including radiofrequency and microwave ablation, was considered. Still, there were concerns regarding the potential damage to the surrounding portal vascular structures due to heat transmission to surrounding vital structures. There were additional concerns about microwave ablation owing to the patient's low body mass index, which increases the risk of cutaneous injury. Despite the safety profile, IRE was not chosen owing to the proximity of the surgical clips and concern regarding energy arcing.[5] Also, the lesion size was 28 mm, which was deemed slightly too large for IRE local treatment efficacy. Cryoablation was the only ablative technology available that offered a good local treatment effect and the ability to visualize the ice ball during treatment to minimize local ablation to surrounding vital structures.

What is the evidence base for the treatment decision?

Liver metastases are a common cause of mortality in patients with colorectal cancer. Surgical resection, when possible, improves survival, but many lesions are deemed unsuitable for surgery. Image-guided ablation, including radiofrequency and microwave ablation, may be considered with curative or palliative intent and as an adjunct to surgical resection. Percutaneous cryoablation is an alternative for patients who are not surgical candidates. Although the procedure is more widely adopted in East Asia,[3] there is limited evidence about its long-term efficacy, as patients treated with this modality generally have a poorer prognosis. Current NICE guidance in England includes information about cryosurgery in an open resection procedure and cryoablation percutaneously (see Further reading). Percutaneous cryoablation should only be used on a case-by-case basis to problem-solve in the carefully selected patient and should be carried out by an expert MDT specialized in image-guided ablative therapies. Cryoablation was chosen as the treatment of choice because of the ability to define the accurate ablation zone during intra-procedural imaging monitoring with reasonable local control and a postulated robust post-ablation immune effect.[6]

How did her surgical and medical history affect the final treatment outcome?

The patient had had previous surgeries and adjuvant chemotherapy, as well as SBRT for recurrent liver metastases. Owing to her immunosuppressed status, she might have been at greater risk of infections, which could have contributed to the formation of an abscess leading to a fistula. However, this is not often observed in cryoablation alone. Cryoablation was selected because it was expected to be beneficial to the patient, as it is postulated to induce an immune-specific reaction, affecting cancer cells outside the ablated tissue. There are currently no consensus guidelines on the course of antibiotics post-ablation in immunocompromised patients. Prophylactic antibiotics for radiofrequency ablation have been discussed for certain groups of patients from personal experience.[7,8] Focused research is needed to explore the benefits of a long course of antibiotics in immunocompromised patients receiving cryoablation or in patients who have undergone multimodal treatment approaches.

What complications of image-guided ablation should one be aware of?

The relative contraindications for thermal ablation of liver metastases include lesions <1 cm from the central biliary duct, coagulopathy and significant ascites. Complications may be broadly divided into puncture- and ablation-related (Table 11.1).[6] 'Cryoshock' syndrome has been reported to occur in 0.3% of patients following cryosurgery to hepatic lesions[9] and cryoablation of kidney cancers.[10]

Most of the available evidence comparing ablation with surgical resection of colorectal liver metastases is from radiofrequency ablation.[11] The current gold standard for colorectal liver

Table 11.1 Complications related to image-guided liver ablation.	
Puncture-related complications	Ablation-related complications
• Pneumothorax/haemothorax • Bowel perforation • Pain • Infection including hepatic abscesses, wound infection and pneumonia • Bile duct damage and related injury including bile leak, biloma, strictures and cholecystitis/cholangitis • Fistula formation	• Post-ablation syndrome with symptoms including fever, nausea and vomiting • Local hepatic parenchymal damage • Liver failure or deranged liver function tests • Cryotherapy-specific: – Ice ball formation in the liver parenchyma that may culminate in major haemorrhage – Cytokine-mediated systemic syndrome 'cryoshock' with symptoms including fever, tachycardia and tachypnoea – Variable ablation zone – Hepatic portal gas – Thrombocytopenia – Acute myocardial infarction and arrhythmias

Case 11: Image-guided cryoablation
for colorectal liver metastases
post-hepatectomy   95

metastasis is surgery, with image-guided thermal ablation reserved for patients with comorbidities or recurrent diseases. However, emerging evidence suggests that image-guided thermal ablation can offer good local oncological durability compared to surgery.[12] To address the evidence gap in the literature, the COLLISION trial (ClinicalTrials.gov NCT03088150) is a two-arm, single-blind, prospective randomized controlled multicentre phase III clinical trial aiming to recruit 618 patients with one or more colorectal liver metastases (≤3 cm) to undergo surgical resection or image-guided thermal ablation.[13] The interim analysis has shown promising results, and the wider interventional oncology community eagerly awaits the final analysis.

Currently, clinicians wishing to offer percutaneous cryoablation should ensure that patients understand the reasoning for choosing one modality over another, the possible complications and any specific management following the procedure. The decision should also have been discussed in an MDT meeting.

Conclusion and learning points

- Percutaneous image-guided ablation for treating colorectal liver metastases remains an area of ongoing research.

- Direct comparisons between surgical resection and image-guided ablation remain challenging, as image-guided ablation is usually reserved for patients deemed unsuitable for surgery. The ongoing COLLISION trial might address the evidence gap.

- There is no evidence-based consensus on the use of prophylactic antibiotics during image-guided ablation. Their use is currently considered on a case-by-case basis by factoring in the patient's immune status. Future research should investigate the optimum course, type and length of antibiotic treatment for immunocompromised patients.

- Several complications may occur after cryoablation, postulated from complications that have arisen from ultrasound-guided cryotherapies. These complications should be explained thoroughly to the patient as part of the consent process.

References

1 Mafeld S, Littler P, Hayhurst H, et al. Liver resection after selective internal radiation therapy with yttrium-90: safety and outcomes. J Gastrointest Cancer 2020; 51: 152–8.

2 Shady W, Petre EN, Do KG, et al. Percutaneous microwave versus radiofrequency ablation of colorectal liver metastases: ablation with clear margins (A0) provides the best local tumor control. J Vasc Interv Radiol 2018; 29: 268–75.e1.

3 Hu J, Chen S, Wang X, et al. Image-guided percutaneous microwave ablation versus cryoablation for hepatocellular carcinoma in high-risk locations: intermediate-term results. Cancer Manage Res 2019; 11: 9801–11.

4 Dunne RM, Shyn PB, Sung JC, et al. Percutaneous treatment of hepatocellular carcinoma in patients with cirrhosis: a comparison of the safety of cryoablation and radiofrequency ablation. Eur J Radiol 2014; 83: 632–8.

5 Ng H, Wang K, Cartledge J, et al. Ureteric injury after image-guided ablation of renal cell cancer with irreversible electroporation. J Vasc Interv Radiol 2021; 32: 322–4.

6 Niu L-Z, Li J-L, Xu K-C. Percutaneous cryoablation for liver cancer. J Clin Transl Hepatol 2014; 2: 182–8.

7 Wah TM, Irving HC. Infectious complications after percutaneous radiofrequency ablation of renal cell carcinoma in patients with ileal conduit. J Vasc Interv Radiol 2008; 19: 1382–5.

8 Ng HHL, Ling L, Lodge P, et al. Mycotic pseudoaneurysm of the hepatic artery as a complication of radiofrequency ablation of hepatic metastases. Radiol Case Rep 2020; 15: 2663–7.

9 Xu K-C, Niu L-Z, He W-B, et al. Percutaneous cryosurgery for the treatment of hepatic colorectal metastases. World J Gastroenterol 2008; 14: 1430–6.

10 Georgiades CS, Hong K, Bizzell C, et al. Safety and efficacy of CT-guided percutaneous cryoablation for renal cell carcinoma. J Vasc Interv Radiol 2008; 19: 1302–10.

11 Kron P, Linecker M, Jones RP, et al. Ablation or resection for colorectal liver metastases? A systematic review of the literature. Front Oncol 2019; 9: 1052.

12 Van Tilborg AAJM, Meijerink MR, Sietses C, et al. Long-term results of radiofrequency ablation for unresectable colorectal liver metastases: a potentially curative intervention. Br J Radiol 2011; 84: 556–65.

13 Puijk RS, Ruarus AH, Vroomen L, et al. Colorectal liver metastases: surgery versus thermal ablation (COLLISION) – a phase III single-blind prospective randomized controlled trial. BMC Cancer 2018; 18: 821.

Further reading

- NICE (2010). Cryotherapy for the treatment of liver metastases. Interventional procedures guidance IPG369. Available from: www.nice.org.uk/guidance/ipg369.

- NICE (2016). Microwave ablation for treating liver metastases. Interventional procedures guidance IPG553. Available from: www.nice.org.uk/guidance/ipg553.

12 Transarterial chemoembolization for the treatment of primary liver tumour

Sadhana Shankar, Dhakshinamoorthy Vijayanand

Case history

A 69-year-old man with type 2 diabetes mellitus and a history of hepatitis B cirrhosis and excessive alcohol use underwent hepatocellular carcinoma (HCC) screening because of a high alpha-fetoprotein (AFP) level. He was generally fatigued but was otherwise able to carry on with his activities of daily living. A triphasic CT scan revealed cirrhotic liver morphology with a 6.4×5.1 cm tumour in segment VII of the liver showing arterial enhancement and venous washout compatible with HCC. There were two smaller satellite nodules around it, but there was no vascular invasion or extrahepatic spread. Haematological investigation revealed haemoglobin 104 g/l, albumin 38 g/l, total bilirubin 23.9 μmol/l, elevated liver enzymes (aspartate aminotransferase [AST] 139 U/l and alanine aminotransferase [ALT] 47 U/l), international normalized ratio (INR) 1.2, serum creatinine 97.2 μmol/l, positive hepatitis B surface antigen (HBsAg), non-reactive anti-hepatitis C virus (HCV) and AFP 680 μg/l.

After discussion in the HCC multidisciplinary team (MDT) meeting, the decision was made to offer transarterial chemoembolization (TACE). Via a 5 Fr right common femoral artery access, a selective celiac and mesenteric artery angiogram demonstrated patent vessels with no variant anatomy. Selective cannulation of the artery supplying the tumour and subsequent chemoembolization using drug-eluting beads (epirubicin microspheres) were performed. Post-embolization angiography was satisfactory, with patent branches providing the remnant liver and no evidence of tumour blush or extravasation.

The patient was admitted for routine overnight observation and was discharged home the next day. Two days later, he presented to A&E with high-grade fever, abdominal pain and confusion. On examination, he was delirious, dehydrated and tachycardic, with a temperature of 39.5°C. He was admitted immediately. Investigations showed haemoglobin 98 g/l, white blood cell count (WCC) 19.3×10⁹/l, C-reactive protein (CRP) 275 mg/l, total bilirubin 44.5 μmol/l, AST 336 U/l, ALT 213 U/l, INR 1.3, serum creatinine 159 μmol/l and serum potassium 6.3 mmol/l. An emergency CT scan showed an intact tumour, patent hepatic vasculature and no intraperitoneal free fluid or gas. He was treated for hyperkalaemia and acute kidney injury and gradually recovered over the next few days.

What was the evidence for treating this patient with TACE?

What complication occurred in this patient and how was it managed?

What are the other known complications following TACE?

How do we assess the response to TACE?

What are the other indications for TACE in primary hepatic tumours?

What was the evidence for treating this patient with TACE?

The Barcelona Clinic Liver Cancer (BCLC) staging system is the most widely used protocol for the management of HCC.[1] Our patient had Child–Pugh class A cirrhosis attributed to a combination of chronic hepatitis B infection and alcohol, as evidenced by his blood results. His ECOG performance status was 1. He had multifocal HCC with no vascular involvement or extrahepatic disease and had stable liver function with no evidence of decompensation. His disease was therefore classified as BCLC stage B (intermediate-stage HCC). Hence, the most appropriate treatment strategy would be to offer him TACE.

Several factors influenced this decision, the most important being the patient's physical condition, underlying liver function, tumour size and number, and discrete tumour-feeding vessels. The best response is observed in patients with good residual synthetic function and smaller tumour volume as well as an absence of aberrant arterial feeders supplying the tumour. This enables super-selective embolization of the tumour, thereby maximizing the tumoricidal effect and minimizing systemic toxicity.

What complication occurred in this patient and how was it managed?

The patient developed symptoms of tumour lysis syndrome (TLS), also known as a post-embolization syndrome. TLS occurs as a result of rapid tumour destruction following cytotoxic therapy. The classic symptoms include abdominal pain, vomiting and fever due to a systemic inflammatory response. The biochemical picture is that of hyperkalaemia, hyperphosphataemia, hyperuricaemia, hypocalcaemia and elevated inflammatory markers. In severe cases, it can lead to obstructive uropathy, acute renal failure, cardiac arrhythmias and cardiac arrest. Therefore, early identification and prevention of TLS in at-risk patients are crucial. Cairo–Bishop is the most widely used system for classifying and grading TLS.[2] Traditionally, patients with a significant tumour burden, rapidly dividing and chemosensitive tumours, and pretreatment renal dysfunction are at increased risk. Such patients should be monitored intensively.

Of the electrolyte abnormalities, hyperuricaemia, as a result of catabolism of rapidly released intracellular nucleic acids, is the most devastating complication as it causes renal vasoconstriction and impaired autoregulation. In addition, urate crystals precipitate in renal tubules causing obstructive uropathy. Furthermore, hyperkalaemia causes muscle weakness, cramps and cardiac arrhythmias, whereas hyperphosphataemia leads to the precipitation of calcium in renal tubules, causing hypocalcaemia and exacerbating muscle weakness, tetany and arrhythmogenic potential.

The treatment principles include rehydration, correction of electrolyte and acid-base abnormalities and aggressive treatment of renal failure. Peri-procedural hydration is often recommended, especially in patients with borderline renal function, as contrast-induced nephrotoxicity can further aggravate renal failure. Allopurinol and rasburicase have been used for the correction of hyperuricaemia as well as forced alkaline diuresis. Early haemodialysis is necessary to avoid irreversible renal failure in case of progressive renal impairment.

What are the other known complications following TACE?

Some additional well-known complications following TACE and their management are outlined in Table 12.1. They also serve as a crucial differential diagnosis for patients developing complications following TACE.

Table 12.1   Complications following TACE.

Complication	Pathophysiology	Management
Tumour rupture causing intraperitoneal bleed	Local vasculopathy due to malignancy, combined with rapidly expanding tissue oedema	Volume replacement Embolization of bleeding vessel Surgical resection or tamponade as last resort
Access site haematoma/pseudoaneurysm/AV fistula	Iatrogenic injury to vessel wall	Meticulous puncture site planning and gel foam to seal tract to avoid haematoma Pressure occlusion for pseudoaneurysm
Hepatic artery injury	Catheter-directed injury can lead to dissection or thrombosis leading to hepatic ischaemia	Vasodilators to minimize vasospasm Stenting to avoid pseudoaneurysm formation and rupture Systemic anticoagulation in case of thrombosis
Portal or hepatic vein thrombosis	Can lead to hepatic ischaemia or congestion and aggravate liver failure	Systemic anticoagulation Supportive treatment
Non-target embolization	Cystic artery: gallbladder necrosis	Cholecystectomy or percutaneous cholecystostomy
	Short gastric vessels: gastric mucosal necrosis and ulcers	PPI Sucralfate
	Gastroduodenal artery: duodenal ulcer and perforation	Difficult to manage with PPI Surgical management for perforation peritonitis
	Pancreatico-duodenal artery: pancreatitis	Conservative management, drainage of peri-pancreatic collections
	Inferior phrenic artery: pleuritis and effusion	Adequate analgesics, percutaneous drainage of pleural effusion
	Pulmonary embolism and chemical pneumonitis occurring in the presence of intratumoral AV fistula or tumours supplied by extrahepatic vessels	Conservative management
Liver failure	Due to decompensated function in pre-existing cirrhosis	Usually transient and managed conservatively Can be minimized by appropriate patient selection (avoid TACE in patients with Child–Pugh class C cirrhosis)

(Continued)

Complication	Pathophysiology	Management
Hepatic abscess and biloma	Due to ischaemic necrosis of peri-biliary capillary plexus causing bile leak; subsequent infection causes abscess formation	Antibiotics Percutaneous drainage of abscess or biloma
Bacteraemia and sepsis	Bacterial translocation due to instrumentation or breakdown of vascular plexus	Prophylactic or treatment dose of antibiotics
Renal failure	Due to contrast nephropathy or TLS	Adequate hydration Renal replacement therapy if needed

AV, arteriovenous; PPI, proton pump inhibitors.

How do we assess the response to TACE?

Repeating a contrast-enhanced CT scan after 4 weeks enables evaluation of the response to TACE. The modified Response Evaluation Criteria in Solid Tumors (mRECIST), based on the arterial enhancement of residual tumour, are used to classify the response.[3] This is because a reduction in size does not immediately accompany tumour necrosis. Therefore, arterial enhancement serves as a good indicator of viable residual disease. Tumours may show a complete or partial response, or there may be stable or progressive disease following TACE. The treatment algorithm is summarized in Figure 12.1.

What are the other indications for TACE in primary hepatic tumours?

In HCC, the concept of tumour stage migration may be applied to offer TACE to patients in whom recommended treatment options according to BCLC criteria are not feasible or have failed. This applies to patients in BCLC stage 0/A who are unfit for surgery or ablation; hence, TACE can be an effective treatment option. Similarly, patients with BCLC stage C suffering from severe adverse

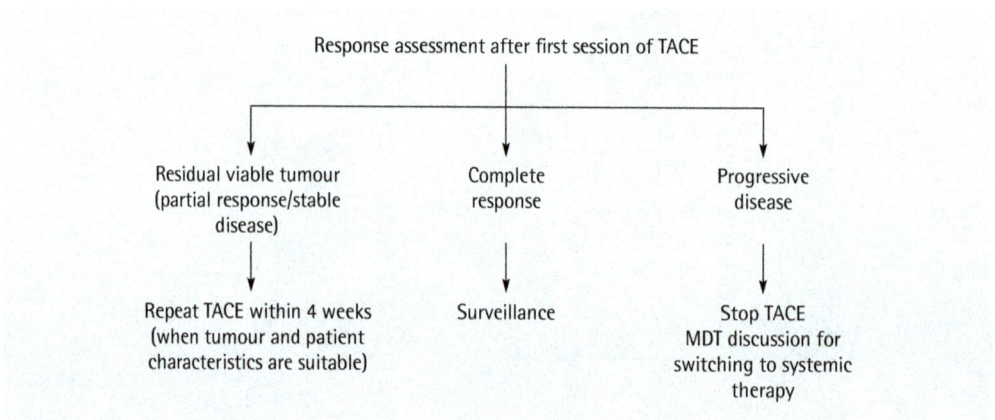

Response assessment after first session of TACE

Residual viable tumour (partial response/stable disease) → Repeat TACE within 4 weeks (when tumour and patient characteristics are suitable)

Complete response → Surveillance

Progressive disease → Stop TACE MDT discussion for switching to systemic therapy

Figure 12.1 Assessment of response and further management following TACE.

effects of systemic therapy may be offered TACE for loco-regional control. Another indication for TACE outside the BCLC criteria is before liver transplantation. It can be used as 'bridging TACE' for the local management of tumours in patients on the waiting list for liver transplants. It can also be used as 'downstaging TACE' in patients who do not fulfil transplant criteria owing to tumour size and extent. TACE may effectively downstage tumour burden in these patients and make them eligible for a liver transplant.

Apart from HCC, TACE has also been used for disease control in the case of inoperable peripheral cholangiocarcinoma.[4] However, the treatment strategy, response and survival rates are highly variable, and a case-based MDT discussion is necessary before offering treatment.

Conclusion and learning points

- Thorough patient evaluation, MDT discussion and appropriate patient selection are necessary before offering TACE for hepatic malignancy. The BCLC criteria serve as guidelines for the treatment of HCC.

- A thorough knowledge of the procedure is necessary to anticipate the associated complications, as most patients receiving this treatment are at high risk of developing organ failure.

- Multiple factors may contribute to complications following TACE and must be thoroughly investigated and appropriately treated.

- The response to TACE is assessed using mRECIST criteria, which also guide further management.

- TACE is also used for bridging or downstaging HCC before liver transplantation and for inoperable peripheral cholangiocarcinoma.

References

1   Reig M, Forner A, Rimola J, et al. BCLC strategy for prognosis prediction and treatment recommendation: the 2022 update. J Hepatol 2022; 76: 681–93.

2   Cairo MS, Coiffier B, Reiter A, et al. Recommendations for the evaluation of risk and prophylaxis of tumour lysis syndrome (TLS) in adults and children with malignant diseases: an expert TLS panel consensus. Br J Haematol 2010; 149: 578–86.

3   Lencioni R, Llovet JM. Modified RECIST (mRECIST) assessment for hepatocellular carcinoma. Semin Liver Dis 2010; 30: 52–60.

4   Park SY, Kim JH, Yoon HJ, et al. Transarterial chemoembolization versus supportive therapy in the palliative treatment of unresectable intrahepatic cholangiocarcinoma. Clin Radiol 2011; 66: 322–8.

13 Recurrent colorectal liver metastases in a young patient

James Walcott, Dhakshinamoorthy Vijayanand

Case history

A 39-year-old man was diagnosed with rectosigmoid cancer after a 3 month history of rectal bleeding. He proceeded directly to laparoscopic anterior resection. He made an uneventful recovery from his colorectal procedure. The pathology showed a pT4N1 moderately differentiated adenocarcinoma with three out of 14 positive nodes, evidence of extramural vascular invasion and clear margins.

A contrast-enhanced MRI scan of his liver after surgery showed multiple subcentimetre metastatic deposits, mainly within the left lobe of the liver, and a right-sided deposit in segment VI (Figure 13.1). An FDG PET scan showed no evidence of extrahepatic disease. The case was discussed at a hepatobiliary multidisciplinary team (MDT) meeting; although the liver metastases were resectable, the MDT decided on systemic therapy for 3 months before considering liver resection.

The patient proceeded through five cycles of fluorouracil and oxaliplatin with grade 2 peripheral neuropathies. A restaging MRI scan showed an excellent response to chemotherapy with a reduction in the size of all lesions; some lesions (including the lesion in segment VI) were no longer visible. He went on to have an open left hepatectomy and cholecystectomy. No right-sided lesions were evident at the surgery. Pathology revealed a partial response to chemotherapy and clear margins.

He went on to have six cycles of adjuvant capecitabine, which were tolerated well. He had 3 years of surveillance with no evidence of disease recurrence. A surveillance scan performed towards the end of the third year revealed multiple recurrent deposits in the remnant liver (Figure 13.2). He underwent surgery to resect the largest lesion and radiofrequency ablation to three other metastases throughout the remnant liver. He continued on a surveillance programme with no further chemotherapy.

Three years after his last surgery, a CT scan showed a 2.1 cm recurrence in segment VII of the liver, close to the right hepatic vein (Figure 13.3). MRI with Primovist confirmed a solitary recurrence. Given the proximity to a significant vessel, he was referred for stereotactic body radiotherapy (SBRT). He received a total of 45 Gy in five treatments, which were tolerated well. Follow-up MRI showed a satisfactory response to radiotherapy with a reduced size and diffusion restriction. His most recent imaging at the time of writing showed no evidence of disease recurrence. He remains clinically well 8 years after his synchronous metastatic colorectal cancer presentation.

What is the benefit of surgical resection for colorectal liver metastases?

What are the risk factors for recurrence after resection for colorectal liver metastases?

What are the limitations of resection and what alternative local therapies are available?

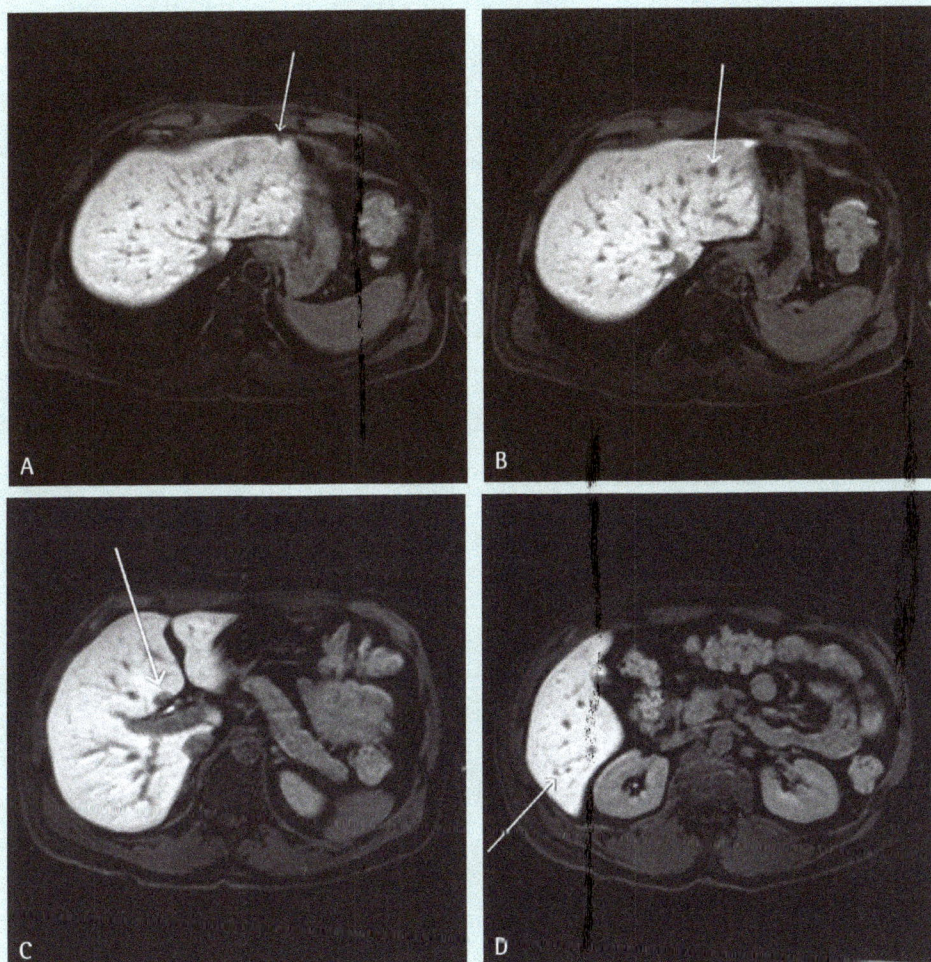

Figure 13.1 Contrast-enhanced MRI with Primovist showing multiple small metastatic deposits.
(A) Segment II peripheral lesion; (B) segment II deeper lesion (C); segment IVb deep lesion;
(D) segment VI lesion.

What is the benefit of surgical resection for colorectal liver metastases?

Colorectal cancer is a common disease, with almost half of cases developing metastases at some point after diagnosis.[1] The treatment of metastatic colorectal cancer has changed dramatically over the last 30 years with improved systemic and surgical treatments and a wide array of loco-regional therapies available. Before the advent of modern chemotherapy, survival for metastatic colorectal cancer was typically measured in months; however, in the contemporary era, studies often present 5 year survival data in the order of 50%.[2] While many of those survivors will have recurrent disease, potentially as many as 25% will survive to 10 years and achieve a 'cure' from their stage IV disease.[3]

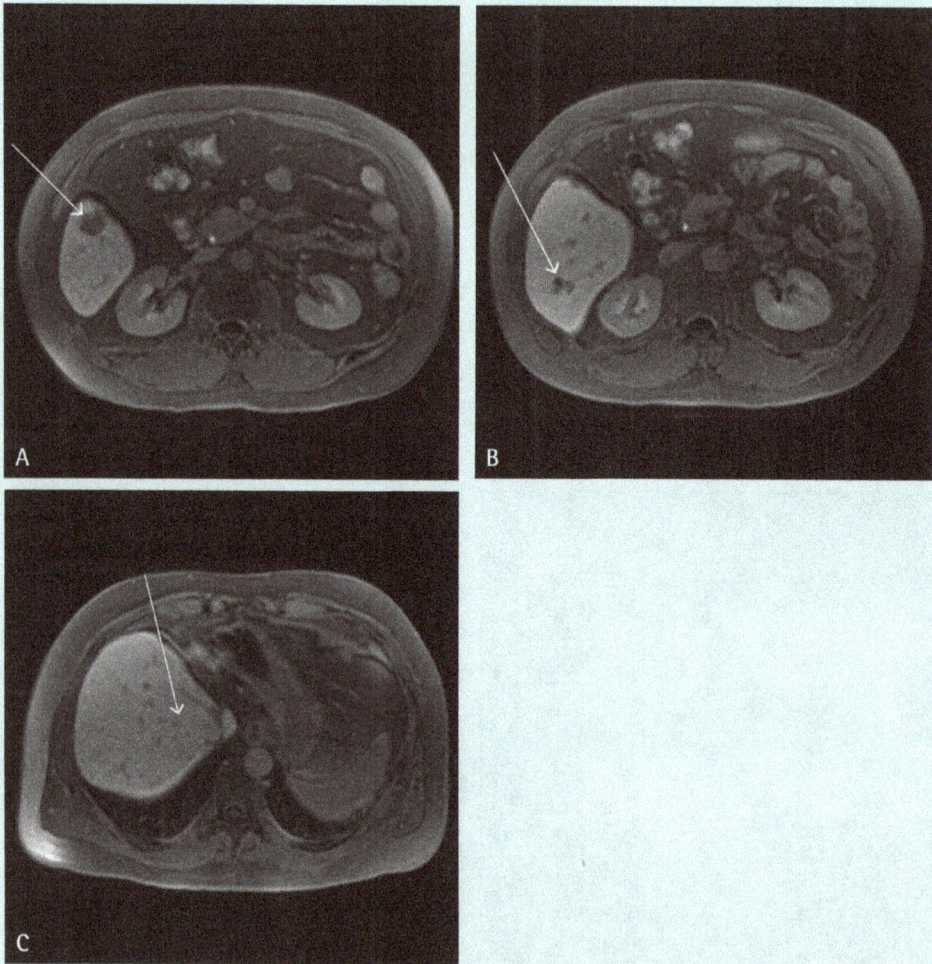

Figure 13.2 Contrast-enhanced MRI with Primovist showing multiple sites of recurrence in liver remnant. (A) Segment V lesion; (B) segment VI lesion; (C) segment VIII lesion.

The rationale for resecting colorectal liver metastases has evolved gradually, notably in the absence of randomized evidence. Retrospective case series conducted as early as the 1970s showed the benefits of liver resection for colorectal liver metastases, which seemed to be greater for those with single rather than multiple metastases.[4] In the 1980s, proposed indications for resection of colorectal liver metastases included fewer than four metastases, no extrahepatic disease, single lobe distribution and resection margins >10 mm.[5] Fast-forward 30 years, and extended criteria were used, including resections for those with more than four metastases, bilobar distribution, centrally located disease, and extrahepatic disease so long as it was resectable.[6] Even though patients with extended criteria had shorter 5 year survival compared with more traditional criteria, the overall outcome of 41 months' median survival in extended criteria resections seemed to justify its use.[6]

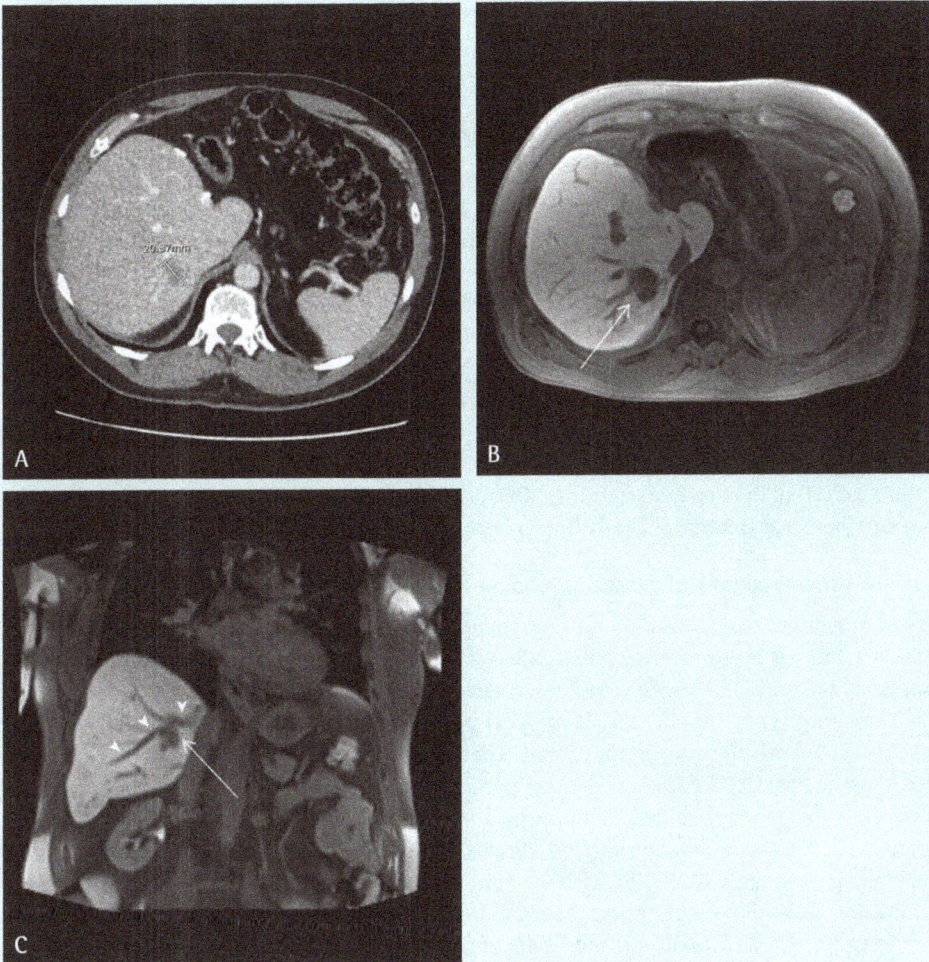

Figure 13.3 Contrast-enhanced CT and MRI showing solitary segment VII recurrence. (A) Axial CT showing segment VII recurrence; (B) axial MRI with Primovist showing segment VII recurrence; (C) coronal MRI with Primovist showing segment VII recurrence (arrow) related to right hepatic vein (arrowheads).

Additionally, along with more effective systemic and loco-regional therapies, patients with a high burden of liver disease may still be considered potentially resectable depending on their response to systemic or loco-regional treatment. This allows the concept of 'converting' a potentially non-resectable condition to a resectable disease. That is to say, resectability can be determined by technical and oncological factors. From an oncological perspective, the rate of progression and response to systemic treatment are essential determinants of cancer biology. But this is not necessarily an entity that is easily measured or known at the outset of the disease. From a technical perspective, with the advancements in modern hepatobiliary surgery almost anything that is considered oligometastatic can be resected as long as the following conditions are met: there must be a sufficient future liver remnant to support life (typically >20–30%), there must be adequate inflow and outflow of the remnant, and an R0 resection should be reasonably achievable.[7] Oligometastatic disease refers to a state of metastatic disease where the number and distribution of the metastases are limited and can be treated using loco-regional techniques, including surgery, to increase overall survival (OS).

What are the risk factors for recurrence after resection for colorectal liver metastases?

Many risk factors and scoring systems are described for recurrence after resection of colorectal liver metastases, and these are typically based on large retrospective cohorts. The clinical risk score described by Fong et al.[8] is the most widely known, but there are others. In this scoring system, the risk factors for recurrence include a positive margin on the primary tumour, extra-hepatic disease, node-positive disease, a short disease-free interval from primary to metastases, number of liver metastases, size of liver metastases and carcinoembryonic antigen level.

These clinical factors help to predict the prognosis of patients with colorectal metastases and may influence the decision to operate on such patients; however, in practice, features such as fitness, response to (and tolerance of) chemotherapy, tumour biology and the patient's wishes often play a more significant role in holistic management. Furthermore, in modern practice, molecular profiling, gene typing of cancers and the addition of immunotherapeutic agents allow for personalized and 'bespoke' treatment algorithms tailored to the individual patient.

What are the limitations of resection and what alternative local therapies are available?

Surgical resection may seem an attractive option for many patients with colorectal liver metastases, but it is by no means a panacea. As mentioned above, there are limitations to what can be achieved technically through resection, which in its simplest form revolves around the ability of the remnant liver to support life. While it is possible to resect substantial portions of the liver (up to 70–80% with the use of additional techniques to promote remnant liver hypertrophy), in the case of colorectal liver metastases, parenchymal sparing methods are preferred. In the present case, the patient had treatment for his liver disease on three occasions after two instances of recurrence. This is not uncommon in long-surviving patients (and hence the tendency towards parenchymal preserving strategies, with the anticipation that further treatments may be necessary in the future). For this patient, the treatment of his liver metastases was different on each occasion. After neoadjuvant chemotherapy, the first treatment consisted of anatomical liver resection of the left lobe of the liver. An intended right-sided non-anatomical resection was not performed owing to a disappearing lesion. The second treatment involved a non-anatomical resection (or wedge resection) combined with image-guided thermal ablation using radiofrequency ablation. A third recurrence was treated quite differently, using SBRT, because the lesion's proximity to a major outflow vessel precluded it from surgical or ablative techniques. Non-surgical techniques intended to treat liver metastases directly may be grouped as loco-regional therapies and are summarized below.

Loco-regional therapies

Loco-regional therapies are generally considered when surgery is not possible or not appropriate or when the patient has a strong preference. There are ongoing randomized controlled trials to evaluate the use of local ablative treatments as first line vs surgery (for example, the COLLISION trial; ClinicalTrials.gov NCT03088150). Historically, studies in this area find it difficult to recruit patients owing to patient and clinician equipoise. That is not to say that loco-regional therapies are ineffective; indeed they form a large arm of treatment options for colorectal liver metastases.

Thermal ablation

Thermal ablative therapies use heat to destroy tissue through coagulative necrosis. They are usually percutaneous procedures performed with imaging guidance but may be completed in the operating theatre, often in combination with a standard resection, as demonstrated in this case. Radiofrequency and microwave ablation are the most commonly used ablative techniques.[9] Both use heat to achieve their aim, although their probes and how they deliver the energy are slightly different. In radiofrequency ablation, an electrode is inserted into the tumour, which uses an alternating current to generate heat by a radiofrequency wave, whereas microwave ablation causes water oscillation to create heat and necrosis leading to cell death. Microwave ablation has become the first-line option in patients suitable for ablative treatment. Its advantages are that it is much quicker to perform and less susceptible to the heat sink effect. However, both are limited in the size and volume that can be ablated and cannot be used near significant structures such as vessels or other organs such as the gallbladder, bowel or diaphragm, although microwaves may be used slightly closer to structures compared with radiofrequency.

Non-thermal ablation

Irreversible electroporation is a newer technology that achieves a non-thermal ablation by providing an electric current through an area, leading to cellular death by apoptosis rather than necrosis. The advantage of electroporation is that it may be used near important structures, such as major vessels, as these are preserved. In addition, it is safe in tumours <5 cm that are unsuitable for resection, ablation or other chemotherapy.[10]

SBRT is a form of external beam radiotherapy where a high dose of focal radiotherapy is applied to a region to achieve an ablative dose. It also has the advantage of preserving vessels and other vital structures, which explains its use in this case. However, SBRT has the disadvantage compared with other ablative techniques of requiring multiple sessions over a period of time and, in the randomized setting, performs worse than thermal ablation with respect to OS and local recurrence.[11] Its use is therefore restricted to the location where thermal ablation is contraindicated owing to size or proximity to major structures.

Transarterial chemoembolization

Transarterial chemoembolization (TACE) is an angiographic method of delivering targeted chemotherapy to tumours in the liver and has been used since the 1970s.[12] In colorectal metastases it is generally considered after failure of systemic chemotherapy when surgery is not a preferred option. TACE is not considered a modality of curative intent in the way surgery and ablative treatments are. Angiographic access is usually via a femoral artery, which allows catheters to be inserted into arteries of the liver where the chemoembolization medications are delivered. In TACE, various embolic agents are available such as gelatine-based or lipiodol. Lipiodol is commonly used as it is lipophilic in nature, which helps in the delivery of lipid-based chemotherapy. In addition, mitomycin, cisplatin and doxorubicin are widely used chemotherapeutic agents in TACE. TACE is generally well tolerated and may be performed as a day procedure.

Conclusion and learning points

- The management of colorectal liver metastases is a complex and evolving area with many options and strategies that can be tailored to the individual patient.

- With the advances in surgical, systemic and loco-regional techniques, many patients with metastatic colorectal cancers can expect to achieve prolonged survival and even a cure that was not thought possible only 20 years ago.
- Owing to the variety of treatment options available, the optimal management strategy is best achieved in a multidisciplinary environment where experts in different fields can collaborate for the patient's best interests.

References

1 Manfredi S, Lepage C, Hatem C, et al. Epidemiology and management of liver metastases from colorectal cancer. Ann Surg 2006; 244: 254–9.

2 Nordlinger B, Sorbye H, Glimelius B, et al. Perioperative FOLFOX4 chemotherapy and surgery versus surgery alone for resectable liver metastases from colorectal cancer (EORTC 40983): long-term results of a randomised, controlled, phase 3 trial. Lancet Oncol 2013; 14: 1208–15.

3 Tomlinson JS, Jarnagin WR, DeMatteo RP, et al. Actual 10-year survival after resection of colorectal liver metastases defines cure. J Clin Oncol 2007; 25: 4575–80.

4 Wilson SM, Adson MA. Surgical treatment of hepatic metastases from colorectal cancers. Arch Surg 1976; 111: 330–4.

5 Ekberg H, Tranberg KG, Andersson R, et al. Determinants of survival in liver resection for colorectal secondaries. Br J Surg 1986; 73: 727–31.

6 van Dam RM, Lodewick TM, van den Broek MA, et al. Outcomes of extended versus limited indications for patients undergoing a liver resection for colorectal cancer liver metastases. HPB (Oxford) 2014; 16: 550–9.

7 Chakedis J, Squires MH, Beal EW, et al. Update on current problems in colorectal liver metastasis. Curr Probl Surg 2017; 54: 554–602.

8 Fong Y, Fortner J, Sun RL, et al. Clinical score for predicting recurrence after hepatic resection for metastatic colorectal cancer: analysis of 1001 consecutive cases. Ann Surg 1999; 230: 309–18; discussion 318–21.

9 Nieuwenhuizen S, Dijkstra M, Puijk RS, et al. Microwave ablation, radiofrequency ablation, irreversible electroporation, and stereotactic ablative body radiotherapy for intermediate size (3–5 cm) unresectable colorectal liver metastases: a systematic review and meta-analysis. Curr Oncol Rep 2022; 24: 793–808.

10 Meijerink MR, Ruarus AH, Vroomen LGPH, et al. Irreversible electroporation to treat unresectable colorectal liver metastases (COLDFIRE-2): a phase II, two-center, single-arm clinical trial. Radiology 2021; 299: 470–80.

11 Nieuwenhuizen S, Dijkstra M, Puijk RS, et al. Thermal ablation versus stereotactic ablative body radiotherapy to treat unresectable colorectal liver metastases: a comparative analysis from the prospective Amsterdam CORE registry. Cancers (Basel) 2021; 13: 4303.

12 Albert M, Kiefer MV, Sun W, et al. Chemoembolization of colorectal liver metastases with cisplatin, doxorubicin, mitomycin C, ethiodol, and polyvinyl alcohol. Cancer 2011; 117: 343–52.

CASE STUDY

14 Recurrent metastatic gastrointestinal stromal tumours in the liver

Dharmadev Trivedi, Dhakshinamoorthy Vijayanand, Magdy Attia

Case history

A 43-year-old man presented to the colorectal surgical team with new-onset constipation in the early spring of 2010. He had a background of hereditary haemorrhagic telangiectasia and a spinal cyst at the level of the L1 vertebra. He did not take any routine medication. In addition, there was a family history of bowel cancer in the maternal grandmother and lung cancer in the paternal uncle. *Per rectum* examination revealed a bulky rectal mass. A biopsy confirmed a gastrointestinal stromal tumour (GIST). A staging CT scan and MRI scan were performed (Figure 14.1).

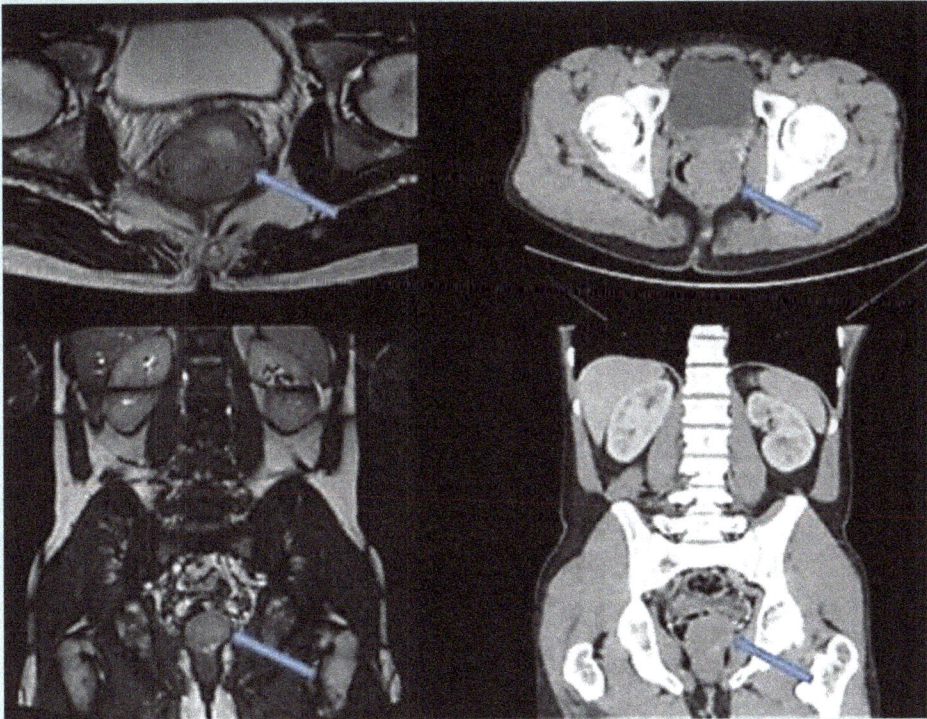

Figure 14.1 Initial CT and MRI images showing large rectal lesion (arrows).

The patient underwent a laparoscopic abdominal-perineal resection with extra-levator completion. Histopathology confirmed GIST pT3N0 (0/2), G2, 40 mitoses per 50 high-power fields (HPFs) and R0 resection. The multidisciplinary team (MDT) advised surveillance and considering imatinib if recurrence was identified. A surveillance CT scan in May 2012 and subsequent liver MRI in July 2012 demonstrated multiple liver metastases (Figure 14.2). The patient started taking imatinib and maintained good treatment response for the next 5 years. In June 2018, the surveillance imaging showed an increased size of left liver lesions and nodular regenerative changes (Figure 14.3). A laparoscopic converted to open segment III metastasectomy was performed. Histopathology confirmed metastatic GIST with *KIT* exon 13 mutations. The patient continued on imatinib. An MRI scan 11 months later demonstrated the increased size of the lesions in segments II, VI and VII of the liver (Figure 14.4).

The MDT considered the options of second-line systemic therapy, ablation or enrolling the patient in the INTRIGUE trial (ripretinib vs sunitinib; ClinicalTrials.gov NCT03673501). The patient enrolled in the trial and commenced ripretinib in November 2019. Owing to disease progression, the treatment was stopped in June 2020 (Figure 14.5).

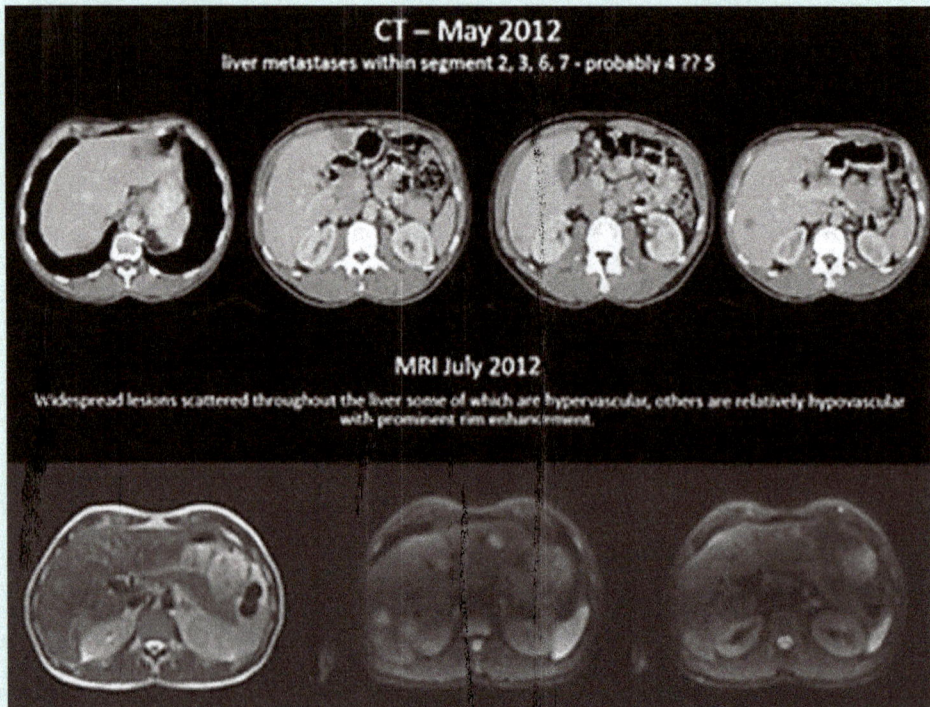

Figure 14.2 CT and MRI showing multiple bilobar liver metastases (May–July 2012).

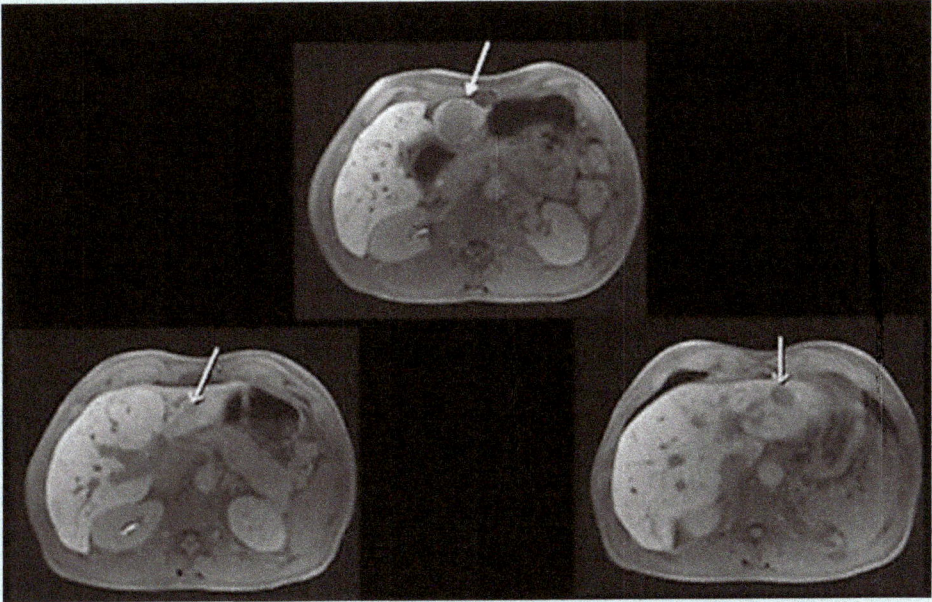

Figure 14.3 Liver MRI (June 2018) showing increased size of left liver lesions (arrows).

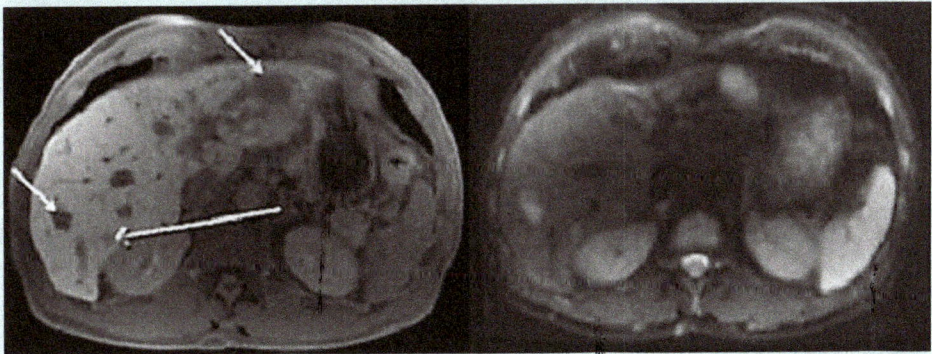

Figure 14.4 Liver MRI (September 2019) showing enlargement of lesions in segments II, VI and VII (arrows).

The MDT considered the options of second-line immunotherapy and resection. A further MRI scan in August 2020 showed enlarging liver metastases (Figure 14.6). The MDT agreed with the patient to proceed with surgical resection of the liver metastases either as a single-stage or a two-stage approach. The patient underwent an open left lateral sectionectomy and right posterior sectionectomy in October 2020. The histology confirmed metastatic GISTs on the background of nodular

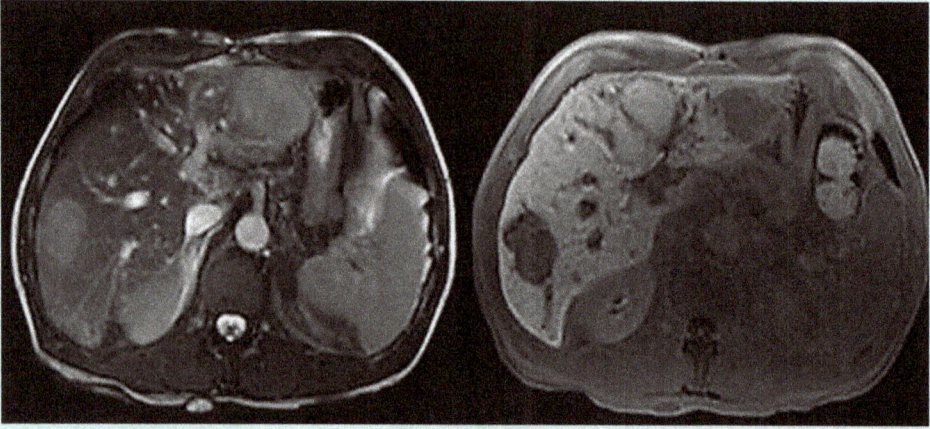

Figure 14.5 Liver MRI (June 2020) showed enlarging lesions in segments II and VII.

regeneration in the liver. Surveillance CT and MRI scans in May 2021 demonstrated a solitary metastasis in segment VIII (Figure 14.7).

The MDT considered options of ablation or repeat surgery. The patient chose to have ablation because he feared that surgery might not work. Percutaneous microwave ablation was performed in September 2021 without any procedural complications (Figure 14.8).

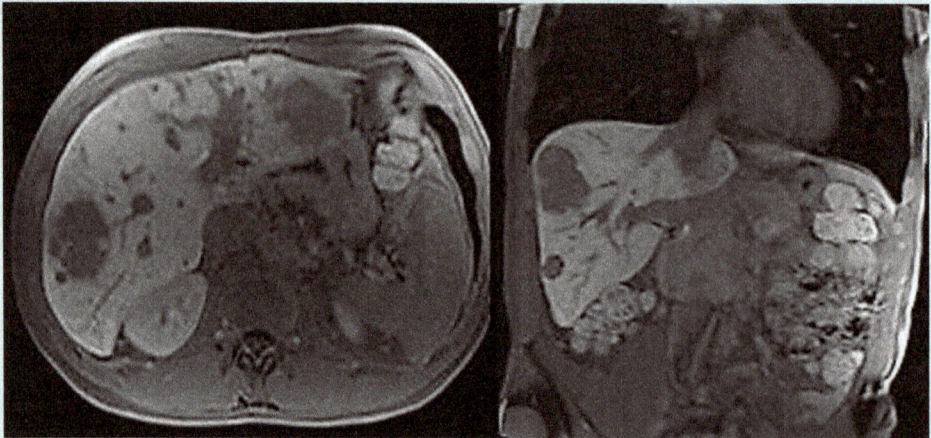

Figure 14.6 Liver MRI (August 2020) showing enlarging metastases in segments II and VII along with nodular regeneration in the liver.

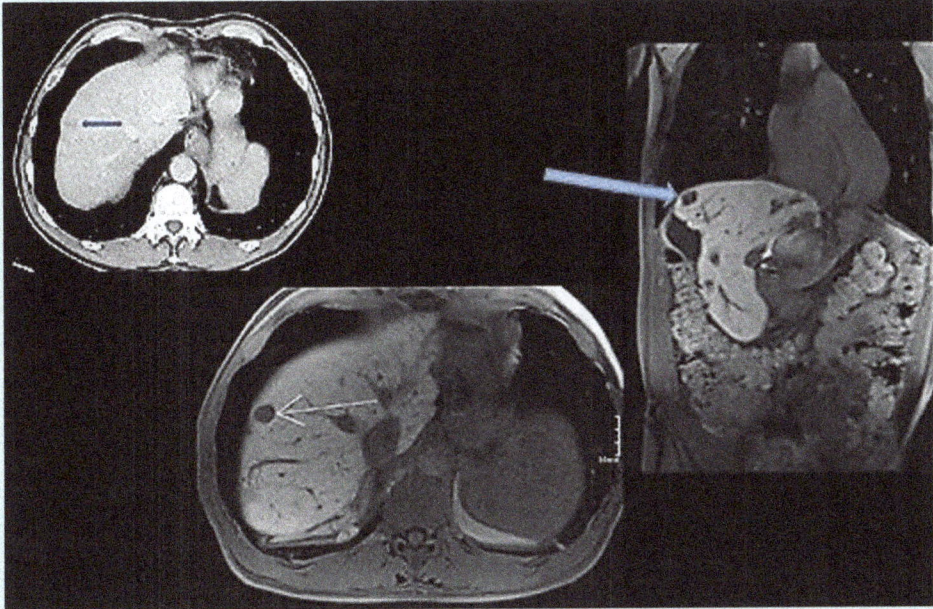

Figure 14.7 CT and MRI (May 2021) showing solitary liver metastasis in segment VIII (arrows).

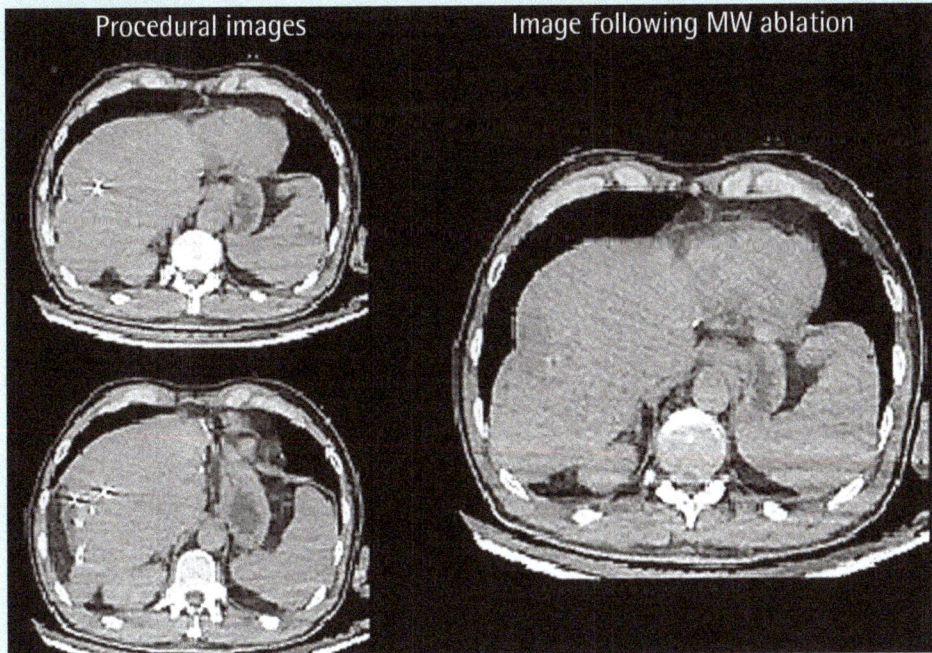

Procedural images   Image following MW ablation

Figure 14.8 Percutaneous microwave (MW) ablation of solitary liver metastasis.

What are GISTs and what are their peculiar features?

How are GISTs risk-stratified?

What should be the follow-up plan for metastatic GIST patients?

What is the evidence base for adjuvant therapy and its length?

What are the second-line tyrosine kinase inhibitors (TKIs) and the evidence for their efficacy?

What are GISTs and what are their peculiar features?

GISTs are rare but still the most common mesenchymal tumours of the elementary tract. They originate from the interstitial cells of Cajal.[1] Globally, the incidence rate of GIST is around 4–5 cases per million population. The stomach is the most common site (55.6%), followed by small intestinal (31.8%), colorectal (6.0%), oesophageal (0.7%) and other sites (5.5%).[2]

The immunohistochemical characteristics of GISTs involve the identification of mutations of c-*KIT* in exon 11 (the most common) but also in exon 9 (the most aggressive) and exons 8, 13 and 17, in around 80% of GISTs, and *PDGFRA* in exon 18 (the most common) and exons 12 and 14, in 8–10% of all GISTs; 12–15% of GISTs are wild-type without mutations.[1,3] *KIT* and *PDGFRA* mutations are mutually exclusive. Among the c-*KIT/PDGFRA* wild-type GISTs, further genetic classification based on either succinate dehydrogenase (SDH) competency or deficiency is possible. SDH-deficient GISTs are seen in the Carney triad or Carney–Stratakis syndrome; SDH-competent GISTs are identified with other mutations such as *BRAF* and *NF1*.[3] The identification of genetic mutations has changed the overall outlook of the treatment of GISTs since the beginning of the new millennium.[1,2,4]

How are GISTs risk-stratified?

GISTs are classified into very-low, low-, intermediate- and high-risk tumours according to tumour size, mitoses/HPF and primary tumour site (Table 14.1).[4]

Table 14.1 Risk stratification of GIST (adapted from Judson et al.[4]).

Risk category	Tumour size (cm)	Mitotic index (per 50 HPFs)	Primary tumour site
Very low risk	<2.0	≤5	Any
Low risk	2.1–5.0	≤5	Any
Intermediate risk	2.1–5.0	>5	Gastric
	≤5.0	6–10	Any
	5.1–10.0	≤5	Gastric
High risk	Any	Any	Tumour rupture
	>10.0	Any	Any
	>5.0	>5.0	Any
	2.1–5.0	>5.0	Non-gastric
	5.1–10.0	≤5.0	Non-gastric

Current UK guidelines for the management of GIST advise considering surveillance for very-low-risk GISTs, excision and surveillance of GISTs >2 cm in size, and complete oncological excision of larger GISTs.[4] For larger and moderate- to high-risk GISTs, neoadjuvant imatinib is also advised to downstage the disease safely with possible survival benefits.[4,5]

What should be the follow-up plan for metastatic GIST patients?

The primary imaging modality for GISTs is high-resolution CT supplemented by MRI as a problem-solving tool and a PET-CT scan in the event of equivocal findings from CT and MRI. The ultrasound scan with or without contrast enhancement is mainly recommended for surveillance of liver lesions and obtaining a biopsy of indeterminate lesions. The current national guidelines advise the following[4]:

- Cross-sectional imaging every 3–6 months while on adjuvant therapy for high-risk GISTs (usually 3 years), followed by:
  - cross-sectional imaging every 3 months for initial 2 years, followed by
  - every 6 months for the next 3 years, and
  - annually for 5 years thereafter.
- Patients with high-risk GISTs not receiving adjuvant treatment should follow the imaging protocol as per the post-adjuvant imaging schedule outlined above.
- Patients with intermediate-risk GISTs should have a CT or MRI scan every 6 months for the first 5 years, followed by annual imaging as per the patient's condition and age (no consensus).
- Less frequent and shorter follow-up for low- or very-low-risk GISTs (no consensus).

What is the evidence base for adjuvant therapy and its length?

Three years of adjuvant imatinib is recommended unless the tumour genetics suggest resistance to TKIs (*PDGFRA* exon 18 mutation D842V).[4] This recommendation is supported chiefly by the results of the Scandinavian Sarcoma Group phase III trial (ClinicalTrials.gov NCT00116935). The trial's long-term (10 years) outcomes showed a significant survival benefit for patients with high-risk GISTs receiving 3 years vs 1 year of adjuvant imatinib (Table 14.2).[6] Other larger studies have also reported increased recurrence-free survival after 1 year[7] or 2 years[8] of adjuvant imatinib compared with placebo for high-risk GIST patients. The beneficial effect of imatinib in an adjuvant setting is well established as a result.

There is no convincing evidence supporting the use of adjuvant TKI beyond 3 years. A multi-centre prospective phase II open-label study (PERSIST-5; ClinicalTrials.gov NCT00867113) explored the safety and efficacy of imatinib for 5 years in an adjuvant setting.[9] The authors noted that the safety profile of imatinib was acceptable, and the survival outcomes were similar to those reported in previous studies. However, 49% (45 of 91) of patients stopped the imatinib before 5 years and 26% were intermediate-risk patients. A prospective randomized phase III trial (ClinicalTrials.gov NCT02413736) is underway based on the findings of the PERSIST-5 trial, comparing 3 vs 5 years of adjuvant imatinib in patients with operable GISTs at high risk of recurrence, which will conclude in 2028.

What are the second-line TKIs and the evidence for their efficacy?

The standard second-line medical therapy is sunitinib, and the third line is regorafenib. Isolated recurrence can be managed with repeat surgery and ablation.[4] Sunitinib and regorafenib

Table 14.2 Key long-term results from the Scandinavian Sarcoma Group trial (*N*=397).[6]

Survival	1 year adjuvant imatinib (%)	3 year adjuvant imatinib (%)	Significance
Overall survival			HR 0.55
			95% CI 0.37, 0.83
			p=0.004
5 years	85.5	92.0	
10 years	65.3	79.0	
Recurrence-free survival			HR 0.66
			95% CI 0.49, 0.87
			p=0.003
5 years	53.0	71.4	
10 years	41.8	52.5	

as second- and third-line treatments have improved survival in patients with advanced GISTs. Additional survival benefit is also noted for patients with surgical metastasectomy in addition to the second-line (66.1 vs 32.4 months; *p*=0.0008) and third-line (37.4 vs 19.7 months; *p*=0.0008) therapy.[10] The INTRIGUE phase III open-label trial compared ripretinib with sunitinib after imatinib failure. In its pivotal study, the trial concluded that the ripretinib group had less severe side effects and better progression-free survival compared with the sunitinib group.[11]

Conclusion and learning points

- The case history and the treatments offered to the patient highlight the importance of a thorough understanding of the management of GISTs, referring to contemporary national and international guidelines with multimodal management.
- Management of GIST patients should involve a specialist MDT.
- The tumour's genetic profile should be obtained for every GIST patient, especially in case of primary and secondary resistance to TKIs.
- Neoadjuvant therapies are now considered in locally advanced cases to attempt downstaging/tumour shrinkage.
- Surgical resection, with or without ablation, in addition to second- and third-line therapies, offers survival benefits in selected patients.

References

1 Rubin BP, Heinrich MC, Corless CL. Gastrointestinal stromal tumour. Lancet 2007; 369: 1731–41.

2 Søreide K, Sandvik OM, Søreide JA, et al. Global epidemiology of gastrointestinal stromal tumours (GIST): a systematic review of population-based cohort studies. Cancer Epidemiol 2016; 40: 39–46.

3   Wu CE, Tzen CY, Wang SY, Yeh CN. Clinical diagnosis of gastrointestinal stromal tumour (GIST): from the molecular genetic point of view. Cancers 2019; 11: 679.

4   Judson I, Bulusu R, Seddon B, et al. UK clinical practice guidelines for the management of gastrointestinal stromal tumours (GIST). Clin Sarcoma Res 2017; 7: 1–10.

5   Iwatsuki M, Harada K, Iwagami S, et al. Neoadjuvant and adjuvant therapy for gastrointestinal stromal tumours. Ann Gastroenterol Surg 2019; 3: 43–9.

6   Joensuu H, Eriksson M, Hall KS, et al. Survival outcomes associated with three years vs one year of adjuvant imatinib for patients with high-risk gastrointestinal stromal tumours: an analysis of a randomized clinical trial after 10-year follow-up. JAMA Oncol 2020; 6: 1–6.

7   Corless CL, Ballman KV, Antonescu CR, et al. Pathologic and molecular features correlate with long-term outcome after adjuvant therapy of resected primary GI stromal tumor: the ACOSOG Z9001 trial. J Clin Oncol 2014; 32: 1563.

8   Casali P, Le Cesne A, Poveda Velasco A, et al. Time to definitive failure to the first tyrosine kinase inhibitor in localized GI stromal tumors treated with imatinib as an adjuvant: a European Organisation for Research and Treatment of Cancer Soft Tissue and Bone Sarcoma Group intergroup randomized trial in collaboration with the Australasian Gastro-Intestinal Trials Group, UNICANCER, French Sar coma Group, Italian Sarcoma Group, and Spanish Group for Research on Sarcomas. J Clin Oncol 2015; 33: 4276–83.

9   Raut CP, Espat NJ, Maki RG, et al. Efficacy and tolerability of 5-year adjuvant imatinib treatment for patients with resected intermediate- or high-risk primary gastrointestinal stromal tumor: the PERSIST-5 clinical trial. JAMA Oncol 2018; 4: e184060.

10 Call JW, Wang Y, Montoya D, et al. Survival in advanced GIST has improved over time and correlates with increased access to post-imatinib tyrosine kinase inhibitors: results from Life Raft Group Registry. Clin Sarcoma Res 2019; 9: 1–4.

11 Heinrich MC, Jones RL, Gelderblom H, et al. INTRIGUE: a phase III, randomized, open-label study to evaluate the efficacy and safety of ripretinib versus sunitinib in patients with advanced gastrointestinal stromal tumor previously treated with imatinib. J Clin Oncol 2022; 40 (36 suppl): 359881.

15 Liver-predominant metastatic uveal melanoma treated with melphalan percutaneous hepatic perfusion

Ganesh Vigneswaran, Brian Stedman, Sachin Modi

Case history

A 65-year-old woman presented with some irregularities in her vision. She had no other significant medical history and was otherwise fit (ECOG performance status 0). An ophthalmic assessment revealed a 6 mm lesion on the iris. The lesion was biopsied and confirmed as uveal melanoma. The patient was referred to an ocular oncology centre and the primary lesion was treated with enucleation. The patient recovered from this treatment and began a surveillance programme. CT of the chest, abdomen and pelvis and MRI of the liver were performed at 6 month intervals.

Eighteen months after the primary diagnosis, a 4 mm subcapsular lesion was found on the left lobe of the liver. After a discussion at the multidisciplinary team (MDT) meeting, the patient was listed for laparoscopic biopsy and resection. At the time of surgery, a month later, she was found to have several subcentimetre metastases in both lobes of the liver. A biopsy of one of the lesions confirmed metastatic uveal melanoma. A repeat MRI scan confirmed at least 12 metastases in the liver; the largest lesion was 5 mm (Figure 15.1).

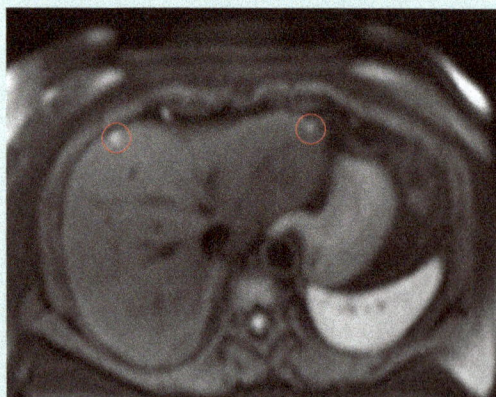

Figure 15.1 Diffusion-weighted MRI scan showing multiple small liver lesions in both lobes.

The patient was referred for chemosaturation to treat her liver disease. She had three cycles of chemosaturation 6–8 weeks apart. After the first two treatments, she had an excellent partial response, with the disappearance of all her right-sided lesions and a reduction of the left-sided lesions. However, after a further treatment, follow-up imaging revealed a complete response in her liver (Figure 15.2).

She continues with 6 monthly surveillance scans and remains disease-free 24 months after her first chemosaturation and 4 years after her primary diagnosis.

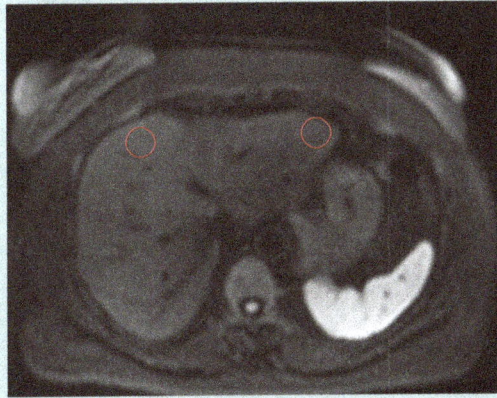

Figure 15.2 Diffusion-weighted MRI scan showing complete response with disappearance of the previously seen liver lesions.

What was the goal of cancer treatment in this patient?

What is melphalan percutaneous hepatic perfusion (M-PHP)?

What are the rationale and evidence for M-PHP in patients with metastatic uveal melanoma?

Which patients should not be treated with M-PHP?

What was the goal of cancer treatment in this patient?

The goal of treatment was hepatic disease control to improve overall survival (OS). The treatment options were limited given the extent of hepatic disease which precluded a definitive surgical approach. Systemic therapies including chemotherapy, immunotherapy or combination therapy were also considered but have limited efficacy in liver-only disease. The selection regarding the eventual treatment approach was determined by the extent of the patient's liver disease, her physical fitness and her personal values as discussed at the MDT meeting.

What is M-PHP?

M-PHP allows targeting the liver with high-dose chemotherapy without exposing peripheral non-target tissues to unsafe doses. Furthermore, the technique takes advantage of the relative

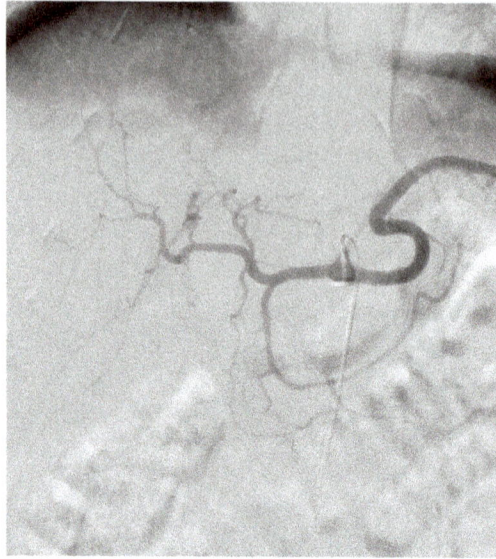

Figure 15.3 Angiogram showing arterial liver vessels to plan delivery of melphalan.

tumoral arterial hyperperfusion compared with that of normal liver parenchyma.[1] It is achieved by introducing melphalan via an arterial catheter into the hepatic artery (Figure 15.3) and filtering the hepatic venous blood via a double balloon catheter placed in the hepatic inferior vena cava (Figure 15.4).[2] The procedure is performed under general anaesthesia at specialist centres with significant interventional radiology, anaesthesia and oncological expertise.

What are the rationale and evidence for M–PHP in patients with metastatic uveal melanoma?

Uveal melanoma, while a relatively uncommon form of melanoma, is the most common intraocular malignancy of adulthood.[3] Metastatic spread is common at the time of initial diagnosis[4] and occurs in 25–34% of patients after initial local treatment.[5] At 1 year, median survival in metastatic disease is poor[5,6] but is notably worse in cases with hepatic metastases (the most prevalent site of metastasis),[7] where median survival can be as low as 3 months,[6,8] even though many patients are diagnosed with only a single site of disease.[7]

Systemic chemotherapy has limited survival benefits.[9,10] Given the poor prognosis and the scope for significant symptomatic and prognostic improvements in treatment, there have been significant efforts and advances in recent years in understanding the underlying molecular tumour biology of metastatic uveal melanoma.[5,11,12] This has led to the introduction of a variety of new systemic immunotherapy and chemoimmunotherapy treatments now being evaluated in clinical trials.[9] Although chemoimmunotherapy has shown promising evidence of efficacy, there is still a substantial proportion of patients who gain no improved survival benefit.[13] As a result, liver-targeted therapies have risen to the forefront in treating patients with liver-only metastatic uveal melanoma, either as monotherapy[1] or in conjunction with immunotherapy.[14] There is a growing body of evidence demonstrating the safety of chemosaturation in terms of peripheral non-target melphalan dose and clinical outcomes, with excellent radiological response and survival improvement.[1,15–18] For example, the

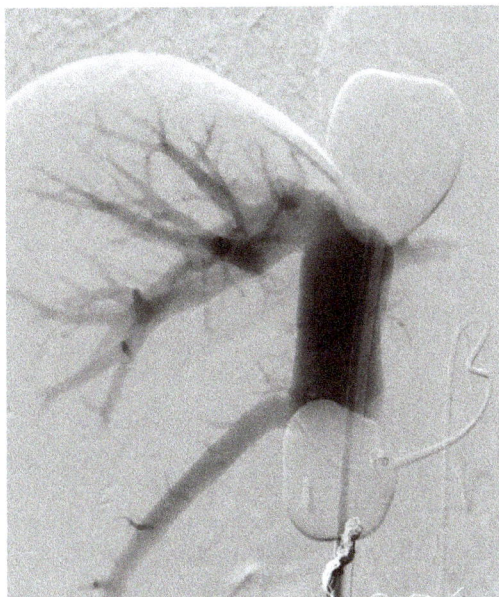

Figure 15.4 Venogram showing double balloon catheter in inferior vena cava with isolation of hepatic venous return.

largest retrospective cohort study involving 250 treatments in 81 patients in the UK has shown a median OS of 14.9 months.[1] Importantly, while retrospective, the study showed excellent hepatic disease control rates (88.9%). In addition, sub-analysis revealed a disparity in survival according to response in the liver: patients obtaining hepatic disease control (complete responders) had significantly longer survival than those with progressive disease (34.7 months vs 7.7 months). There were no fatal treatment-related adverse events and the overwhelming majority of adverse events were limited to grade 1 or 2 (72.3%). Other studies have shown longer median survival (>27 months) following M–PHP treatment but are limited by heterogeneous patient characteristics and low patient numbers.[19,20]

Other liver-directed therapies such as selective internal radiation therapy have also shown some promise; a recent phase II study showed a median survival of 18.5 months but was limited by small cohort sizes.[21] Transarterial chemoembolization has also been explored, but again the evidence is very much limited by non-randomization, variable procedural techniques and chemo-embolic agent used.[22-24]

Which patients should not be treated with M–PHP?

M-PHP is suitable for many patients with liver-predominant metastatic disease but requires careful clinical assessment and workup to ensure tolerability of general anaesthesia and haemo-filtration.[1] Patients are recommended to be between 18 and 80 years of age, have an ECOG performance status <1 and be without significant cardiac or respiratory disease. Furthermore, pre-procedural imaging is required to evaluate hepatic arterial and venous anatomy to ensure no significant anomaly would preclude technical success. The reliance on haemofiltration also means that patients with clotting or bleeding disorders or abnormal haematological parameters are unsuitable. Lastly, significant background liver disease (Child–Pugh class >A), >60% disease

Problem Solving in Interventional Oncology

replacement in the liver or more than one site of extrahepatic disease would also preclude treatment given the likely limited benefit in these patients.

Conclusion and learning points

- For liver-predominant metastatic disease in the setting of uveal melanoma, controlling the hepatic disease burden improves OS. However, surgical management is often not possible and conventional systemic therapies such as immunotherapy have shown limited efficacy.
- Of the liver-directed therapies, M-PHP has a growing body of evidence and is suitable if the patient has a sufficient reserve to undergo general anaesthesia and haemofiltration.
- M-PHP involves isolating the hepatic circulation with a double balloon catheter and delivering melphalan via the hepatic artery. Filtration ensures that high doses may be administered without inducing systemic toxicity.
- Evidence for M-PHP in this setting has demonstrated reasonable response rates in controlling the hepatic disease and improving OS. Still, it is somewhat limited by the retrospective nature of most studies.
- Research is ongoing comparing combination therapies involving M-PHP with immunological therapies to improve OS further.

References

1 Modi S, Gibson T, Vigneswaran G, et al. Chemosaturation with percutaneous hepatic perfusion of melphalan for metastatic uveal melanoma. Melanoma Res 2022; 32: 103–11.
2 Pingpank JF, Libutti SK, Chang R, et al. Phase I study of hepatic arterial melphalan infusion and hepatic venous hemofiltration using percutaneously placed catheters in patients with unresectable hepatic malignancies. J Clin Oncol 2005; 23: 3465–74.
3 Singh AD, Turell ME, Topham AK. Uveal melanoma: trends in incidence, treatment, and survival. Ophthalmology 2011; 118: 1881–5.
4 Kujala E, Mäkitie T, Kivelä T. Very long-term prognosis of patients with malignant uveal melanoma. Invest Ophthalmol Vis Sci 2003; 44: 4651–9.
5 Amaro A, Gangemi R, Piaggio F, et al. The biology of uveal melanoma. Cancer Metastasis Rev 2017; 36: 109–40.
6 Gragoudas ES, Egan KM, Seddon JM, et al. Survival of patients with metastases from uveal melanoma. Ophthalmology 1991; 98: 383–90.
7 Rietschel P, Panageas KS, Hanlon C, et al. Variates of survival in metastatic uveal melanoma. J Clin Oncol 2005; 23: 8076–80.
8 Khoja L, Atenafu EG, Suciu S, et al. Meta-analysis in metastatic uveal melanoma to determine progression free and overall survival benchmarks: an International Rare Cancers Initiative (IRCI) ocular melanoma study. Ann Oncol 2019; 30: 1370–80.
9 Buder K, Gesierich A, Gelbrich G, Goebeler M. Systemic treatment of metastatic uveal melanoma: review of literature and future perspectives. Cancer Med 2013; 2: 674–86.
10 Rantala ES, Hernberg M, Kivelä TT. Overall survival after treatment for metastatic uveal melanoma: a systematic review and meta-analysis. Melanoma Res 2019; 29: 561–8.

11 Vidwans SJ, Flaherty KT, Fisher DE, et al. A melanoma molecular disease model. PLoS One 2011; 6: e18257.

12 Karlsson J, Nilsson LM, Mitra S, et al. Molecular profiling of driver events in metastatic uveal melanoma. Nat Commun 2020; 11: 1894.

13 Wang X, Ji Q, Yan X, et al. The impact of liver metastasis on anti-PD-1 monoclonal antibody monotherapy in advanced melanoma: analysis of five clinical studies. Front Oncol 2020; 10: 546604.

14 Tong TML, van der Kooij MK, Speetjens FM, et al. Combining Hepatic Percutaneous Perfusion with Ipilimumab plus Nivolumab in Advanced Uveal Melanoma (CHOPIN): study protocol for a phase Ib/randomized phase II trial. Trials 2022; 23: 137.

15 Hughes MS, Zager J, Faries M, et al. Results of a randomized controlled multicenter phase III trial of percutaneous hepatic perfusion compared with best available care for patients with melanoma liver metastases. Ann Surg Oncol 2016; 23: 1309–19.

16 de Leede EM, Burgmans MC, Meijer TS, et al. Prospective clinical and pharmacological evaluation of the Delcath System's second-generation (GEN2) hemofiltration system in patients undergoing percutaneous hepatic perfusion with melphalan. Cardiovasc Radiol 2017; 40: 1196–205.

17 Karydis I, Gangi A, Wheater MJ, et al. Percutaneous hepatic perfusion with melphalan in uveal melanoma: a safe and effective treatment modality in an orphan disease. J Surg Oncol 2018; 117: 1170–8.

18 Meijer TS, Burgmans MC, Fiocco M, et al. Safety of percutaneous hepatic perfusion with melphalan in patients with unresectable liver metastases from ocular melanoma using the Delcath Systems' second-generation hemofiltration system: a prospective non-randomized phase II trial. Cardiovasc Radiol 2019; 42: 841–52.

19 Artzner C, Mossakowski O, Hefferman G, et al. Chemosaturation with percutaneous hepatic perfusion of melphalan for liver-dominant metastatic uveal melanoma: a single center experience. Cancer Imaging 2019; 19: 31.

20 Meijer TS, Burgmans MC, de Leede EM, et al. Percutaneous hepatic perfusion with melphalan in patients with unresectable ocular melanoma metastases confined to the liver: a prospective phase II study. Ann Surg Oncol 2021; 28: 1130–41.

21 Gonsalves CF, Eschelman DJ, Thornburg B, et al. Uveal melanoma metastatic to the liver: chemoembolization with 1,3-bis-(2 chloroethyl)-1-nitrosourea. Am J Roentgenol 2015; 205: 429–33.

22 Carling U, Dorenberg EJ, Haugvik SP, et al. Transarterial chemoembolization of liver metastases from uveal melanoma using irinotecan-loaded beads: treatment response and complications. Cardiovasc Intervent Radiol 2015; 38: 1532–41.

23 Valpione S, Aliberti C, Parrozzani R, et al. A retrospective analysis of 141 patients with liver metastases from uveal melanoma: a two-cohort study comparing transarterial chemoembolization with CPT-11 charged microbeads and historical treatments. Melanoma Res 2015; 25: 164–8.

24 Shibayama Y, Namikawa K, Sone M, et al. Efficacy and toxicity of transarterial chemoembolization therapy using cisplatin and gelatin sponge in patients with liver metastases from uveal melanoma in an Asian population. Int J Clin Oncol 2017; 22: 577–84.

Further reading

• NICE (2021). Melphalan chemosaturation with percutaneous hepatic artery perfusion and hepatic vein isolation for primary or metastatic cancer in the liver. Interventional procedures guidance IPG691. Available from: www.nice.org.uk/guidance/ipg691.

16 A diagnostic conundrum: an incidental small renal mass

Ashley Thorpe, John Spillane, Lawrence Bell

Case history

57-year-old man presented with abdominal pain. A portal venous phase contrast-enhanced CT scan of his abdomen and pelvis revealed an incidental 12 mm left-sided renal lesion (Figure 16.1A). After discussion at the urology multidisciplinary team (MDT) meeting, a decision was made to perform a follow-up CT scan with and without intravenous contrast 6 months later to formally characterize the lesion and assess its growth.

Unfortunately, when the follow-up CT scan was performed 6 months later, only a single phase (portal venous) scan was acquired. It demonstrated an indeterminate renal lesion that had increased in size by 4 mm to 16 mm (Figure 16.1B). A repeat discussion by the urology MDT noted that the lesion was solitary and had no definite aggressive malignant features (lymphadenopathy or local invasion); it was therefore

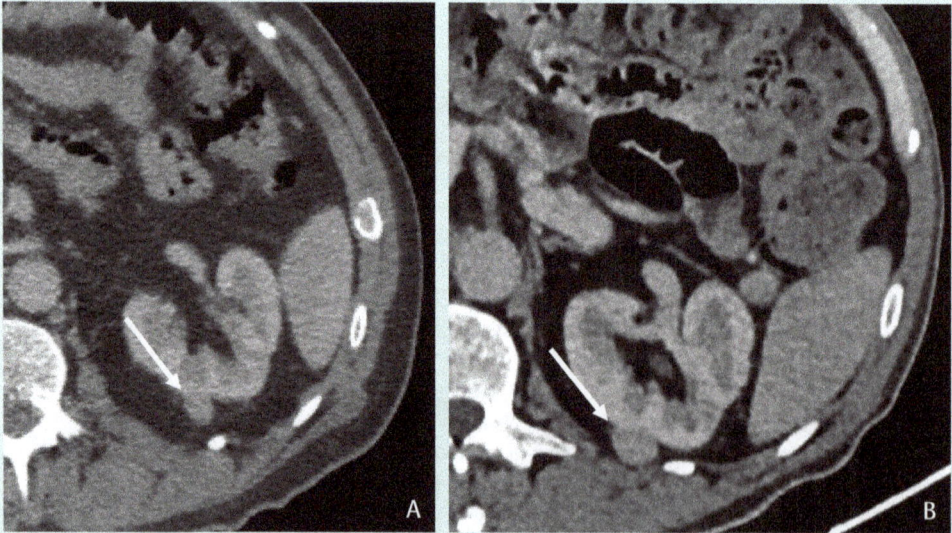

Figure 16.1 Single axial slice through a portal venous phase contrast-enhanced CT scan. (A) The patient's initial presentation shows a 12 mm exophytic lesion arising from the posterior aspect of the left kidney (arrow). (B) The same renal lesion 6 months later shows it has grown by 4 mm to 16 mm (arrow).

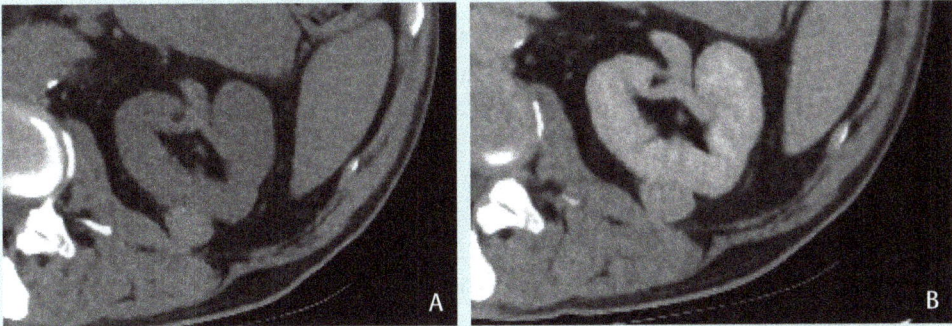

Figure 16.2 Non-contrast and nephrographic phase contrast-enhanced CT scan images 18 months after
initial presentation. (A) Single axial slice from a non-contrast CT scan shows the exophytic lesion arising
from the posterior aspect of the left kidney; its attenuation value was 58 HU. (B) A nephrographic (120 s)
post-contrast image, obtained at the same sitting, which shows subjective enhancement and an attenuation
value of 88 HU.

decided to follow up with a CT scan with and without intravenous contrast in
1 year's time.

This subsequent CT scan demonstrated enhancement of the renal lesion by
30 Hounsfield units (HU) and a further increase in size by 7 mm to 23 mm
(Figure 16.2). After an MDT discussion, it was decided to proceed with a biopsy,
which was subsequently performed and the results were consistent with a benign
angiomyolipoma.

How often are renal masses detected on imaging as an incidental finding?

What is the differential diagnosis of an incidental small renal mass?

What imaging features favour a benign vs a malignant cause?

What is the role of percutaneous renal biopsy?

Case discussion

How often are renal masses detected on imaging as an incidental finding?

Renal lesions have been detected with increasing incidence over the last two decades, particularly
in the older population, owing to the increased availability and use of cross-sectional imaging.[1-4]
Studies estimate that between 14% and 27% of adults undergoing abdominal imaging will be
found to have a renal lesion, either cystic or solid,[5,6] and more than half of patients over the age of
50 will have at least one renal lesion.[7]

What is the differential diagnosis of an incidental small renal mass?

A small renal mass is defined as a renal neoplasm that measures <4 cm and shows some contrast
enhancement. Simple renal cysts do not show enhancement and are a very common finding, seen
in 11–40% of patients.[8,9]

Small renal masses pose a diagnostic conundrum because despite earlier detection the mortality rate associated with renal cell carcinoma (RCC) has not significantly changed.[1,3,4] This is

likely because 20–30% of small renal masses are found to have benign histology (including onco-cytomas, metanephric adenomas and angiomyolipomas). Of the remaining 70–80% that are malignant, 70–80% are low-grade RCCs with low metastatic potential and an indolent growth rate of 0–0.3 cm/year.[1-4] Although there are several subtypes of RCC, 90% are one of three subtypes: clear cell RCC is the most common, followed by papillary RCC and then chromophobe RCC. They have different prognoses but cannot be accurately differentiated by imaging (although some subtypes do have characteristic imaging features).

What imaging features favour a benign vs a malignant cause?

There are three possibilities when evaluating an incidental small renal lesion[10]:

- it has been fully characterized on the imaging study and a management plan can be suggested;
- it has been inadequately characterized on the imaging study and further imaging is required before a definitive management plan can be suggested;
- it is inadequately characterized but demonstrates features which make it highly likely to be benign and further imaging studies are unlikely to aid decision making.

In the present case, a single portal venous phase CT scan of the abdomen and pelvis had been performed, which fits with the second possibility above. On this single phase scan we can evaluate two main imaging features:

- Size of the mass: a renal mass <1 cm has an over 40% chance of being benign.[11] Small renal masses <4 cm have a 20–30% chance of being benign. As the mass enlarges to over 4 cm the rate of malignancy increases to over 95%.[12]
- Homogeneity and attenuation: a homogenous lesion (i.e. one without internal variation of attenuation values) with a thin, smooth wall and between −9 and 20 HU may be safely characterized as a benign simple cyst requiring no further follow-up. A mass which contains macroscopic fat with attenuation values below −20 HU is strongly suggestive of an angiomyolipoma (a benign mass).[13] It is important to note, however, that a small percentage of angiomyolipomas are fat-poor and the absence of fat does not rule out this diagnosis.[14] Adding further complexity, a small percentage of RCCs contain fat, but the presence of intralesional calcification may point towards a malignant mass.[15]

Unfortunately, in many cases an incidental lesion is inadequately characterized for the simple reason that the imaging protocol was not aimed specifically at the urinary tract.

Imaging features which require pre- and post-contrast protocols and sequential imaging in-clude the following.

Enhancement

Enhancement is defined as an increase in attenuation of >20 HU between a non-contrast and a contrast phase study.[10] In the present case, non-contrast and nephrographic phase CT scans were organized in order to evaluate enhancement. The patient's renal mass demonstrated a 30 HU increase in the nephrographic phase and was therefore considered to be an enhancing lesion. En-hancement of a renal lesion is considered one of the important criteria for identifying malignant masses, although it still does not reliably differentiate between a malignant and a benign mass.[16] There are also different enhancement characteristics between the main subtypes of RCC. Clear cell RCCs are hypervascular and therefore typically enhance; papillary and chromophobe RCCs are typically less vascular and may be poorly enhancing.[17] Other imaging modalities can also be used to assess for enhancement such as MRI and contrast-enhanced ultrasound. These can be particularly useful as problem-solving tools or in younger patients where less radiation exposure is desirable.

Growth and change in appearance

Sequential imaging is needed to determine the growth rate of a mass. Several papers have suggested that lesions with a slow growth rate (<0.5 cm/year) have an insignificant (although not zero) risk of developing metastases. In one such meta-analysis, which followed 286 renal masses with a mean size of 2.6 cm and a mean follow-up of 34 months, the mean growth rate was 0.28 cm per year and progression to metastatic disease was seen in only 1% of cases.[18] Masses that grow faster than 0.5 cm/year may be characterized as progressive and with a higher likelihood of being aggressive.[2] Additionally, if the mass changes in appearance over the surveillance time frame, i.e. it becomes more heterogeneous or demonstrates invasion into nearby structures, this also points towards a malignant pathology.

What is the role of percutaneous renal biopsy?

Renal biopsy can be useful in characterizing renal masses as benign or malignant, with sensitivities ranging between 80% and 92% and specificities between 83% and 100%.[19] Complications from renal biopsy are uncommon: the reported risk of major complications, including major haemorrhage requiring arterial embolization or blood transfusion, is reported to be between 6% and 7%, with life-threatening complications 0.1%.[20]

Biopsy is being increasingly used as a problem-solving tool in patients with small renal masses and has been shown to alter clinical management in up to 60% of cases.[21]

Case discussion

There is no definitive strategy for managing small renal masses. Guidelines offered by both the European Association of Urology[16] and the American Urological Association[22] do exist, but no definitive management protocol is provided by either. They both go through the evidence for the different management strategies, which may include active surveillance, percutaneous biopsy and active management (ablation, partial nephrectomy, radical nephrectomy). Deciding between these strategies will depend on the patient's age and performance status, their personal preferences and the specific characteristics of the small renal mass. Practices can therefore vary between hospitals, and local protocols should be taken into account.

Looking more closely at our patient's case, we incidentally found an indeterminate renal lesion. It was decided that, although uncharacterized at this point, it could be followed up at 6 months; this is because many renal lesions are benign, or if they are malignant many have an indolent course. Some may ask why we did not immediately characterize the lesion; the reason is because follow-up was required anyway and immediately characterizing the lesion in an additional CT scan would have had no tangible benefit. Although the initial follow-up CT scan at 6 months unfortunately did not fully characterize the lesion, we did gain some useful information: the lesion remained small with no agressive malignant features but had increased in size by 4 mm.

The second CT scan carried out 18 months after presentation with and without contrast confirmed a solid lesion and also showed a further increase in size by 7 mm (i.e. an 11 mm increase in size over a period of 18 months). This corresponds to a growth rate of 0.7 cm/year and it places the lesion in a higher risk group. After MDT discussion, and in conjunction with the patient, a biopsy was performed which showed that the mass was a benign angiomyolipoma. The biopsy in this case potentially avoided a partial nephrectomy and gave peace of mind to the patient.

Conclusion and learning points

- Incidental renal masses are very common.
- Differentiating benign and malignant causes can be challenging on imaging alone.
- Malignant small renal masses are often low grade, have low metastatic potential and are indolent; therefore, a period of monitoring is often appropriate (depending on patient factors and local protocol).
- Imaging features that may be helpful in characterizing a small renal mass include:
  - size;
  - heterogeneity and attenuation;
  - enhancement;
  - growth and morphological change.
- Biopsy can be helpful in determining the diagnosis and can change clinical decision making.

References

1 Pierorazio PM, Hyams ES, Mullins JK, et al. Active surveillance for small renal masses. Rev Urol 2012; 14: 13–19.

2 Sebastià S, Corominas D, Musquera M, et al. Active surveillance of small renal masses. Insights Imaging 2020; 11: 63.

3 Sohlberg EM, Metzner TJ, Leppert JT. The harms of overdiagnosis and overtreatment in patients with small renal masses: a mini-review. Eur Urol Focus 2019; 5: 943–5.

4 Volpe A. The role of active surveillance of small renal masses. Int J Surg 2016; 36: 518–24.

5 O'Connor SD, Pickhardt PJ, Kim DH, et al. Incidental finding of renal masses at unenhanced CT: prevalence and analysis of features for guiding management. Am J Roentgenol 2011; 197: 139–45.

6 Gill IS, Aron M, Gervais DA, et al. Clinical practice. Small renal mass. N Engl J Med 2010; 362: 624–34.

7 Di Vece F, Tombesi P, Ermili F, et al. Management of incidental renal masses: time to consider contrast-enhanced ultrasonography. Ultrasound 2016; 24: 34–40.

8 Carrim ZI, Murchison JT. The prevalence of simple renal and hepatic cysts detected by spiral computed tomography. Clin Radiol 2003; 58: 626–9.

9 Chang CC, Kuo JY, Chan WL, et al. Prevalence and clinical characteristics of simple renal cyst. J Chin Med Assoc 2007; 70: 486–91.

10 Herts BR, Silverman SG, Hindman NM, et al. Management of the incidental renal mass on CT: a white paper of the ACR Incidental Findings Committee. J Am Coll Radiol 2018; 15: 264–73.

11 Frank I, Blute ML, Cheville JC, et al. Solid renal tumors: an analysis of pathological features related to tumor size. J Urol 2003; 170 (6 pt 1): 2217–20.

12 Kurban LAS, Vosough A, Jacob P, et al. Pathological nature of renal tumors – does size matter? Urol Ann 2017; 9: 330–4.

13 Silverman SG, Pedrosa I, Ellis JH, et al. Bosniak classification of cystic renal masses, version 2019: an update proposal and needs assessment. Radiology 2019; 292: 475–88.

14 Jinzaki M, Tanimoto A, Narimatsu Y, et al. Angiomyolipoma: imaging findings in lesions with minimal fat. Radiology 1997; 205: 497–502.

15 Rossi SH, Prezzi D, Kelly-Morland C, et al. Imaging for the diagnosis and response assessment of renal tumours. World J Urol 2018; 36: 1927–42.

16 Ljungberg B, Albiges L, Bedke J, et al. (2022). EAU guidelines on renal cell carcinoma. Available from: https://d56bochluxqnz.cloudfront.net/documents/full-guideline/EAU-Guidelines-on-Renal-Cell-Carinoma-2022.pdf (accessed 10 February 2022).

17 Sun MR, Ngo L, Genega EM, et al. Renal cell carcinoma: dynamic contrast-enhanced MR imaging for differentiation of tumor subtypes – correlation with pathologic findings. Radiology 2009; 250: 793–802.

18 Chawla SN, Crispen PL, Hanlon AL, et al. The natural history of observed enhancing renal masses: meta-analysis and review of the world literature. J Urol 2006; 175: 425–31.

19 Sahni VA, Silverman SG. Biopsy of renal masses: when and why. Cancer Imaging 2009; 9: 44–55.

20 Lefaucheur C, Nochy D, Bariety J. Renal biopsy: procedures, contraindications, complications [in French]. Néphrol Thér 2009; 5: 331–9.

21 Maturen KE, Nghiem HV, Caoili EM, et al. Renal mass core biopsy: accuracy and impact on clinical management. Am J Roentgenol 2007; 188: 563–70.

22 Campbell S, Uzzo RG, Allaf ME, et al. Renal mass and localized renal cancer: AUA guideline. J Urol 2017; 198: 520–9.

17 Managing T1a renal cell carcinoma in von Hippel–Lindau syndrome: the interventional oncology approach

Vinson Wai-Shun Chan, Tze Min Wah

Case history

Annual screening in 2008 of a 53-year-old woman with a history of von Hippel–Lindau (VHL) syndrome revealed a new (*de novo*), small, right-sided renal mass. In 1988, she had received laser treatment for haemangioblastoma in her right eye. In 1989, she had had a partial nephrectomy for a right-sided renal cell carcinoma (RCC). Later that year, she had also had a right adrenalectomy for a renal adenoma. In 2004, she received image-guided radiofrequency ablation with a retrograde cold pyeloperfusion technique for a central RCC in the left kidney. Unfortunately, she experienced a ureteric stricture.

The *de novo* T1a RCC measured 11 mm (Figure 17.1) and was found to be in close proximity to the right pelvic–ureteric junction at the lower pole of the right kidney. Image-guided cryoablation under CT guidance was used under general anaesthesia with curative intent. Owing to the close proximity of the tumour to the

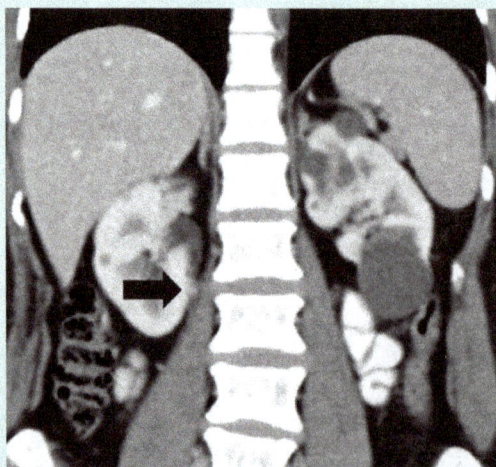

Figure 17.1   Coronal CT scan, performed prior to image-guided cryoablation, showing an 11 mm mass in close proximity to the right pelvic–ureteric junction and proximal ureter (arrow).

pelvic–ureteric junction, a retrograde ureteric stent was inserted on the advice of the urologists to protect the ureter; unfortunately, the patient still experienced a proximal ureteric stricture, managed long term by biannual retrograde ureteric stent replacement.

She manages well with the stents and had three further cryoablation treatments in the right kidney for *de novo* RCCs. To date, she is free of recurrence, metastasis and dialysis. Her stabilized estimated glomerular filtration rate is 38 ml/min per 1.73 m².

What is VHL syndrome and how does it affect the lifetime risk of RCC?

What is the evidence base for image-guided ablation compared with surgical resection (partial or radical nephrectomy) for T1a RCC?

What are the potential advantages of using image-guided ablation over surgical resection in patients with RCC associated with VHL syndrome?

What are the latest developments in interventional oncology for the treatment of small renal masses and how might they benefit people in the future?

What is VHL syndrome and how does it affect the lifetime risk of RCC?

VHL syndrome has an estimated incidence of between 1 in 27,000 and 1 in 43,000 live births.[1] It is characterized by a germline mutation on the short arm of chromosome 3 (cytoband 3p25-26), notably named the *VHL* gene.[2] People with VHL syndrome are at risk of both benign and malignant tumours, including phaeochromocytomas, neuroendocrine pancreatic tumours and haemangioblastomas of the central nervous system and retina.[3] Specifically, they are also at risk of multiple, recurring RCCs, ultimately leading often to death from metastatic RCC.[4] Two major phenotypes of VHL syndrome have been described, with further subdivisions of the second type[5]:

- type 1 is associated with development of all VHL syndrome-associated tumours except for phaeochromocytomas;
- type 2A is associated with a low risk of development of RCC;
- type 2B is associated with a high risk of development of RCC;
- type 2C is not associated with development of RCC but is characterized by haemangioblastomas and phaeochromocytomas.

The lifetime cumulative risk of individuals with VHL syndrome going on to develop RCC is around 24–45%, with a mean age at onset age of 37 years,[6,7] compared with less than 1% for the general population.[8]

What is the evidence base for image-guided ablation compared with surgical resection (partial or radical nephrectomy) for T1a RCC?

Historically, radical nephrectomy was the gold standard for management of small renal masses.[9] The development of partial nephrectomy (i.e. removal of only the disease-containing segment of the kidney) was originally advocated as a good alternative for those with bilateral masses, poor renal function or a high risk of developing subsequent tumours.

As techniques improved and complication rates fell, partial nephrectomy became the accepted gold standard, particularly for T1a lesions, owing to the improved preservation of renal function. Nephron preservation was postulated as the reason why, in some studies, those undergoing radical nephrectomy appeared to have a higher incidence of late cardiovascular complications and higher overall mortality.[10]

More recently, image-guided ablation was introduced as an alternative to surgical management owing to its perceived reduced invasiveness, reduced complications and improved preservation of renal function. Initially it was used in individuals who were not fit for surgery, but latterly its indications have expanded.[11]

Image-guided ablation has been hampered by a lack of head-to-head data. A review by the European Association of Urology Renal Cell Cancer Guideline Panel concluded that because of significant heterogeneity in the data, together with the limited number and quality of primary studies in the literature, it was impossible to draw reliable conclusions comparing partial nephrectomy with ablation.[12] The panel found that only nine retrospective studies had specifically compared image-guided ablation with partial nephrectomy. Only four of these had a sufficient sample size to allow for any meaningful comparison of oncological and perioperative outcomes between ablation and partial nephrectomy.

Historically, ablation has been reserved for older, frailer patients considered poor candidates for surgery, thus clouding the data. In a recent systematic review and meta-analysis comparing generic ablative therapies (including laparoscopic ablation) and partial nephrectomy in individuals with T1a RCC, the ablation groups were on average 5.7 years older and had more comorbidities and higher tumour complexity, suggesting some bias towards a partial nephrectomy population in the literature.[13] This inevitably leads to the poorer overall survival (OS) in the ablation group being attributed to selection bias. In spite of this, the potential for image-guided ablation to prove itself to be non-inferior to partial nephrectomy is suggested by the similar cancer-specific survival rates in both groups, with no differences in local recurrence-free or metastasis-free survival. The analysis suggested fewer complications and a smaller drop in renal function in those undergoing ablative therapies. This meta-analysis suggests an exciting trend towards non-inferiority of oncological ablative therapies, with the potential for reduced complication rates.

Two recent large single institution retrospective datasets directly compared partial nephrectomy and image-guided ablation.[14,15] The first, a single-centre retrospective analysis from the Mayo Clinic, probably represents the best direct comparison currently available.[14] The clinic reviewed the outcomes of patients who underwent partial nephrectomy (n=1055), radiofrequency ablation (n=180) or cryoablation (n=187) for T1a lesions. Median follow-up was 9.4 years for partial nephrectomy, 7.5 years for radiofrequency ablation and 6.3 years for cryoablation. Local recurrence-free survival, metastasis-free survival and cancer-specific survival were similar in all groups. OS was worse in the image-guided ablation groups compared with the partial nephrectomy group, which was attributed to the higher comorbidity scores and ages in the former. Complications and renal function outcomes were not reported.

The second study was a retrospective series from Leeds that compared the outcomes of patients who had undergone image-guided cryoablation (n=103), radiofrequency ablation (n=100) or laparoscopic partial nephrectomy (n=93).[15] The results showed similar oncological outcomes (local recurrence-free survival, metastasis-free survival and cancer-specific survival) in the three groups. The number of postoperative complications was also similar in the three groups, at around 15%, reflecting mostly complications from general anaesthesia. Interestingly however, the image-guided ablation groups demonstrated a significantly lower drop in renal function: the median percentage fall was 2.2% in the radiofrequency ablation group, 3.4% in the cryoablation group and 9.4% in the partial nephrectomy group.

Overall, the current evidence base is of low quality because of significant selection bias, small sample sizes and mostly short follow-up periods. There have been attempts to rectify this with prospective trials, but to date these have been unable to recruit.[16,17]

The maturing retrospective datasets indicate a trend suggesting at least non-inferiority of image-guided ablation compared with partial nephrectomy because of similar oncological durability. When combined with a potentially better complication profile and the possibility of improved preservation of renal function, image-guided ablation has a potentially exciting future, but there remains a need for level 1 evidence.

What are the potential advantages of using image–guided ablation over surgical resection in patients with RCC associated with VHL syndrome?

RCC associated with VHL syndrome is linked to multiple *de novo* recurrent tumours. Repeated partial nephrectomy for recurrent RCC is prone to high complication rates and reduces renal function significantly over time.[18] The main challenge in managing patients with RCC associated with VHL syndrome is to balance both optimal oncological outcomes and long-term renal function. In a series of 51 tumours, repeated partial nephrectomy was associated with a major complication rate of almost 20%, and as many as 64.7% of patients received intraoperative transfusions.[18] Of the 47 patients included in the study, two (3.9%) required long-term dialysis at a median follow-up of 56 months.

By comparison, the largest published series for image-guided ablation comprised 54 tumours in 17 patients with VHL syndrome undergoing multimodal image-guided ablation.[2] Among the 50 treatment sessions, only one major complication (2%) was observed. No blood transfusions were required, and no patients required long-term dialysis at a median follow-up of 79 months. At 10 years, local recurrence-free survival was 97.87%, metastasis-free survival and cancer-specific survival were 100% and OS was 90%, suggesting that multimodal image-guided ablation achieves excellent oncological durability and preservation of renal function.

What are the latest developments in interventional oncology for the treatment of small renal masses and how might they benefit people in the future?

Multiple innovative technologies are being introduced for image-guided ablation of small RCCs. Microwave[19] and irreversible electroporation[20] are newer energy sources currently in practice. In the future, it is hoped that non-invasive technologies such as histotripsy, a non-thermal focused ultrasound technology, could further reduce the invasiveness if image-guided ablations improve oncological outcomes in small RCCs.[21]

Before new technologies are put to use, however, it is important to standardize and establish best current practice. Historically, some lesions have been treated on the basis of imaging criteria alone, further clouding the data. One key to standardization will be confirming malignancy prior to treatment using renal tumour biopsy, which will both guide treatment and provide robust data.[22,23]

The (albeit limited) studies discussed introduce enough doubt as to what is truly the best strategy for small renal masses to warrant pursuing difficult to perform randomized controlled trials comparing surveillance, surgery and ablation. It is hoped that the highly anticipated results of the NEST feasibility study (Nephron-Sparing Treatment for Small Renal Masses; ISRCTN18156881) will be the first step to achieving this.[24]

Conclusion and learning points

- VHL syndrome increases the lifetime risk of multiple *de novo* recurrent RCCs; clinicians must balance optimal oncological durability and renal function preservation with minimal invasiveness. Image-guided ablation has been proven to be safe and have good oncological durability and preservation of renal function in patients with VHL syndrome requiring repeated treatment sessions.

- The current evidence base for the use of image-guided ablation in VHL syndrome is limited by small sample sizes, short follow-up periods and difficulty in prospective recruitment.

- Retrospective evidence suggests that image-guided ablation has similar oncological durability compared with partial nephrectomy; however, complication rates and drop in renal function may be significantly lower with image-guided ablation compared with partial nephrectomy, suggesting potential non-inferiority of the former vs the latter.

- Ongoing research may establish image-guided ablation as an equivalent gold standard to partial nephrectomy for small RCCs, with new technologies down the line having the potential to further improve the outcomes of image-guided ablation for RCCs.

References

1 National Cancer Institute (updated 28 December 2022). Von Hippel–Lindau disease. Available from: www.cancer.gov/types/kidney/hp/renal-cell-carcinoma-genetics/vhl-syndrome (accessed 5 January 2023).

2 Chan VW, Lenton J, Smith J, et al. Multimodal image-guided ablation on management of renal cancer in von Hippel–Lindau syndrome patients from 2004 to 2021 at a specialist centre: a longitudinal observational study. Eur J Surg Oncol 2022; 48: 672–9.

3 Ng H, Chan VW-S, Cartledge J, et al. Iatrogenic ureteric stricture post image guided renal cryoablation in a patient with von Hippel–Lindau syndrome. Radiol Case Rep 2021; 16: 2057.

4 Duffey BG, Choyke PL, Glenn G, et al. The relationship between renal tumor size and metastases in patients with von Hippel–Lindau disease. J Urol 2004; 172: 63–5.

5 Zbar B, Kishida T, Chen F, et al. Germline mutations in the von Hippel–Lindau disease (VHL) gene in families from North America, Europe, and Japan. Hum Mutat 1996; 8: 348–57.

6 Lonser RR, Glenn GM, Walther M, et al. von Hippel–Lindau disease. Lancet 2003; 361: 2059–67.

7 Choyke PL, Glenn GM, Walther MM, et al. von Hippel–Lindau disease: genetic, clinical, and imaging features. Radiology 1995; 194: 629–42.

8 Padala SA, Barsouk A, Thandra KC, et al. Epidemiology of renal cell carcinoma. World J Oncol 2020; 11: 79–87.

9 Manikandan R, Srinivasan V, Rané A. Which is the real gold standard for small-volume renal tumors? Radical nephrectomy versus nephron-sparing surgery. J Endourol 2004; 18: 39–44.

10 Huang WC, Elkin EB, Levey AS, et al. Partial nephrectomy versus radical nephrectomy in patients with small renal tumors – is there a difference in mortality and cardiovascular outcomes? J Urol 2009; 181: 55–61.

11 Wah TM, Irving HC, Gregory W, et al. Radiofrequency ablation (RFA) of renal cell carcinoma (RCC): experience in 200 tumours. BJU Int 2014; 113: 416–28.

12 Abu-Ghanem Y, Fernández-Pello S, Bex A, et al. Limitations of available studies prevent reliable comparison between tumour ablation and partial nephrectomy for patients with localised renal masses: a systematic review from the European Association of Urology Renal Cell Cancer Guideline Panel. Eur Urol Oncol 2020; 3: 433–52.

13 Chan VW-S, Abul A, Osman FH, et al. Ablative therapies versus partial nephrectomy for small renal masses – a systematic review and meta-analysis. Int J Surg 2022; 97: 106194.

14 Andrews JR, Atwell T, Schmit G, et al. Oncologic outcomes following partial nephrectomy and percutaneous ablation for cT1 renal masses. Eur Urol 2019; 76: 244–51.

15 Chan VW-S, Osman FH, Cartledge J, et al. Long-term outcomes of image-guided ablation and laparoscopic partial nephrectomy for T1 renal cell carcinoma. Eur Radiol 2022; 32: 5811–20.

16 Soomro N, Lecouturier J, Stocken DD, et al. Surveillance versus ablation for incidentally diagnosed small renal tumours: the SURAB feasibility RCT. Health Technol Assess 2017; 21: 1–68.

17 Lee CT, Katz J, Fearn PA, Russo P. Mode of presentation of renal cell carcinoma provides prognostic information. Urol Oncol 2002; 7: 135–40.

18 Johnson A, Sudarshan S, Liu J, et al. Feasibility and outcomes of repeat partial nephrectomy. J Urol 2008; 180: 89–93.

19 Cornelis FH, Marcelin C, Bernhard JC. Microwave ablation of renal tumors: a narrative review of technical considerations and clinical results. Diagn Interv Imaging 2017; 98: 287–97.

20 Wah TM, Lenton J, Smith J, et al. Irreversible electroporation (IRE) in renal cell carcinoma (RCC): a mid-term clinical experience. Eur Radiol 2021; 31: 7491–9.

21 Knott EA, Swietlik JF, Longo KC, et al. Robotically-assisted sonic therapy for renal ablation in a live porcine model: initial preclinical results. J Vasc Interv Radiol 2019; 30: 1293–302.

22 Chan VW, Keeley FX Jr, Lagerveld B, et al. The changing trends of image-guided biopsy of small renal masses before intervention – an analysis of European multinational prospective EuRECA registry. Eur Radiol 2022; 32: 4667–78.

23 Chan VW-S, Tan WS, Leow JJ, et al. Delayed surgery for localised and metastatic renal cell carcinoma: a systematic review and meta-analysis for the COVID-19 pandemic. World J Urol 2021; 39: 4295–303.

24 Neves JB, Cullen D, Grant L, Walkden M, et al. Protocol for a feasibility study of a cohort embedded randomised controlled trial comparing nephron sparing treatment (NEST) for small renal masses. BMJ Open 2019; 9: e030965.

18 A 5.5 cm incidental renal mass: balancing the risks

Amy Greenwood, Guy Hickson

Case history

A 60-year-old woman was found to have an incidental 5.5 cm left renal lesion on CT colonoscopy. At presentation she had well-controlled type 2 diabetes, with a baseline estimated glomerular filtration rate of 50 ml/min per 1.73 m² and an even split of function between her kidneys on dimercaptosuccinic acid scan. In addition to working full time, she helped to care for her elderly parents. Her brother developed renal failure requiring dialysis in his early 50s. Biopsy confirmed renal cell carcinoma (RCC).

The woman's case was reviewed at the renal cancer multidisciplinary team (MDT) meeting; the lesion was deemed technically unsuitable for a partial nephrectomy but she would be fit for nephrectomy.

During a subsequent consultation she expressed her concerns about major surgery, in terms of recovery time, its implications for the care of her parents and also her anxiety about the possibility of needing dialysis in the future. The risk of needing dialysis after surgery was estimated to be approximately 50%. She was reluctant to pursue surgical resection given the risks and recovery time.

Is there a role for surveillance in an individual with a T1b RCC?

Is there any evidence supporting the use of thermo-ablative treatments in T1b RCC?

In what circumstances would thermo-ablative therapy be considered?

Is there a role for surveillance in an individual with a T1b RCC?

A small proportion of small renal cancers will progress to metastases. Tumours which demonstrate rapid growth are at higher risk of systemic disease.[1] Surveillance is a reasonable option for older people and those at high risk for intervention. If the person were to develop metastatic disease within the surveillance window, however, treatment options would be less likely to be curative. The risk of disease progression while undergoing active surveillance should be understood by the patient. At a size of 5.5 cm the statistical likelihood of metastasis is approximately 2%.[1] While this woman could elect for active surveillance, treatment would be recommended to maximize the likelihood of cancer-free survival.

Is there any evidence supporting the use of thermo-ablative treatments in T1b RCC?

Current NICE guidance recommends a maximum renal tumour size of approximately 4 cm for percutaneous ablative therapies, while noting they have been successfully used in larger tumours.[2,3]

Based on the presentation scan, this woman had stage T1b disease. In the absence of a surgical resection, histology is limited to that obtained at pretreatment biopsy. Heterogeneity within the tumour may therefore result in biopsy results that may not reflect the complete lesion; for example, some areas of the tumour may potentially have higher grade features that could be missed on focal biopsy. As this makes it difficult to risk stratify lesions on the basis of a biopsy, surrogate measures must be used to risk stratify into treatment options.

The malignant potential of renal tumours increases with their size. For this reason, surgery is still considered to be the gold standard for T1b lesions: it ensures confirmed surgical margins and allows risk stratification for follow-up with complete histology. As in this case, however, the risks of surgery are sometimes increased, making it reasonable to consider other options.

The evidence for ablative cure being achieved in T1a lesions is reasonably solid (though possibly partly due to the higher incidence of lower grade tumours in this patient population); however, there is emerging evidence that T1b lesions can also be treated successfully.[4,5] In a study reviewing outcomes of microwave ablation and partial or radical nephrectomy for T1b disease, there was no difference in 5 year metastasis-free survival or cancer-specific survival, although comorbidity scores in the ablation group were higher than in the surgical groups, so overall survival (OS) was lower (attributed to death from other causes). Length of stay for ablation was shorter compared with surgery.[6]

Further studies demonstrate 5 year local recurrence and metastasis-free survival rates similar to those associated with partial nephrectomy; differences in OS are likely due to selection bias (partial nephrectomy cohorts being younger with lower comorbidity scores).[4] One study focusing on outcomes of cryoablation for T1 disease found both 5 year local recurrence and metastasis-free survival to be in the region of 94%.[7] In this study, no significant difference was found between the treated T1a and T1b lesions.

Renal function is better preserved with either partial nephrectomy or tumour ablation; larger drops in renal function are observed with radical nephrectomy, carrying with it a higher risk of endstage renal failure.[8] It might therefore be reasonable to consider ablation in cases where this risk is higher than normal and where partial nephrectomy is not an option or is considered high risk.

Residual or recurrent disease is a risk with ablative technologies and it increases with the size of the tumour. The risk appears to be lower with cryoablation compared with radiofrequency ablation, with some retrospective analyses suggesting that longer term oncological outcomes such as cancer-specific survival are equal to those with partial nephrectomy.[4-7,9] The patient would need to acknowledge and accept the need for careful follow-up and potentially repeated procedures.[9] It should also be noted that pursuing ablation in the first instance would not preclude radical nephrectomy at a later date.

In what circumstances would thermo-ablative therapy be considered?

Thermo-ablative therapy could be considered for this woman, given that she has T1b disease that is not suitable for partial nephrectomy and for whom radical nephrectomy would pose a higher risk of endstage renal failure – something which she is keen to avoid.[5] The evidence for ablation of T1b lesions from the Mayo clinic group only included cryoablation, presumably as it offers larger single treatment ablation zones in comparison with radiofrequency and microwave ablation.[4]

There needs to be careful discussion regarding the risks of residual or recurrent local disease requiring further treatment, either via further ablation or surgical resection. However, the risks of repeat procedures remain low even in T1b lesions[10] and the potential life-shortening consequences of renal replacement therapy[11] need to be carefully included in the consent process. The patient should be offered all available options, even if it means referral to another unit.

Conclusion and learning points

- Surgery is still considered the gold standard for treatment of T1b lesions; however, there may be cases where the risks of surgery outweigh the potential small downsides of ablation. For larger lesions, cryotherapy is the preferred method of ablation.

- Ablation of T1b lesions can be an effective and curative treatment; however, as it currently falls outside NICE guidelines, a careful analysis of the risks and benefits should be undertaken, in both the MDT setting and in subsequent consultation with the patient, and documented in the consent process.

- Further evidence is required to clarify these grey areas; as such, careful audit should be undertaken of ablations performed for T1b lesions.

References

1 Smaldone MC, Kutikov A, Egleston BL, et al. Small renal masses progressing to metastases under active surveillance: a systematic review and pooled analysis. Cancer 2012; 118: 997–1006.

2 NICE (2011). Percutaneous cryotherapy for renal cancer. Interventional procedures guidance IPG402. Available from: www.nice.org.uk/Guidance/IPG402 (accessed 16 December 2022).

3 NICE (2010). Percutaneous radiofrequency ablation for renal cancer. Interventional procedures guidance IPG353. Available from: www.nice.org.uk/guidance/ipg353 (accessed 16 December 2022).

4 Thompson RH, Atwell T, Schmit G, et al. Comparison of partial nephrectomy and percutaneous ablation for cT1 renal masses. Eur Urol 2015; 67: 252–9.

5 Georgiades CS, Rodriguez R. Efficacy and safety of percutaneous cryoablation for stage 1A/B renal cell carcinoma: results of a prospective, single-arm, 5-year study. Cardiovasc Intervent Radiol 2014; 37: 1494–9.

6 Shapiro DD, Wells SA, Best SL, et al. Comparing outcomes for patients with clinical T1b renal cell carcinoma treated with either percutaneous microwave ablation or surgery. J Urol 2020; 135: 88–94.

7 Breen DJ, King AJ, Patel N, et al. Image-guided cryoablation for sporadic renal cell carcinoma: three- and 5-year outcomes in 220 patients with biopsy-proven renal cell carcinoma. Radiology 2018; 289: 554–61.

8 Patel HD, Pierorazio PM, Johnson MH, et al. Renal functional outcomes after surgery ablation and active surveillance of localized renal tumors: a systematic review and meta-analysis. Clin J Am Soc Nephrol 2017; 12: 1057–69.

9 Kunkle DA, Uzzo RG. Cryoablation or radiofrequency ablation of the small renal mass: a meta-analysis. Cancer 2008; 113: 2671–80.

10 Wessendorf J, König A, Heers H, et al. Repeat percutaneous radiofrequency ablation of T1 renal cell carcinomas is safe in patients with von Hippel–Lindau disease. Cardiovasc Intervent Radiol 2021; 44: 2022–5.

11 Hemke AC, Heemskerk MB, van Diepen M, et al. Survival prognosis after the start of a renal replacement therapy in the Netherlands: a retrospective cohort study. BMC Nephrol 2013; 14: 258.

19 A fit 65 year old with a 7 cm renal tumour

Rebecca Smith, Jeremy Nettleton

Case history

A 65-year-old man was referred by his GP to the 2 week wait haematuria clinic with a 1 month history of unexplained persistent macroscopic haematuria without dysuria or lower urinary tract symptoms. His medical history included hypertension and obesity; there was no family history of renal cancer. He was an ex-smoker but was otherwise fit and had a performance status of 1. Urinalysis was positive for blood only; blood tests showed mild anaemia and a normal estimated glomerular filtration rate. Flexible cystoscopy did not reveal a lower tract tumour or any prostatic pathology.

A triple-phase renal CT scan showed a left-sided, enhancing, solid, 7 cm, exophytic, lower pole tumour confined to the kidney. No other abnormality of the renal tract was identified. A staging CT scan of the chest showed no evidence of metastatic disease. The urology multidisciplinary team (MDT) recommended a left partial nephrectomy for a T1bN0M0 renal mass.

Surgery was performed as a robot-assisted laparoscopic procedure without complication. The man's postoperative recovery was unremarkable and he was discharged from hospital after 3 days. Histology confirmed a clear cell T1N0M0 renal cell carcinoma (RCC) with clear resection margins; the results were discussed with him in clinic 6 weeks postoperatively. Aside from a small, asymptomatic incisional hernia, no complications were identified.

As he was deemed to be at intermediate risk of recurrence his surveillance schedule consisted of a CT scan of the chest, abdomen and pelvis every 6 months for a year, annually for the following 2 years, and then once every 2 years thereafter. His renal function remains normal and there has been no evidence of recurrence or distant metastases.

What are the surgical management options?

What are the considerations for partial nephrectomy vs radical nephrectomy?

Which surgical techniques may be used?

What follow-up is required?

What are the surgical management options?

Surgery should be offered with curative intent if the patient has a localized cancer and is fit for surgery. Biopsy was not recommended in this case as the radiological findings (i.e. a large, solid, contrast-enhancing tumour) were highly suspicious for an RCC. Counselling should be provided on the risk of benign histology following nephrectomy (e.g. renal oncocytoma, which represents 3–7% of all solid renal tumours).[1]

What are the considerations for partial nephrectomy vs radical nephrectomy?

Partial nephrectomy is synonymous with nephron-sparing surgery, whereas radical nephrectomy involves removal of the entire kidney, the surrounding fat and lymph nodes, as well as the upper part of the ureter. Both options, regardless of the technique used, demonstrate oncological equivalence in terms of overall survival.[2] Compared with radical nephrectomy, partial nephrectomy results in better preservation of renal function and reduction in the long-term incidence of cardiovascular and metabolic disease and morbidity, but it has a slightly higher rate of complications such as perioperative bleeding and postoperative urinary fistulae.[3]

As well as patient choice and fitness for surgery, decision making regarding appropriate surgical management involves the following considerations.

What is technically feasible?

- Tumour stage: the larger the tumour, the more difficult it is to perform partial nephrectomy safely and effectively. The European Association of Urology guidelines recommend that partial nephrectomy should be offered to all patients with T1 tumours, and may be considered in patients with T2 tumours with a solitary kidney or chronic kidney disease.[4]

- Tumour location: partial nephrectomy is more technically challenging for centrally located or endophytic tumours compared with peripheral or exophytic tumours.

Is preservation of renal function essential or desirable?

- Bilateral renal tumours or solitary kidney: this is an absolute indication for partial nephrectomy, as radical nephrectomy would render the patient anephric.

- Chronic kidney disease: partial nephrectomy should be offered to individuals who are at risk of developing endstage renal failure following radical nephrectomy, which would necessitate postoperative renal replacement therapy. Renal scintigraphy (e.g. dimercaptosuccinic acid [DMSA] scan) is recommended in patients with a reduction in estimated glomerular filtration rate, to assess split renal function prior to surgical intervention.

As our patient had a T1 tumour in a favourable anatomical location, he was offered a partial nephrectomy. Normal renal function and anatomy meant that a preoperative DMSA scan was not required. Other associated procedures, such as ipsilateral adrenalectomy and extended lymph node dissection, are not routinely performed unless clinically indicated (e.g. evidence of invasion on preoperative imaging or as an intraoperative finding).[5,6] There is no benefit of tumour embolization prior to routine nephrectomy.[7]

Which surgical techniques may be used?

Both radical nephrectomy and partial nephrectomy may be performed using an open, laparoscopic or robot-assisted technique. The surgical approach for these techniques may be either transperitoneal or retroperitoneal; the choice of approach depends on surgeon experience and patient factors, as there is no significant difference in clinical outcome between the two. Laparoscopic or robot-assisted nephrectomy is a minimally invasive technique which results in lower overall morbidity as well as a shorter hospital stay and convalescence, but it has a longer operation time compared with open nephrectomy. Oncological outcomes for T1–T2a tumours are similar regardless of surgical technique.[8] In light of this, the European Association of Urology recommends the following:

- The indications for partial nephrectomy supersede those for a minimally invasive radical nephrectomy, i.e. a patient with a T1 tumour should be offered a partial nephrectomy using any feasible technique, rather than a radical nephrectomy using a minimally invasive technique.
- A minimally invasive radical nephrectomy should be offered to patients with T2 tumours if partial nephrectomy is not feasible.
- A minimally invasive technique must not be offered if it may compromise oncological, functional or perioperative outcomes.

There is no clear evidence of one technique or approach being superior to another. Selection of an appropriate technique depends on tumour factors (e.g. size, location, relationship to surrounding organs), patient factors (e.g. comorbidities, previous surgery, preference), surgeon factors (e.g. expertise) and health service factors (e.g. facilities, staff, funding).

What follow-up is required?

The purpose of surveillance after treatment for localized RCC is to identify postoperative complications, diagnose disease recurrence and limit possible long-term sequelae such as cardiovascular events and renal impairment. There is currently no evidence-based standard surveillance schedule; however, most centres will follow patients up using regular cross-sectional imaging postoperatively for at least 5 years. The timing of surveillance imaging depends on a patient's risk of recurrence, which can be determined using validated prognostic models such as the Leibovich score.[9] There is no consensus on the optimal length of follow-up, but it may be decided based on risk of recurrence, cost-effectiveness and survival benefit of ongoing surveillance. A proposed surveillance schedule suggested by the European Association of Urology is presented in Table 19.1.

Surveillance renal and chest CT allows for the detection of local recurrence, contralateral kidney recurrence and distant metastases. Targeted imaging may be considered in patients with organ-specific symptoms (e.g. CT scan of the brain in patients with new-onset focal neurology). Chest radiography is less sensitive than CT in detecting metastases, and PET-CT is not routinely recommended. Patients who develop recurrence may be considered for further surgery, ablative or systemic therapy, and their case should be discussed again by the MDT.

Table 19.1 Proposed follow-up schedule following treatment for localized RCC (adapted from Ljungberg et al.[9]).

Risk profile	Oncological follow-up after date of surgery								
	3 months	6 months	12 months	18 months	24 months	30 months	36 months	>3 years	>5 years
Low	–	CT	–	CT	–	CT	–	CT once every 2 years	–
Intermediate	–	CT	CT	–	CT	–	CT	CT once a year	CT once every 2 years
High	CT	CT	CT	CT	CT	–	CT	CT once a year	CT once every 2 years

Conclusion and learning points

- Localized renal cancer should be surgically treated with curative intent if the patient is fit for surgery and has non-metastatic disease.
- All patients with T1 tumours should be offered partial nephrectomy, if feasible, using any surgical technique.
- Minimally invasive nephrectomy, which includes laparoscopic and robot-assisted surgery, results in quicker recovery and lower postoperative morbidity, with no difference in oncological outcome compared with open nephrectomy.
- Follow-up should consist of regular CT scans of the chest, abdomen and pelvis. The frequency, timing and length of follow-up depend on the risk of disease recurrence, likely survival benefit and cost-effectiveness of surveillance.

References

1 Williams GM, Lynch DT. Renal oncocytoma. Treasure Island, FL: StatPearls Publishing, 2022.

2 Kunath F, Schmidt S, Krabbe LM, et al. Partial nephrectomy versus radical nephrectomy for clinical localized renal masses. Cochrane Database Syst Rev 2017; 5: CD012045.

3 Van Poppel H, Da Pozzo L, Albrecht W, et al. A prospective randomized EORTC intergroup phase 3 study comparing the complications of elective nephron-sparing surgery and radical nephrectomy for low-stage renal cell carcinoma. Eur Urol 2007; 51: 1606–15.

4 Ljungberg B, Albiges L, Bedke J, et al. (2022). EAU guidelines on renal cell carcinoma. Available from: https://d56bochluxqnz.cloudfront.net/documents/full-guideline/EAU-Guidelines-on-Renal-Cell-Carinoma-2022.pdf (accessed 15 April 2022).

5 Lane BR, Tiong HY, Campbell SC, et al. Management of the adrenal gland during partial nephrectomy. J Urol 2009; 181: 2430–7.

6 Capitanio U, Becker F, Blute ML, et al. Lymph node dissection in renal cell carcinoma. Eur Urol 2011; 60: 1212–20.

7 May M, Brookman-Amissah S, Pflanz S, et al. Pre-operative renal arterial embolisation does not provide survival benefit in patients with radical nephrectomy for renal cell carcinoma. Br J Radiol 2009; 82: 724–31.

8 MacLennan S, Imamura M, Lapitan MC, et al. Systematic review of perioperative and quality-of-life outcomes following surgical management of localized renal cancer. Eur Urol 2012; 62: 1097–117.

9 Leibovich BC, Blute ML, Cheville JC, et al. Prediction of progression after radical nephrectomy for patients with clear cell renal cell carcinoma: a stratification tool for prospective clinical trials. Cancer 2003; 97: 1663–71.

20 Metastatic renal cancer and its management options

Henry Delacave, Faith McMeekin

Case history

A 74-year-old man presented to his GP with fatigue, leg pain and weight loss. He was an ex-smoker and had a background of hypertension and osteoarthritis. His Karnofsky performance status was 80%.[1] A urine test at the GP surgery demonstrated non-visible haematuria and he was referred to urology under the 2 week wait rule.

At the one-stop fast track urology clinic, blood tests showed C-reactive protein (CRP) 43 mg/l and haemoglobin 115 g/l; flexible cystoscopy was normal. Renal tract ultrasound revealed a significant mass in the right kidney. The urologist explained to the man the probability of malignancy and that further investigations were required. A CT scan of the chest was done and contrast renal CT performed with a urographic phase. Given the bony pain, a bone scan was also done. These investigations showed a large (8 cm) mass in the right kidney which was avid on the arterial phase, as well as evidence of metastases in the left femoral shaft and a nodule in the lung, suspicious for a further metastasis.

The man's case was discussed at the specialist multidisciplinary team meeting. Given his intermediate-risk profile (as measured by the presence of metastases and symptoms consistent with cancer), it was decided that the priority should be to start systemic therapy after a renal biopsy, with possible consideration of cytoreductive nephrectomy in the future. His histology was consistent with clear cell renal cell carcinoma (RCC), the commonest histological subtype in RCCs.

The man returned to clinic anxious about his diagnosis: his friend had died of a similar metastatic RCC 10 years ago, only 6 months after diagnosis. It was explained that while his cancer was incurable, there have been significant advances in the treatment of metastatic RCC over the last 15 years and his best option was to start treatment with an immune checkpoint inhibitor (ICPI) plus a tyrosine kinase inhibitor (TKI), neither of which were available for his friend. Nivolumab/cabozantinib was chosen. A few months later, he experienced redness and swelling of his hands and feet. He was diagnosed with palmar–plantar erythrodysaesthesia, which was successfully treated with a short course of glucocorticoids.

At 1 year follow-up, the patient's tumour had decreased by 30% in size and there was no evidence of further metastases. He was offered cytoreductive nephrectomy but considered the risks too high and opted to continue with immunotherapy. At 2 year follow-up, scans showed progression in the number and size of metastases accompanied by a rise in CRP; sunitinib was therefore chosen as second-line therapy.

At 3 year follow-up, scans showed further progression. Because of his poor quality of life and the adverse effects of systemic therapy, the patient opted for palliation.

How should RCCs be investigated initially?

What risk calculators are available to help prognosticate and counsel this patient?

What is the evidence base for his treatment options?

Is there any evidence to support cytoreductive nephrectomy?

How should his metastases be managed?

How should RCCs be investigated initially?

Over 50% of RCCs are detected incidentally when investigating other pathologies such as abdominal pain and non-specific symptoms.[2] As a result, a large proportion of patients have already undergone a contrast-enhanced CT scan of their abdomen and pelvis by the time they reach urology. The radiological findings may or may not be enough to fully characterize the renal pathology and in many cases a further CT scan with arterial and urographic phases may need to be carried out, either to help surgical planning or to clarify the pathology. In addition, a CT scan of the thorax should be carried out to check for lung metastases.

In cases where CT is contraindicated (i.e. pregnancy or contrast allergy), MRI can provide similar information, albeit at a higher resource cost. MRI may also provide additional information on venous thrombus extent and can delineate renal cysts with greater sensitivity compared with contrast-enhanced CT.[3]

In the present case, the patient had had no previous imaging and was investigated for haematuria with cystoscopy and upper tract imaging (ultrasound scan), which prompted further investigations. As he was also suffering from bone pain, he underwent a bone scan. Asymptomatic patients do not, however, need to be screened for bone or brain metastases.[4,5] PET-CT is not currently recommended in the investigation of metastatic RCC, owing to the lack of appropriate biomarkers.[6]

Patients who have metastases but are fit enough to be treated should undergo a coaxial renal biopsy of the solid component of the tumour, avoiding areas of fluid or central necrosis to assess histological subtype (accuracy is around 90%) and allow planning of systemic therapy. It should be a core biopsy, rather than fine needle aspiration, and for large tumours (>T2) the practitioner should aim to sample at least four separately enhancing areas.[7,8] Finally, in young patients (<46 years) or in those with a strong family history of RCC, a referral for genetic assessment should be made.[9]

What risk calculators are available to help prognosticate and counsel this patient?

Two prognostic models have been validated in the metastatic RCC population. These are the Memorial Sloan Kettering Cancer Center model[10] and the International Metastatic Renal Cell Carcinoma Database Consortium model.[11] The latter has featured in recent trials and is therefore useful in advising patients and prognosticating. The model uses six variables, although the addition of a seventh has been suggested.[12] The presence of no factors indicates favourable-risk disease; one or two factors indicates intermediate-risk disease; three or more factors indicates poor-risk disease:

- Karnofsky performance status <80%;
- interval from diagnosis to treatment <1 year;

- haemoglobin below the lower limit of normal;
- corrected calcium level above the upper limit of normal;
- neutrophil count above the upper limit of normal;
- platelet count above the upper limit of normal;
- presence of bone, brain or liver metastases (possible seventh variable).

Our patient scored for his haemoglobin and for the interval between diagnosis and initiation of treatment. He could also have scored for his metastases if this variable were included. He therefore had at least intermediate-risk disease, if not poor-risk disease. The relative risk of disease can be reflected in the prognosis and, until recently, median survival values had been ascribed to each risk profile. However, given the array of new therapies available (see below), those values are now being recalculated.

What is the evidence base for his treatment options?

Over the last 15 years, the treatment of metastatic RCCs has dramatically shifted. We now know that inactivation of the *VHL* gene is common in clear cell RCCs and that it leads to build-up of hypoxia-inducible factor and subsequent upregulation of vascular endothelial growth factor (VEGF) – key in the progression and pathogenesis of RCCs. In the late 2000s, targeted TKIs aimed at inhibiting VEGF demonstrated overall survival (OS) and progression-free survival (PFS) benefit when compared with placebo or interferon-alpha. Specifically, a strong body of evidence supports the use of sunitinib in metastatic RCCs.[13] Other anti-VEGF TKIs include sorafenib, pazopanib, axitinib, cabozantinib, lenvatinib and tivozanib. Classes of drugs such as monoclonal VEGF antibodies and mechanistic target of rapamycin (mTOR) inhibitors are no longer used first line because there are more attractive alternatives, but they may be considered as second- or third-line treatments.

Over the last 5 years, ICPIs have come to the fore and, although none have demonstrated an OS or PFS benefit as monotherapy, many have shown benefit in combination with TKIs. ICPIs are monoclonal antibodies that help to reverse tumour-induced immunosuppression by inhibiting immune checkpoints, e.g. programmed cell death protein 1 (PD-1) and cytotoxic T lymphocyte-associated protein 4 (CTLA-4).

CheckMate 214,[14] CheckMate 9ER,[15] JAVELIN Renal 101,[16] CLEAR[17] and Keynote-426[18] are key trials. All these trials have shown superiority of an ICPI+TKI when compared with sunitinib alone and their results represent a paradigm shift in the treatment of metastatic RCCs. Updates and further analyses are still in the process of being published but there are enough data surrounding OS and PFS benefits that they have been unilaterally recommended as first-line treatments for metastatic RCC in the recent update to the European Association of Urology guidelines.[19] In addition, all trials seem to show a small (~10%) proportion of complete response, which brings much hope to patients. Given this rapid change in treatment, second-line therapies and pathways are still very much in flux and should be determined at an experienced centre.

In short, the current evidence demonstrates significant benefit of combination therapies (ICPI+TKI or ICPI+ICPI) and, although the depth of research continues to develop, patients should now be started on combination therapies as first line.

Is there any evidence to support cytoreductive nephrectomy?

The beneficial evidence for cytoreductive nephrectomy was gathered nearly 20 years ago in the age of interferon-based therapies[20] and yet it remains a part of the treatment pathway of metastatic

RCC in many centres despite a relative paucity of evidence with targeted therapies. Two large randomized controlled trials – CARMENA (ClinicalTrials.gov NCT00930033) and SURTIME (ClinicalTrials.gov NCT01099423) – aimed to rectify this. The CARMENA trial showed that sunitinib alone was not inferior to cytoreductive nephrectomy followed by sunitinib.[21] Similarly, the SURTIME trial demonstrated that the timing of cytoreductive nephrectomy pre- or post-sunitinib did not change PFS.[22] These results raised questions about the role of cytoreductive nephrectomy in the context of metastatic RCC. However, a secondary endpoint was reached in the SURTIME trial, which showed an OS benefit in patients who had cytoreductive nephrectomy after systemic therapy, rather than before, and when combined with other retrospective studies also showed OS benefit of upfront cytoreductive nephrectomy.[22] The use of cytoreductive nephrectomy in metastatic RCC continues to be debated.

The inconclusive evidence makes it difficult for healthcare practitioners to know whether their patient would benefit from cytoreductive nephrectomy; this is especially true for patients in the intermediate-risk group. Further trials assessing cytoreductive nephrectomy using ICPIs+TKIs are eagerly awaited: the NORDIC-SUN trial (ClinicalTrials.gov NCT03977571) and the PROBE trial (ClinicalTrials.gov NCT04510597). Nevertheless, there appears still to be a role for cytoreductive nephrectomy in two groups of patients. First, in those at intermediate risk who have responded well to systemic therapy (or at least not progressed); and, second, in those with favourable-risk profiles who do not require immediate systemic therapy.[23] In the current climate of ICPIs, it is important to remember that cytoreductive nephrectomy should not delay the initiation of systemic therapy, nor should it be performed in those with poor-risk disease or a prognosis <12 months. This is reflected in the most recent European Association of Urology RCC guidelines.[24–26]

As our patient had symptomatic metastatic RCC it was treated with systemic therapy at the point of diagnosis. He could have been considered for cytoreductive nephrectomy later, depending on his response.

How should his metastases be managed?

Historically, surgical removal of the primary tumour and of the metastatic deposits was seen to be the only way to render a patient disease-free. This adage was backed up by a systematic review which consistently demonstrated improved OS and PFS in patients who underwent complete metastasectomy compared with those who had incomplete metastasectomy or no metastasectomy at all.[27] However, the evidence base for the review was retrospective and non-randomized in nature, using small numbers of patients, which resulted in a high risk of bias. Therefore, while there may indeed be a benefit associated with metastasectomy, further trials must be carried out before it can be recommended. Certainly, the evidence is much weaker than the evidence for systemic therapy. In patients where there is an intention to treat (such as in our patient), systemic therapy should be prioritized. There is also an argument for active surveillance of patients without starting them on systemic therapy at all. This seems to be most appropriate course in patients with favourable-risk disease and only one or two metastatic deposits.[28]

Alternatively, ablative therapy can help with control of local symptoms. This can be achieved through a variety of modalities such as embolization, metastasectomy, cryotherapy, microwave or radiofrequency ablation and radiotherapy. As our patient had a metastatic deposit in his femur, pain secondary to this deposit could either be managed by metastasectomy/curettage or by image-guided radiotherapy.[29]

Conclusion and learning points

- Patients who presented with metastatic RCC 20 years ago could expect a short lifespan and a range of surgical interventions.

- In patients who present with metastatic RCC now the outlook is much more positive owing to the advent of ICPIs and their use in combination with TKIs, which has transformed the management of metastatic RCCs.

- There remain several uncertainties in the treatment pathway, specifically over the use of metastasectomy, cytoreductive nephrectomy and the most appropriate second-line therapies. Further trials are underway to help guide management. Nevertheless, there appears to be a place for surgical intervention, but surgery should be reserved for a carefully selected and informed patient group.

References

1 Schag CC, Heinrich RL, Ganz PA. Karnofsky performance status revisited: reliability, validity, and guidelines. J Clin Oncol 1984; 2: 187–93.

2 Jayson M, Sanders H. Increased incidence of serendipitously discovered renal cell carcinoma. Urology 1998; 51: 203–5.

3 Defortescu G, Cornu JN, Ejar SB, et al. Diagnostic performance of contrast-enhanced ultrasonography and magnetic resonance imaging for the assessment of complex renal cysts: a prospective study. Int J Urol 2017; 24: 184–9.

4 Marshall ME, Pearson T, Simpson W, et al. Low incidence of asymptomatic brain metastases in patients with renal cell carcinoma. Urology 1990; 36: 300–2.

5 Koga S, Tsuda S, Nishikido M, et al. The diagnostic value of bone scan in patients with renal cell carcinoma. J Urol 2001; 166: 2126–8.

6 Vig SVL, Zan E, Kang SK. Imaging for metastatic renal cell carcinoma. Urol Clin North Am 2020; 47: 281–91.

7 Marconi L, Dabestani S, Lam TB, et al. Systematic review and meta-analysis of diagnostic accuracy of percutaneous renal tumour biopsy. Eur Urol 2016; 69: 660–73.

8 Abel EJ, Heckman JE, Hinshaw L, et al. Multi-quadrant biopsy technique improves diagnostic ability in large heterogeneous renal masses. J Urol 2015; 194: 886–91.

9 Shuch B, Vourganti S, Ricketts CJ, et al. Defining early-onset kidney cancer: implications for germline and somatic mutation testing and clinical management. J Clin Oncol 2014; 32: 431–7.

10 Sorbellini M, Kattan M, Snyder M, et al. A postoperative prognostic nomogram predicting recurrence for patients with conventional clear cell renal cell carcinoma. J Urol 2005; 173; 48–51.

11 Heng DY, Xie W, Regan MM, et al. External validation and comparison with other models of the International Metastatic Renal Cell Carcinoma Database Consortium prognostic model: a population-based study. Lancet Oncol 2013; 14: 141–8.

12 Massari F, di Nunno V, Guida A, et al. Addition of primary metastatic site on bone, brain, and liver to IMDC criteria in patients with metastatic renal cell carcinoma: a validation study. Clin Genitourin Cancer 2021; 19: 32–40.

13 Motzer RJ, Hutson TE, Tomczak P, et al. Overall survival and updated results for sunitinib compared with interferon alfa in patients with metastatic renal cell carcinoma. J Clin Oncol 2009; 27: 3584–90.

14 Motzer RJ, Tannir NM, McDermott DF, et al. Nivolumab plus ipilimumab versus sunitinib in advanced renal-cell carcinoma. N Engl J Med 2018; 378: 1277–90.

15 Choueiri TK, Powles T, Burotto M, et al. Nivolumab plus cabozantinib versus sunitinib for advanced renal-cell carcinoma. N Engl J Med 2021; 384: 829–41.

16 Motzer RJ, Penkov K, Haanen J, et al. Avelumab plus axitinib versus sunitinib for advanced renal-cell carcinoma. N Engl J Med 2019; 380: 1103–15.

17 Motzer RJ, Porta C, Eto M, et al. Phase 3 trial of lenvatinib (LEN) plus pembrolizumab (PEMBRO) or everolimus (EVE) versus sunitinib (SUN) monotherapy as a first-line treatment for patients (pts) with advanced renal cell carcinoma (RCC) (CLEAR study). J Clin Oncol 2021; 39 (6 suppl): 269.

18 Rini BI, Plimack ER, Stus V, et al. Pembrolizumab plus axitinib versus sunitinib for advanced renal-cell carcinoma. N Engl J Med 2019; 380: 1116–27.

19 Bedke J, Albiges L, Capitanio U, et al. The 2021 updated European Association of Urology guidelines on renal cell carcinoma: immune checkpoint inhibitor-based combination therapies for treatment-naive metastatic clear-cell renal cell carcinoma are standard of care. Eur Urol 2021; 80: 393–7.

20 Flanigan RC, Mickisch G, Sylvester R, et al. Cytoreductive nephrectomy in patients with metastatic renal cancer: a combined analysis. J Urol 2004; 171: 1071–6.

21 Méjean A, Ravaud A, Thezenas S, Colas S, et al. Sunitinib alone or after nephrectomy in metastatic renal-cell carcinoma. N Engl J Med 2018; 379: 417–27.

22 Ljungberg B, Sundqvist P, Lindblad P, et al. Survival advantage of upfront cytoreductive nephrectomy in patients with primary metastatic renal cell carcinoma compared with systemic and palliative treatments in a real-world setting. Scand J Urol 2020; 54: 487–92.

23 Bhindi B, Abel EJ, Albiges L, et al. Systematic review of the role of cytoreductive nephrectomy in the targeted therapy era and beyond: an individualized approach to metastatic renal cell carcinoma. Eur Urol 2019; 75: 111–28.

24 Heng DYC, Wells JC, Rini BI, et al. Cytoreductive nephrectomy in patients with synchronous metastases from renal cell carcinoma: results from the International Metastatic Renal Cell Carcinoma Database Consortium. Eur Urol 2014; 66: 704–10.

25 Bex A, Albiges L, Ljungberg B, et al. Updated European Association of Urology guidelines for cytoreductive nephrectomy in patients with synchronous metastatic clear-cell renal cell carcinoma. Eur Urol 2018; 74: 805–9.

26 Ljungberg B, Albiges L, Abu-Ghanem Y, et al. European Association of Urology guidelines on renal cell carcinoma: the 2022 update. Eur Urol 2022; 82: 399–410.

27 Dabestani S, Marconi L, Hofmann F, et al. Local treatments for metastases of renal cell carcinoma: a systematic review. Lancet Oncol 2014; 15: e549–61.

28 Harrison MR, Costello BA, Bhavsar NA, et al. Active surveillance of metastatic renal cell carcinoma: results from a prospective observational study (MaRCC). Cancer 2021; 127: 2204–12.

29 Zelefsky MJ, Greco C, Motzer R, et al. Tumour control outcomes following hypofractionated and single-dose stereotactic image-guided intensity-modulated radiotherapy for extracranial metastases from renal cell carcinoma. Int J Radiat Oncol Biol Phys 2014; 82: 1744–8.

21 Management options in recurrent renal cell carcinoma

Caitlin Bowden, Marios P. Decatris

Case history

A 66-year-old man presented with recurrent urinary tract infections and ongoing microscopic haematuria. He reported no systemic symptoms such as weight loss. CT of the kidneys, ureter and bladder showed a 10 cm enhancing right upper pole renal tumour. Flexible cystoscopy showed no lower urinary tract pathology, and a completion CT of the chest showed no metastases. His medical history included hypertension and a left-sided knee replacement. He had no family history of malignancy, was a non-smoker and continued to work. His ECOG performance status was 1. Further investigations included blood tests, which showed a haemoglobin level of 100 g/l and normal estimated glomerular filtration rate level. Urinalysis confirmed microscopic haematuria.

His case was discussed by the urology multidisciplinary team (MDT) and it was agreed that an open radical right nephro-ureterectomy was indicated. He underwent surgery without any complications. Final histology confirmed that he had a right-sided pT3aN0M0 clear cell renal cell carcinoma (RCC).

He underwent follow-up CT scans at 6 months, 12 months and 24 months, which showed no signs of recurrence. A CT scan at 3 years showed a possible lung nodule. Review by the respiratory MDT advised to repeat the scan in 3 months' time. The repeat CT scan showed further nodules and a right iliac bone metastasis. The patient was well and remained at performance status 1; repeat blood tests showed a haemoglobin level of 94 g/l. All other blood test results were within normal limits.

What is the best practice follow-up for high- and low-risk patients following nephrectomy?

What is the management for local recurrence?

What is the evidence for ablation in recurrent RCC?

How is distant disease managed?

What is the optimal time to start systemic treatment?

What is the best practice follow-up for high- and low-risk patients following nephrectomy?

Post-nephrectomy follow-up of patients with RCC is commonly based on European Association of Urology guidelines (Table 21.1), which advise a CT scan of the chest, abdomen and pelvis at regular intervals as well as regular clinical assessment.[1] The timing of surveillance imaging

Table 21.1 European Association of Urology guidelines for post-nephrectomy follow-up.[1]

Risk profile	Oncological follow-up after date of surgery								
	3 months	6 months	12 months	18 months	24 months	30 months	36 months	>3 years	>5 years
Low risk of recurrence Clear cell RCC Leibovich score 0–2 Non-clear cell RCC pT1a–T1b pNx–0 M0 and histological grade 1 or 2	–	CT	–	CT	–	CT	–	CT once every 2 years	–
Intermediate risk of recurrence Clear cell RCC Leibovich score 3–5 Non-clear cell RCC pT1b pNx–0 and/or histological grade 3 or 4	–	CT	CT	–	CT	–	CT	CT once a year	CT once every 2 years
High risk of recurrence Clear cell RCC Leibovich score ≥6 Non-clear cell RCC pT2–pT4 with any histological grade or pT any, pN1 cM0 with any histological grade	CT	CT	CT	CT	CT	–	CT	CT once a year	CT once every 2 years

depends on the risk of disease recurrence as well as the cost-effectiveness and survival benefit of ongoing surveillance (e.g. future treatment options).

The Leibovich score is a validated prognostic model that is commonly used to predict the risk of disease recurrence and therefore the required frequency of imaging (Table 21.2). It derives from a study by Leibovich et al.[2] which examined the clinical and pathological features of 1671 patients with clinically localized clear cell RCC who had undergone radical nephrectomy. A multivariate Cox proportional hazards regression model was used to determine the associations between clinical and pathological features and the occurrence of distant metastases. The scoring system that was developed is used to estimate metastasis-free survival after radical nephrectomy for clear cell RCC according to risk scores (Table 21.3). This in turn influences follow-up, as shown in Table 21.1.

What is the management for local recurrence?

Local fossa recurrence of RCC is uncommon (prevalence 1–3%).[1] Such patients pose a significant surgical and therapeutic challenge as they are at high risk of metastatic disease and have a poor prognosis (28% survival at 5 years).[3] The time to recurrence is likely to be important. Recurrence before 5 years (most cases) is considered 'early' recurrence and after 5 years, 'late' recurrence, the latter being associated with a better prognosis. In one study late recurrence (either local or distant)

Table 21.2 The Leibovich score (adapted from Leibovich et al.[2]).

Feature	Score
T category of primary tumour	
pT1a	0
pT1b	2
pT2	3
pT3a–4	4
Regional lymph node status	
pNx and pN0	0
pN1 and pN2	2
Tumour size (cm)	
<10	0
≥10	1
Nuclear grade	
1 and 2	0
3	1
4	3
Histological tumour necrosis	
No	0
Yes	1

Table 21.3 Estimated metastasis-free survival after radical nephrectomy for clear cell RCC by risk group (adapted from Leibovich et al.[2]).

Risk group	Score	Estimated metastasis-free survival rate (%)		
		Year 1	Year 5	Year 10
Low	0–2	99.5	97.1	92.5
Intermediate	3–5	90.4	73.6	64.3
High	6–11	57.7	31.2	23.6

was observed in ~9% of radically resected patients who were cancer-free for >5 years.[4] Itano et al.[3] found the median time to recurrence was 19–36 months in isolated local recurrence.

Evidence suggests that an approach using aggressive local resection offers the best chance of durable local tumour control and improves survival.[5–7] One study found that patients who underwent surgical resection had a 5 year cause-specific survival rate of 51%, compared with a rate of 18% in patients who received adjuvant medical therapy.[3] Adverse prognostic factors include a short time interval since initial surgery (less than 12 months), sarcomatoid differentiation of the recurrent lesion and incomplete surgical resection.[8] In patients with contraindications to surgery, such as comorbidities, a palliative approach using radiotherapy to alleviate symptoms may be appropriate.

As there is a lack of data for the use of stereotactic body radiotherapy (SBRT) for local recurrence in RCC, patients should be considered for clinical trials where possible. SBRT has shown efficacy in unresectable localized RCC, but data are lacking for recurrent localized disease.[9]

What is the evidence for ablation in recurrent RCC?

Thermal ablation using microwaves can have durable oncological outcomes in patients with solitary T1a kidney tumours. There is very limited trial evidence to support thermal ablation in recurrent tumours and metastatic disease, but case studies highlight that it may be a good alternative treatment option for patients who are not surgical candidates.[10] Ablation may allow patients to delay the initiation of systemic treatments in oligometastatic and locally recurrent disease; however, as there are currently no solid data to support this, it must be carefully discussed by the MDT and the best oncological principles applied.[11]

How is distant disease managed?

Patients with metastatic disease are risk-stratified prior to consideration of systemic treatments. The International Metastatic Renal Cell Carcinoma Database Consortium (IMDC)[12] prognostic model integrates six adverse factors:

- Karnofsky performance status <80% (ECOG performance status ≥1);
- time from diagnosis to treatment <1 year;
- haemoglobin concentration less than the lower limit of normal;
- adjusted serum calcium greater than the upper limit of normal;
- neutrophil count greater than the upper limit of normal;
- platelet count above the upper limit of normal.

The IMDC model divides patients into low-, intermediate- and poor-risk groups (Table 21.4). The patient in the present case study would have had an IMDC score of 1 (because of his haemoglobin level), putting him into the intermediate-risk group.

Sequencing of systemic treatments in metastatic renal cancer has become a challenge as an increasing number of drugs and combination treatments become available. Below is an overview of available treatments.

Favourable risk

Table 21.5 shows the systemic therapy options in low-risk metastatic RCC.

Table 21.4 Median OS by risk category using the IMDC prognostic model.[12]

	Level of risk		
Survival by risk group	Low	Intermediate	Poor
No. of IMDC risk factors	0	1–2	≥3
Median OS (months)	43.2	22.5	7.8

Table 21.5 Systemic therapy options in favourable-risk disease.

IMDC risk level	Standard of care	Alternative[a]
Favourable	Pembrolizumab/lenvatinib[b]	Sunitinib[c]
	Avelumab/axitinib[c]	Pazopanib[c]
	Nivolumab/cabozantinib	Tivozanib[c]
	Pembrolizumab/axitinib	

[a]If ICPIs are contraindicated or not funded.
[b]Pembrolizumab/lenvatinib is not NHS-funded for low-risk disease.
[c]Currently NHS-funded regimens.

Low disease burden
Active surveillance is appropriate for this cohort of patients, provided they are asymptomatic, have a slow tumour growth rate and no vital organs are threatened owing to the location of the tumour. This entails surveillance CT scans every 3 months for the first year, every 4 months in the second year and 6 monthly thereafter. Other options include single-agent antiangiogenic (vascular endothelial growth factor receptor [VEGFR]-directed) therapy with tyrosine kinase inhibitors (TKIs) such as sunitinib, pazopanib or tivozanib.

High disease burden/rapid tumour growth/organ compromise
Patients with symptoms and bulky disease that is rapidly progressive or demonstrates organ insult often require early treatment. Increasingly, immunotherapy-based combination treatment is preferred, particularly in patients where a rapid treatment response is required.

   Immune checkpoint inhibitor (ICPI) combinations such as ipilimumab/nivolumab have not been found to be superior to anti-VEGFR therapy in patients with a favourable level of risk.[13] Moreover, the overall survival (OS) results in this risk group are immature in the other studies of immunotherapy/anti-VEGFR combinations such as avelumab/axitinib and not conclusively superior to sunitinib.[14] However, the better response rates and progression-free survival (PFS) outcomes support the use of combination therapy (ipilimumab/nivolumab) in selected patients with a favourable level of risk (i.e. those with a good performance status and no comorbidities).[15]

Intermediate or poor risk
Table 21.6 shows first-line systemic therapy options in intermediate- and poor-risk metastatic RCC. Tables 21.7 and 21.8 show options for subsequent lines of therapy.

Table 21.6 First-line treatment options in intermediate- and poor-risk disease.

IMDC risk level	Standard of care	Alternative[a]
Intermediate or poor	Ipilimumab/nivolumab[b]	Cabozantinib[b]
	Pembrolizumab/lenvatinib[b]	Sunitinib[b]
	Nivolumab/cabozantinib	Pazopanib[b]
	Pembrolizumab/axitinib	

[a]If ICPIs are contraindicated or not funded.
[b]Currently NHS-funded regimens.

Table 21.7 Second-line treatment options in metastatic RCC.

First line	Standard of care	Alternative[a]
Prior immunotherapy	Any anti-VEGFR TKI which has not been used in combination with ICPIs[b] Sunitinib/pazopanib/axitinib Tivozanib[b] (no previous VEGFR therapy except for first-line avelumab/axitinib) Cabozantinib[b] (second- or third-line)	Lenvatinib/everolimus[b]
Prior VEGFR therapy	Nivolumab[b,c] Cabozantinib[b] Lenvatinib/everolimus[b]	Axitinib[b]

[a]If ICPIs are contraindicated or not funded.
[b]Currently NHS-funded regimens.
[c]After one or two lines of previous VEGFR-directed TKI.

Table 21.8 Third-line treatment options in metastatic RCC.

First line	Second line	Third line	
		Standard of care	Alternative[a]
TKI	Nivolumab[b]	Cabozantinib[b]	Axitinib or everolimus[b]
TKI	Cabozantinib[b]	Nivolumab[b]	Axitinib or everolimus[b]
TKI	TKI	Nivolumab[b] or cabozantinib	Everolimus[b]
Ipilimumab/nivolumab	TKI	Another TKI[b] or everolimus	
Pembrolizumab/lenvatinib	TKI	Another TKI[b] or everolimus	

[a]If ICPIs are contraindicated or not funded.
[b]Currently NHS-funded regimens.

Patients with intermediate or poor-risk disease are usually recommended to have immunotherapy combination treatment rather than antiangiogenic therapy in isolation. The choice of combination treatment is guided by the disease burden and patient factors. The immunotherapy combination ipilimumab/nivolumab can achieve major durable responses and is preferred in sarcomatoid histology or if there is no urgent need for cytoreduction.[16,17] Immunotherapy/TKI regimens such as pembrolizumab/lenvatinib with a high response rate and shorter time to response than ipilimumab/nivolumab may be preferred when there is an urgent need to cytoreduce.[18,19] In patients where immunotherapy/VEGFR therapy combinations are not possible (e.g. patients with contraindications or if the combination is not funded), cabozantinib is preferred.[20]

Second-line therapy data after prior immunotherapy doublets or immunotherapy/anti-VEGFR doublets are limited to small phase II studies using sunitinib, pazopanib and axitinib[15] and retrospective analyses for cabozantinib (Table 21.7).[21,22] Lenvatinib/everolimus with a long progression-free survival is also a second-line option.[23]

Sequencing of systemic therapy options

Tables 21.6–21.8 illustrate the sequencing options in advanced disease. Sequencing of treatments for systemic disease has become more complicated as different combinations of treatments have emerged. The choice is often based on toxicity profiles, patient comorbidities and patient preferences, since most combination treatments have demonstrated an improved OS, particularly when compared with single-agent antiangiogenic therapy.[15]

It would be reasonable to treat the present patient with combination systemic treatment such as ipilimumab/nivolumab or combined immunotherapy/TKI, given that he has two sites of metastases, is in the IMDC intermediate-risk group and has disease progression.

Bone metastases

Denosumab, an inhibitor of the receptor activator of nuclear factor kappa-B ligand (RANKL), or a bone resorption inhibitor such as a bisphosphonate, is recommended in order to reduce the risk of pathological fractures or skeletal-related events.[24] Zoledronic acid has been shown to reduce the incidence and delay the occurrence of a first skeletal-related event,[25] while denosumab, which has the advantage of subcutaneous administration, has been shown to be non-inferior to zoledronic acid in delaying a first skeletal-related event.[24] Patients need to be appropriately counselled for side effects such as osteonecrosis of the jaw, and vitamin D levels should be checked and hypovitaminosis corrected before commencement of bisphosphonate therapy. A dental check is also required, as is regular clinical and biochemical monitoring during treatment.[24,25]

Brain metastases

Patients with intracranial metastases (10% of patients with RCC) should be considered for surgery and/or radiotherapy (stereotactic radiosurgery [SRS] is preferable to whole brain radiotherapy) prior to initiation of systemic treatment. Patients have a risk of haemorrhage in untreated intracranial disease. Immunotherapy is favoured after local treatment for treated or asymptomatic patients, provided their disease is stable on the minimum steroid dose (≤10 mg prednisolone or steroid equivalent per day). Most immunotherapy trials excluded patients with active brain metastases. A study comparing SRS alone with whole brain radiotherapy alone or in combination found no statistically significant difference in 2 year OS between SRS and SRS plus whole brain radiotherapy, though intracerebral control was superior for the combination.[26]

Management of non-clear cell RCC

As there are no phase III trials in patients with non-clear cell RCC, data come from expanded access programmes and case studies. The most common subgroup is papillary RCC. Cabozantinib is appropriate treatment based on results of the SWOG PAPMET trial (ClinicalTrials. gov NCT02761057), owing to a superior PFS and response rate.[27] Alternatives are sunitinib and pembrolizumab[28,29]; savolitinib (where available) is an alternative in *MET*-driven tumours.[27] Ipilimumab and nivolumab in intermediate- and poor-risk groups is now also available to treat metastatic non-clear cell RCC.[15]

What is the optimal time to start systemic treatment?

The optimal time to start systemic treatment is not well defined. RCCs form a very heterogeneous group. A period of observation may be suitable for patients with a more indolent disease course, particularly those who are asymptomatic and have a low tumour burden. A prospective trial in 2016 showed that there was a subset of patients (namely, those with a lower number of IMDC risk factors and a lower number of metastatic disease sites) who did not require immediate systemic treatment.[30] The median surveillance period for these patients was over a year with no adverse impact on their quality of life. Patients who had the longest surveillance period were those with zero or one IMDC risk factor and at most two sites of metastatic disease; however, caution is needed on account of the small patient numbers in this trial.

Conclusion and learning points

- Post-nephrectomy follow-up consists of regular CT scans of the chest, abdomen and pelvis. The frequency, timing and length of follow-up depend on the patient's risk of disease recurrence and likely survival benefit.

- Isolated local recurrence of an RCC post-nephrectomy is rare and requires an aggressive surgical approach if the patient has a good performance status; nevertheless, OS remains poor.

- Multiple systemic agents are available to treat patients with metastases. Systemic treatments depend on the patient's IMDC score and comorbidities as well as the burden of disease and survival benefit of treatment. Sequencing is becoming more challenging as combination treatments using immunotherapy and TKIs have become available.

References

1   European Association of Urology (2022). EAU guidelines on renal cell carcinoma. Available from: https://d56bochluxqnz.cloudfront.net/documents/full-guideline/EAU-Guidelines-on-Renal-Cell-Carinoma-2022.pdf (accessed 3 January 2023).

2   Leibovich BC, Blute ML, Cheville JC, et al. Prediction of progression after radical nephrectomy for patients with clear cell renal cell carcinoma: a stratification tool for prospective clinical trials. Cancer 2003; 97: 1663–71.

3   Itano NB, Blute ML, Spotts B, Zincke H. Outcome of isolated renal cell carcinoma fossa recurrence after nephrectomy. J Urol 2000; 164: 322–5.

4   Park YH, Baik KD, Lee YJ, et al. Late recurrence of renal cell carcinoma >5 years after surgery: clinicopathological characteristics and prognosis. BJU Int 2012; 110 (11 pt B): E553–8.

5   Marchioni M, Sountoulides P, Furlan M, et al. Management of local recurrence after radical nephrectomy: surgical removal with or without systemic treatment is still the gold standard. Results from a multicenter international cohort. Int Urol Nephrol 2021; 53: 2273–80.

6   Margulis V, McDonald M, Tamboli P, et al. Predictors of oncological outcome after resection of locally recurrent renal cell carcinoma. J Urol 2009; 181: 2044–51.

7   Thomas AZ, Adibi M, Borregales LD, et al. Surgical management of local retroperitoneal recurrence of renal cell carcinoma after radical nephrectomy. J Urol 2015; 194: 316–22.

8   Herout R, Graff J, Borkowetz A, et al. Surgical resection of locally recurrent renal cell carcinoma after nephrectomy: oncological outcome and predictors of survival. Urol Oncol 2018; 36: 11.e1–6.

9   Siva S, Louie AV, Warner A, et al. Pooled analysis of stereotactic ablative radiotherapy for primary renal cell carcinoma: a report from the International Radiosurgery Oncology Consortium for Kidney (IROCK). Cancer 2018; 124: 934–42.

10 Ierardi AM, Carnevale A, Rossi UG, et al. Percutaneous microwave ablation therapy of a renal cancer local relapse after radical nephrectomy: a feasibility and efficacy study. Med Oncol 2020; 37: 27.

11 Zagoria RJ, Pettus JA, Rogers M, et al. Long-term outcomes after percutaneous radiofrequency ablation for renal cell carcinoma. Urology 2011; 77: 1393–7.

12 Heng DY, Xie W, Regan MM, et al. External validation and comparison with other models of the International Metastatic Renal-Cell Carcinoma Database Consortium prognostic model: a population-based study. Lancet Oncol 2013; 14: 141–8.

13 Motzer RJ, McDermott DF, Escudier B, et al. Conditional survival and long-term efficacy with nivolumab plus ipilimumab versus sunitinib in patients with advanced renal cell carcinoma. Cancer 2022; 128: 2085–97.

14 Choueiri TK, Motzer RJ, Rini BI, et al. Updated efficacy results from the JAVELIN Renal 101 trial: first-line avelumab plus axitinib versus sunitinib in patients with advanced renal cell carcinoma. Ann Oncol 2020; 31: 1030–9.

15 Powles T, Albiges L, Bex A, et al. ESMO clinical practice guideline update on the use of immunotherapy in early stage and advanced renal cell carcinoma. Ann Oncol 2021; 32: 1511–19.

16 Albiges L, Tannir NM, Burotto M, et al. Nivolumab plus ipilimumab versus sunitinib for first-line treatment of advanced renal cell carcinoma: extended 4-year follow-up of the phase III CheckMate 214 trial. ESMO Open 2020; 5: e001079.

17 Tannir NM, Signoretti S, Choueiri TK, et al. Efficacy and safety of nivolumab plus ipilimumab versus sunitinib in first-line treatment of patients with advanced sarcomatoid renal cell carcinoma. Clin Cancer Res 2021; 27: 78–86.

18 Motzer R, Alekseev B, Rha SY, et al. Lenvatinib plus pembrolizumab or everolimus for advanced renal cell carcinoma. N Engl J Med 2021; 384: 1289–300.

19 Motzer RJ, Tannir NM, McDermott DF, et al. Nivolumab plus ipilimumab versus sunitinib in advanced renal cell carcinoma. N Engl J Med 2018; 378: 1277–90.

20 Choueiri TK, Hessel C, Halabi S, et al. Cabozantinib versus sunitinib as initial therapy for metastatic renal cell carcinoma of intermediate or poor risk (Alliance A031203 CABOSUN randomised trial): progression-free survival by independent review and overall survival update. Eur J Cancer 2018; 94: 115–25.

21 Shah AY, Kotecha RR, Lemke EA, et al. Outcomes of patients with metastatic clear cell renal cell carcinoma treated with second-line VEGFR-TKI after first-line immune checkpoint inhibitors. Eur J Cancer 2019; 114: 67–75.

22 Ged Y, Gupta R, Duzgol C, et al. Systemic therapy for advanced clear cell renal cell carcinoma after discontinuation of immune-oncology and VEGF targeted therapy combinations. BMC Urol 2020; 20: 84.

23 Motzer RJ, Hutson TE, Glen H, et al. Lenvatinib, everolimus and the combination in patients with metastatic renal cell carcinoma: a randomised, phase 2, open label, multicentre trial. Lancet Oncol 2015; 16: 1473–82.

24 Henry DH, Costa L, Goldwasser F, et al. Randomised, double-blind study of denosumab versus zoledronic acid in the treatment of bone metastases in patients with advanced cancer (excluding breast and prostate cancer or multiple myeloma). J Clin Oncol 2011; 29: 1125–32.

25 Rosen LS, Gordon D, Tchekmedyian NS, et al. Long-term efficacy of zoledronic acid in the treatment of skeletal metastases in patients with nonsmall cell carcinoma and other solid tumors: a randomised phase III, double-blind, placebo-controlled trial. Cancer 2004; 100: 2613–21.

26 Fokas E, Henzel M, Hamm K, et al. Radiotherapy for brain metastases from renal cell cancer: should whole-brain radiotherapy be added to stereotactic radiosurgery? Analysis of 88 patients. Strahlenther Onkol 2010; 186: 210–17.

27 Pal SK, Tangen C, Thompson IM Jr, et al. A comparison of sunitinib, cabozantinib, crizotinib and savolitinib for treatment of advanced papillary renal cell carcinoma: a randomised, open-label, phase 2 trial. Lancet 2021; 397: 695–703.

28 McDermott DF, Lee JL, Ziobro M, et al. Open-label, single-arm, phase II study of pembrolizumab monotherapy as first-line therapy in patients with advanced non-clear cell renal cell carcinoma. J Clin Oncol 2021; 39: 1029–39.

29 Choueiri TK, Heng DYC, Lee JL, et al. Efficacy of savolitinib vs sunitinib in patients with MET-driven papillary renal cell carcinoma: the SAVOIR phase 3 randomised clinical trial. JAMA Oncol 2020; 6: 1247–55.

30 Rini BI, Dorff TB, Elson P, et al. Active surveillance in metastatic renal-cell carcinoma: a prospective, phase 2 trial. Lancet Oncol 2016; 17: 1317–24.

22 Palliative options in renal cancer

Usman Mahay, Salil Karkhanis

Case history

A 66-year-old man with a known large renal cell carcinoma (RCC) presented with pain in his right arm following minimal trauma. A CT scan showed a right-sided mid-humeral shaft pathological fracture (Figure 22.1A). Subsequent characterization by MRI (Figure 22.1B) showed features in keeping with a metastasis. Management options were considered in a multidisciplinary team (MDT) meeting; a consensus was agreed upon palliative care for the RCC with surgical fixation of the humeral metastasis for symptom control (requiring preoperative embolization owing to the hypervascular nature of the metastasis).

Conventional digital subtraction angiography (DSA) revealed an intense right humerus tumour blush consistent with a hypervascular RCC bone metastasis (Figure 22.1C). Embolization was performed using a combination of coils and a liquid embolic (Figure 22.1D). The patient went on to have successful fixation of the humerus with minimal blood loss.

Unfortunately, the patient re-presented to the emergency department with frank haematuria 2 months later. A repeat CT scan showed aggressive features of the known large RCC (Figure 22.2A), now complicated with tumour thrombus extending into the inferior vena cava. Following a further MDT discussion, the patient was offered palliative embolization of the RCC with a view to controlling episodes of haematuria.

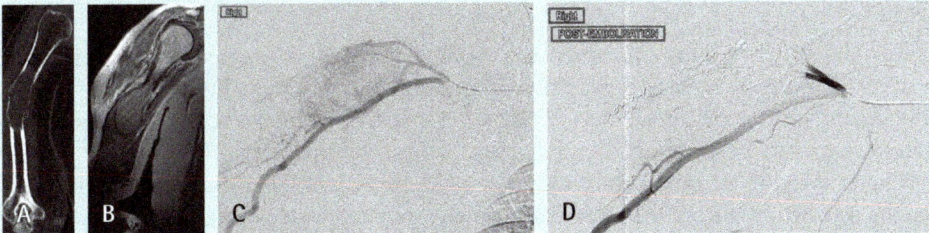

Figure 22.1 (A) CT scan image showing a right mid-humeral shaft pathological fracture. (B) MRI image further characterizing a right humeral metastasis. (C) DSA image showing an intense right humerus tumour blush consistent with a hypervascular RCC bone metastasis. (D) Post-embolization DSA image showing significantly reduced flow to the metastasis. (Images courtesy of Dr Robert Jones.)

The tumour was shown on conventional DSA imaging to be intensely vascular (Figure 22.2B) and was adequately embolized using coils and a liquid embolic (Figure 22.2C). Although not completely free of haematuria, significant control of bleeding was achieved to improve quality of life during palliation and reduce the need for transfusion.

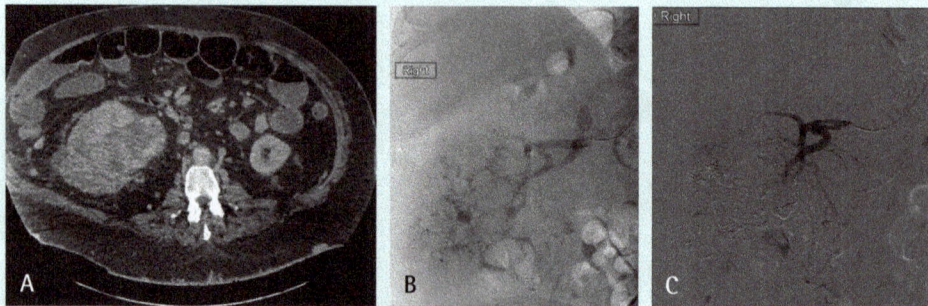

Figure 22.2 (A) CT scan image showing disease progression of the known right RCC. (B) DSA image showing an intensely vascular right RCC. (C) Post-embolization DSA image showing significantly reduced flow to the right RCC. (Images courtesy of Dr Robert Jones.)

What is the role of interventional oncology in the management of a long bone metastasis from RCC?

Is there a role for interventional oncology in pain relief for other metastases from RCC?

What is the role of interventional oncology in the management of haematuria from RCC?

What is the role of interventional oncology in the management of a long bone metastasis from RCC?

Quality of life may be significantly impacted in patients with RCC, particularly those with wide-spread metastatic disease. Several palliative options aim to improve quality of life.

The second most common site for metastases in patients with advanced RCC after lung metastases are bones, most frequently the femur, followed by the humerus.[1,2] Routine staging or surveillance imaging for early identification of bone metastases from RCC is somewhat limited given the osteolytic nature of RCC bone metastases compared with osteoblastic metastases, which can be more readily identified on skeletal scintigraphy.[3] As a result, aggressive osteolytic RCC bone metastases may present late with pathological fractures, resulting in significant morbidity and disabling pain.[4]

A number of options are available to alleviate pain from RCC bone metastases; however, once a fracture is present or imminent, surgical fixation is the mainstay. Given the hypervascular aetiology of RCC bone metastases, perioperative blood loss during fixation is a significant risk. Measures should be taken to attenuate the need for perioperative blood transfusion, which has been shown to adversely affect long-term survival of patients undergoing surgical management of long bone metastases.[5] Preoperative embolization is a safe option to achieve a reduction in intraoperative blood loss, provided it is performed in a timely fashion prior to orthopaedic fixation.[6,7] It is important to discuss this option in an MDT setting to ensure that patients get access to appropriate treatments.

Is there a role for interventional oncology in pain relief for other metastases from RCC?

Spinal metastases account for approximately one-third of bone metastases secondary to RCC and may lead to significant pain and neurological disability.[8] A number of options are available to alleviate pain from RCC spinal metastases other than preoperative embolization discussed above. These include radiotherapy, ablation and kyphoplasty.

Stereotactic body radiotherapy (SBRT) is a minimally invasive option in the loco-regional management of RCC bone metastases, including spinal disease (Figure 22.3). Traditionally RCC has been considered relatively radio-resistant; however, the higher fraction doses permitted by SBRT have recently led to a paradigm shift.[9] SBRT for oligometastatic disease was shown in a phase II randomized controlled trial to improve survival with no detriment to quality of life.[10] Additionally, the use of SBRT may be enhanced when combined with targeted drugs in the management of oligometastatic disease in selected patients.[11,12]

While SBRT is a good option, in some situations it may lead to a paradoxical increased risk of fracture,[13] which may require surgical fixation. Patients receiving palliative care are often not fit for surgery. In such cases, thermal ablation and stabilization may be considered.

Radiofrequency ablation is a minimally invasive option, where small electrodes generate heat within the target metastasis destroying the tumour tissue.[14] It is a particularly effective technique when combined with vertebroplasty to stabilize the inevitable defect left in the bone (Figure 22.4), reducing the chance of vertebral collapse, pain and nerve impingement.[15] While radiofrequency

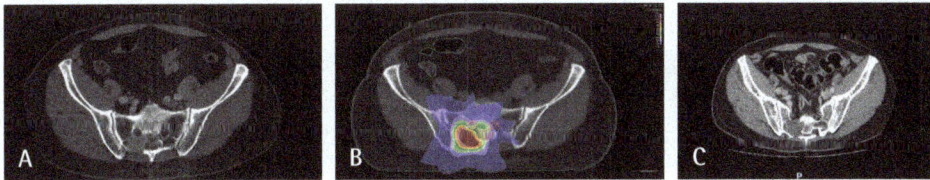

Figure 22.3 (A) CT scan image pre-SBRT showing a right sacral metastasis. (B) SBRT treatment planning image. (C) CT scan image 8 months post-SBRT. (Images courtesy of Dr Anjali Zarkar.)

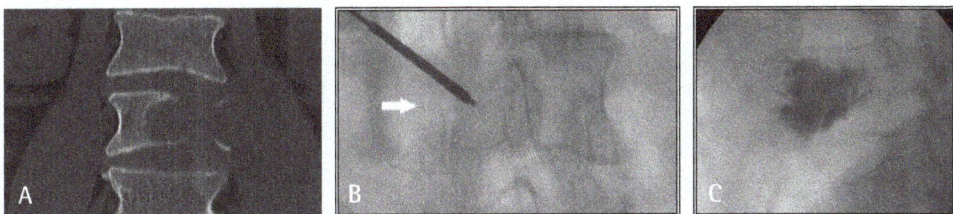

Figure 22.4 (A) CT scan image showing a vertebral metastasis. (B) Image taken during radiofrequency ablation. (C) Post-vertebroplasty image. (Images courtesy of Dr Steven James.)

ablation is well established in many centres, cryoablation is increasingly taking its place in the management of pain secondary to an osteolytic bone metastasis. This is because it is possible to visualize the ice on CT, thus making it easier to avoid nearby critical structures.[16,17]

What is the role of interventional oncology in the management of haematuria from RCC?

Haematuria may limit the quality and length of life of patients with RCC. Haematuria may lead not only to symptomatic anaemia, requiring repeated admissions for transfusion, but also to clot retention, requiring bladder catheterization. For patients with advanced disease and poor performance status, where other options including radiotherapy may be less well tolerated,[18] embolization is a feasible option in the palliative management of haematuria secondary to RCC.[18,19]

Given the minimally invasive nature of embolization, it can potentially be performed as a day case procedure using either a femoral or radial approach.[20] However, patients should be warned of the likely post-embolization syndrome that will follow embolization of a large tumour, with flu-like symptoms and fevers. There is also a risk of necrosis and infection requiring antibiotic therapy.[21,22]

Conclusion and learning points

- Interventional oncology techniques have much to offer in the palliative management of pain from bone metastases secondary to RCC.
- Embolization can play a role in reducing the debilitating effects of haematuria on quality of life in late-stage RCC.
- For the best end-of-life care in RCC an MDT approach is required to make the patient as comfortable as possible. It is essential that the MDT contains all relevant specialties, so that the patient is presented with the best options.

References

1 Bianchi M, Sun M, Jeldres C, et al. Distribution of metastatic sites in renal cell carcinoma: a population-based analysis. Ann Oncol 2012; 23: 973–80.

2 Casadei R, Drago G, Di Pressa F, Donati D. Humeral metastasis of renal cancer: surgical options and review of literature. Orthop Traumatol Surg Res 2018; 104: 533–8.

3 Sohaib SA, Cook G, Allen SD, et al. Comparison of whole-body MRI and bone scintigraphy in the detection of bone metastases in renal cancer. Br J Radiol 2009; 82: 632–9.

4 Woodward E, Jagdev S, McParland L, et al. Skeletal complications and survival in renal cancer patients with bone metastases. Bone 2011; 48: 160–6.

5 Geraets SE, Bos PK, van der Stok J. Preoperative embolization in surgical treatment of long bone metastasis: a systematic literature review. EFORT Open Rev 2020; 5: 17–25.

6 Çelebioğlu EC, Bilgiç S, Merter A, et al. Scheduling surgery after transarterial embolization: does timing make any difference to intraoperative blood loss for renal cell carcinoma bone metastases? Diagn Interv Radiol 2021; 27: 740–5.

7 Cirstoiu C, Cretu B, Iordache S, et al. Surgical management options for long-bone metastasis. EFORT Open Rev 2022; 7: 206–13.

8 Attalla K, Duzgol C, McLaughlin L, et al. The spinal distribution of metastatic renal cell carcinoma: support for locoregional rather than arterial hematogenous mode of early bony dissemination. Urol Oncol 2021; 39: 196.e9–14.

9 De Meerleer G, Khoo V, Escudier B, et al. Radiotherapy for renal-cell carcinoma. Lancet Oncol 2014; 15: e170–7.

10 Palma DA, Olson R, Harrow S, et al. Stereotactic ablative radiotherapy for the comprehensive treatment of oligometastatic cancers: long-term results of the SABR-COMET phase II randomized trial. J Clin Oncol 2020; 38: 2830–8.

11 Grünwald V, Eberhardt B, Bex A, et al. An interdisciplinary consensus on the management of bone metastases from renal cell carcinoma. Nat Rev Urol 2018; 15: 511–21.

12 Onal C, Hurmuz P, Guler OC, et al. The role of stereotactic body radiotherapy in switching systemic therapy for patients with extracranial oligometastatic renal cell carcinoma. Clin Transl Oncol 2022; 24: 1533–41.

13 Vargas E, Susko MS, Mummaneni PV, et al. Vertebral body fracture rates after stereotactic body radiation therapy compared with external-beam radiation therapy for metastatic spine tumors. J Neurosurg Spine 2020; 33: 870–6.

14 Li C, Wu Q, Chang D, et al. State-of-the-art of minimally invasive treatments of bone metastases. J Bone Oncol 2022; 34: 100425.

15 Yildizhan S, Boyaci MG, Rakip U, et al. Role of radiofrequency ablation and cement injection for pain control in patients with spinal metastasis. BMC Musculoskelet Disord 2021; 22: 912.

16 Zugaro L, Di Staso M, Gravina GL, et al. Treatment of osteolytic solitary painful osseous metastases with radiofrequency ablation or cryoablation: a retrospective study by propensity analysis. Oncol Lett 2016; 11: 1948–54.

17 Ryan A, Byrne C, Pusceddu C, et al. CIRSE standards of practice on thermal ablation of bone tumours. Cardiovasc Intervent Radiol 2022; 45: 591–605.

18 Maxwell NJ, Saleem Amer N, Rogers E, et al. Renal artery embolisation in the palliative treatment of renal carcinoma. Br J Radiol 2007; 80: 96–102.

19 Pozzi Mucelli F, Pozzi Mucelli RA, Marrocchio C, et al. Endovascular interventional radiology of the urogenital tract. Medicina 2021; 57: 278.

20 Chu HH, Kim JW, Shin JH, Cho SB. Update on transradial access for percutaneous transcatheter visceral artery embolization. Korean J Radiol 2021; 22: 72.

21 Gunn AJ, Patel AR, Rais-Bahrami S. Role of angio-embolization for renal cell carcinoma. Curr Urol Rep 2018; 19: 76.

22 Wright B, Johnson BS, Vassar M, et al. Trans-arterial embolization of renal cell carcinoma: a systematic review and meta-analysis. Abdom Radiol (NY) 2022; 47: 2238–43.

Further reading

- Wang CJ, Christie A, Lin M-H, et al. Safety and efficacy of stereotactic ablative radiation therapy for renal cell carcinoma extracranial metastases. Int J Radiat Oncol Biol Phys 2017; 98: 91–100.

23 A patient requiring surgery for non-small-cell lung cancer

Nabil Hussein, Richard Milton

Case history

A 67-year-old ex-smoker (30 pack-years) was invited to a newly introduced lung health check. During assessment the man reported no cardiorespiratory symptoms, had adequate exercise tolerance and was fully independent in his activities of daily living. Assessment was followed by a low-dose CT scan of the chest, which demonstrated a 3 cm lesion in the right upper lobe. He was referred to the local lung multidisciplinary team. A PET scan confirmed the lesion was highly avid (maximum standardized uptake value of 10) and showed a mildly enlarged mediastinal lymph node (R4). Subsequent endobronchial ultrasound-guided transbronchial needle aspiration was negative for metastatic disease. CT-guided biopsy of the right upper lobe lesion confirmed adenocarcinoma (T1cN0M0).

On physical assessment the man reported no cardiac risk factors, achieved a distance of >400 m on a shuttle walk test and had normal lung function on spirometry and diffusing capacity for carbon monoxide test. He was subsequently referred to thoracic surgery for consideration of lung cancer resection. One week after review by the surgical team the patient underwent an uneventful elective right video-assisted thoracoscopic (VATS) upper lobectomy with lymph node sampling. The chest drain was removed on postoperative day 2 and he was discharged the following day. Formal histological assessment of the intraoperative specimens (right upper lobe, lymph node samples from stations 2R, 4R, 7 and 10R) confirmed adenocarcinoma with complete resection margins and no evidence of metastatic disease (pT1cN0M0R0).

At 4 weeks' follow-up the patient was informed that his curative surgery had been successful and that he would continue his cancer follow-up in the local survivorship programme.

What was the goal of cancer treatment in this patient?

What is the lung health check?

What are the principles for a right VATS upper lobectomy?

What is the evidence base for lobectomy, and are sublobar resections better?

Are there any benefits of minimally invasive (VATS) over open surgery?

Is there a benefit in performing a mediastinal lymphadenectomy over lymph node sampling?

What was the goal of cancer treatment in this patient?

The goal of cancer treatment was threefold:

- curative intent with complete resection of the lung cancer;
- completion of pathological staging;
- reduction of the risk of cancer recurrence and promotion of disease-free survival.

What is the lung health check?

The NHS lung health check is a service that is offered in some parts of England.[1] People between the ages of 55 and 75 with a history of smoking are invited to have spirometry, smoking cessation advice (if applicable) and an assessment of their lung cancer risk. Those identified as high risk undergo a low-dose CT scan. If a highly suspicious lesion is identified (>300 mm³ or >8 mm maximum diameter and Brock risk >10%) the individual is referred to a rapid access lung clinic for further assessment. If considered intermediate risk, the person will be invited for a repeat scan at specific intervals (3, 12 or 24 months). If no lesion is identified on the initial scan the person will be invited after 24 months for a repeat scan.

What are the principles for a right VATS upper lobectomy?

The patient undergoes general anaesthesia with single lung ventilation to the non-operative lung via a double lumen endotracheal tube. The patient is placed in the left decubitus position with hands placed in the 'prayer' position in front of the face. There are various methods described for VATS lobectomy including the anterior,[2] posterior[3] and uniportal approaches. A 1 cm camera port incision is initially placed just superior to the level of the diaphragm to allow inspection of the pleural cavity and assess whether it is appropriate to continue with the VATS approach. For the anterior approach a 5 cm anterior utility incision is placed between the lower angle of the scapula and the breast in the fourth intercostal space, just anterior to the latissimus dorsi, and an additional 1.5 cm posterior port is made to complete triangulation. This approach gives excellent exposure of the anterior hilum to enable dissection of the main pulmonary vessels and bronchus.[2]

Usually, the right superior pulmonary vein is first dissected and divided with an endoscopic vascular stapler. The truncus anterior and posterior ascending segmental artery are sequentially dissected and divided in the same manner. The bronchus to the upper lobe is dissected and clamped. The lung is then ventilated to ensure that the correct bronchus has been clamped without compromising the remaining lung. Once confirmed, the bronchus is divided with an endostapler. To complete the lobectomy the remaining fissures are completed and the lobe is retrieved.

Pathological staging is completed by lymph node sampling of stations 2R, 4R, 7 and 10R. A water test is performed to assess the bronchial stump and a chest drain is placed into the pleural cavity through one of the small incisions. The remaining incisions are closed in the usual surgical manner.

The posterior approach is an alternative technique that uses the same principles as the anterior approach.[3] A three- or four-port technique gives the surgeon a similar view to that in an open lobectomy. The major difference is the order in which structures are dissected and divided. Usually this is the bronchus, followed by the pulmonary artery branches and the superior pulmonary vein. Uniportal (single port) lobectomies can also be performed safely, with the aim to further minimize the number of incisions required to complete the lobectomy.

What is the evidence base for lobectomy, and are sublobar resections better?

Pulmonary lobectomy is the gold standard in the surgical management of non-small-cell lung cancer (NSCLC). The Lung Cancer Study Group performed a prospective, multi-institutional randomized controlled trial (RCT) comparing limited resection with lobectomy in participants with peripheral early-stage NSCLC.[4] In total, 247 participants were randomized to either lobectomy (n=125) or limited resection (n=122). Limited resection consisted of either wedge resection or segmentectomy. Compared with the lobectomy arm, in the limited resection arm there was an observed 75% increase in recurrence rates (p=0.02), a 30% increase in overall death rate (p=0.08) and a 50% increase in death with cancer rate (p=0.09). The group concluded that lobectomy must be considered the surgical procedure of choice in early-stage NSCLC.

Of note, although the above is an important study, it is now over 25 years old and most likely does not represent modern day practice. There have been attempts to explore whether there are benefits in segmentectomy in early-stage NSCLC. A meta-analysis evaluated the outcomes of segmentectomy vs lobectomy for stage I, stage IA only and stage IA <2 cm NSCLC.[5] The meta-analysis included 28 studies (26 retrospective) that reported overall survival (OS), cancer-specific survival and recurrence-free survival. For stage I lesions <4 cm, segmentectomy was inferior to lobectomy in all three outcomes (p<0.02). For stage IA lesions <3 cm, differences in OS (p=0.04) and cancer-specific survival (p=0.02) favoured lobectomy, but there were no differences in recurrence-free survival (p=0.1). In stage IA lesions <2 cm there was no significant difference among all outcomes (p>0.1).

A large retrospective cohort study (N=16,819) compared survival rates (OS and lung cancer-specific survival) after lobectomy, segmentectomy and wedge resection in early-stage NSCLC (stage IA).[6] The study found that for stage IA lesions <1 cm all techniques were comparable; for lesions measuring 1.1–2 cm segmentectomy was equivalent to lobectomy; but for lesions >2 cm lobectomy was superior.

In the last year, the first phase III RCT has been published comparing segmentectomy vs lobectomy in small-sized peripheral NSCLC (UMIN000002317).[7] In this non-inferiority trial, patients with stage 1A NSCLC were assigned to either segmentectomy (n=522) or lobectomy (n=554), with OS being the primary endpoint. Median follow-up was 7.3 years (range 0.0–10.9 years). The study demonstrated a potential benefit of segmentectomy over lobectomy in patients with small-sized peripheral NSCLC, with a 5 year OS of 94.3% (95% CI 92.1%, 96.0%) vs 91.1% (95% CI 88.4%, 93.2%) (non-inferiority, p<0.0001; superiority, p=0.0082). There was no significant difference in 5 year relapse-free survival in the two groups (p=0.99); however, there was a difference in the proportion of patients with local relapse favouring lobectomy (segmentectomy 10.5% vs lobectomy 5.4%; p=0.0018). Other postoperative complications were similar between the two groups.

The results of these recent studies are likely to lead to a growth in the adoption of segmentectomies, particularly in early-stage lesions <2 cm; however, at present, lobectomy remains the gold standard in such patients.

Are there any benefits of minimally invasive (VATS) over open surgery?

Open lung resection via a thoracotomy has been the gold standard in the surgical management of NSCLC. Over the last two decades there has been a growth of VATS and, more recently, robotic surgery. However, there is limited information from RCTs to assess whether there is a benefit of minimally invasive techniques vs open surgery.

The VIOLET study (ISRCTN13472721) is a UK multicentre, parallel-group RCT with blinding of outcome assessors and participants that aims to compare the effectiveness, cost-effectiveness and acceptability of VATS vs open lobectomy.[8] Over a 4 year period, 503 patients with known or suspected (cT1-3 N0-1) lung cancer were randomized to VATS ($n=247$) or open ($n=256$) lobectomy. Recent 1 year results have shown that VATS patients had less pain, despite lower analgesic consumption (mean ratio 0.90; 95% CI 0.80, 1.01).[9] The VATS arm also demonstrated better functional recovery ($p=0.002$) at 5 weeks and fewer complications (relative risk 0.74; 95% CI 0.66, 0.84; $p<0.001$) as well as no difference in in-hospital serious adverse events ($p=0.9$). Furthermore, median hospital stay was shorter by 1 day in the VATS arm (4 vs 5 days; $p=0.006$). On discharge there was a 19% reduction in serious adverse events ($p=0.053$) and lower readmission rates in the VATS arm. In patients with lymph node disease, 50.9% of those in the VATS arm and 45.9% in the open arms received adjuvant therapy, with no difference in time to therapy ($p=0.7$). Up to 1 year, recurrence rates, progression-free survival and OS were not significantly different ($p>0.2$). Although promising, time will tell if VATS surgery is a better option than open surgery.

Is there a benefit in performing a mediastinal lymphadenectomy over lymph node sampling?

Mediastinal lymphadenectomy (i.e. lymph node dissection) or sampling is performed to assist with the pathological staging of the disease. A lymphadenectomy involves removing all mediastinal tissue containing lymph nodes and may either be systematic or lobe-specific, whereas lymph node sampling only samples lymph node tissue from a particular region. Studies have explored whether there is a survival benefit in lymphadenectomy vs sampling.

The American College of Surgery Oncology Group Z0030 trial was a randomized, multi-institutional prospective trial comparing mediastinal lymph node dissection vs mediastinal lymph node sampling in patients with early-stage NSCLC.[10] Patients with NSCLC underwent lymph node sampling during surgery for frozen section. Lymph node stations 2R, 4R, 7 and 10R were sampled in right-sided, and 5, 6, 7 and 10L in left-sided, tumours. If samples were negative for malignancy, eligible patients ($N=1023$) were randomized to either no further lymph node sampling ($n=498$) or complete mediastinal lymph node dissection ($n=525$). There was no significant difference in median survival between the two groups (8.1 years for lymph node sampling vs 8.5 years for lymph node dissection; $p=0.25$). Five year disease-free survival was similar in both groups (69% vs 68%; $p=0.92$). There was no difference in local, regional or distant recurrence between the groups ($p>0.5$).

A meta-analysis has shown similar rates of OS, local recurrence and distant metastasis between lymph node sampling and lymph node dissection.[11] Despite lymph node dissection being a more invasive procedure, there was no evidence that it increased complications.

Conclusion and learning points

- The surgical goal in patients with early-stage NSCLC is to obtain cure by complete resection, to complete the pathological staging, and to reduce the risk of recurrence and promote disease-free survival.

- The NHS lung health check is a new cancer screening programme that aims to identify early-stage lung cancers that may be amenable to curative treatment.

- Pulmonary lobectomy via either open or minimally invasive approaches is the gold standard in the surgical management of NSCLC, although there is an increasing trend towards segmentectomies, with recent studies demonstrating non-inferiority to lobectomy for small-sized peripheral NSCLC.

- Recent evidence has demonstrated that there are benefits of VATS lobectomy over open lung resection, including reduced pain, shorter in-hospital stay and a reduction in serious adverse events and readmission rates.
- Lobe-specific mediastinal lymph node sampling is equivalent to full mediastinal lymph node dissection in relation to survival and recurrence rates and is appropriate for pathological staging.

References

1 NHS England (2019). Targeted screening for lung cancer with low radiation dose computed tomography. Available from: www.england.nhs.uk/publication/targeted-screening-for-lung-cancer (accessed 14 March 2022).

2 Hansen HJ, Petersen RH, Christensen M. Video-assisted thoracoscopic surgery (VATS) lobectomy using a standardized anterior approach. Surg Endosc 2011; 25: 1263–9.

3 Richards JM, Dunning J, Oparka J, et al. Video-assisted thoracoscopic lobectomy: the Edinburgh posterior approach. Ann Cardiothorac Surg 2012; 1: 61–9.

4 Ginsberg RJ, Rubinstein LV. Randomized trial of lobectomy versus limited resection for T1 N0 non-small cell lung cancer. Lung Cancer Study Group. Ann Thorac Surg 1995; 60: 615–22.

5 Winckelmans T, Decaluwé H, De Leyn P, Van Raemdonck D. Segmentectomy or lobectomy for early-stage non-small-cell lung cancer: a systematic review and meta-analysis. Eur J Cardiothorac Surg 2020; 57: 1051–60.

6 Cao J, Yuan P, Wang Y, et al. Survival rates after lobectomy, segmentectomy, and wedge resection for non-small cell lung cancer. Ann Thorac Surg 2018; 105: 1483–91.

7 Saji H, Okada M, Tsuboi M, et al. Segmentectomy versus lobectomy in small-sized peripheral non-small-cell lung cancer (JCOG0802/WJOG4607L): a multicentre, open-label, phase 3, randomised, controlled, non-inferiority trial. Lancet 2022; 399: 1607–17.

8 Lim E, Batchelor T, Shackcloth M, et al. Study protocol for Video Assisted Thoracoscopic Lobectomy versus Conventional Open Lobectomy for Lung Cancer, a UK multicentre randomised controlled trial with an internal pilot (the VIOLET study). BMJ Open 2019; 9: e029507.

9 Lim EKS, Batchelor TJP, Dunning J, et al. Video-assisted thoracoscopic versus open lobectomy in patients with early-stage lung cancer: one-year results from a randomized controlled trial (VIOLET). J Clin Oncol 2021; 39 (15 suppl): 8504.

10 Darling GE, Allen MS, Decker PA, et al. Randomized trial of mediastinal lymph node sampling versus complete lymphadenectomy during pulmonary resection in the patient with N0 or N1 (less than hilar) non-small cell carcinoma: results of the American College of Surgery Oncology Group Z0030 trial. J Thorac Cardiovasc Surg 2011; 141: 662–70.

11 Huang X, Wang J, Chen Q, Jiang J. Mediastinal lymph node dissection versus mediastinal lymph node sampling for early stage non-small cell lung cancer: a systematic review and meta-analysis. PLoS One 2014; 9: e109979.

Further reading

- McWilliams A, Tammemagi MC, Mayo JR, et al. Probability of cancer in pulmonary nodules detected on first screening CT. N Engl J Med 2013; 369: 910–19.

24 Radiofrequency ablation of a solitary colorectal lung metastasis: a multidisciplinary approach

David Jarosz, Claire Ryan, Jonathan Smith

Case history

A 76-year-old woman presented via the bowel cancer screening programme with a 2 cm sessile rectal polyp. Her medical history included hypertension and she was a smoker. Endorectal ultrasound and MRI confirmed an early-stage polyp. Initial biopsies suggested a tubulovillous adenoma with high-grade dysplasia; however, lymphovascular invasion was seen and the lesion was upgraded to a poorly differentiated adenocarcinoma. She underwent uneventful transanal endoscopic microsurgery to remove the polyp, followed by a 5 week course of chemoradiotherapy.

After 5 years of remission, a rise in carcinoembryonic antigen levels was noted during surveillance and a planned CT scan was expedited. The scan showed a spiculated 16 mm left upper lobe mass. Given her ongoing smoking, the mass was suspected to be a primary lung cancer; however, a CT-guided lung biopsy proved it to be a colorectal adenocarcinoma metastasis.

Following discussion at the local lung multidisciplinary team (MDT) meeting, the woman was referred to thoracic surgery for consideration of resection and booked for a pre-assessment. The thoracic surgeon who saw her in clinic referred her case to interventional oncology, and the lesion was deemed suitable for ablation.

The woman suffered a stroke while awaiting her procedure and was left with an expressive dysphasia. Her quality of life, however, was excellent with no limitations to her activities of daily living. She had a full social life and communicated through writing. The left upper lobe lung mass remained stable on further imaging (Figure 24.1). The surgeon met the patient in clinic again and, given the increased surgical risk from the recent stroke, the decision was made to proceed with ablation.

One year after the initial CT scan, the patient underwent radiofrequency ablation to the left upper lobe lesion, under general anaesthesia. A single probe was placed centrally within the tumour under CT guidance, with the patient positioned supine.

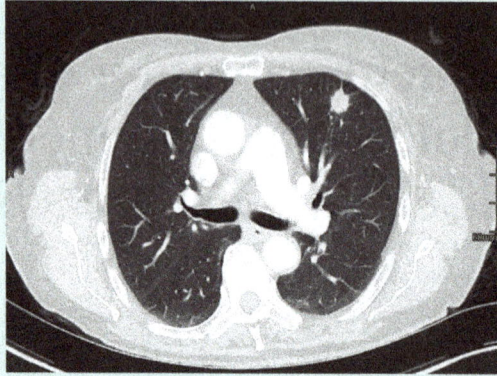

Figure 24.1 Biopsy-proven colorectal metastasis. The image shows a 16 mm spiculated left upper lobe mass.

The total treatment time was 13 min. The procedure was uneventful; there was a small, predicted haematoma surrounding the lesion, but no other immediate complications (Figures 24.2 and 24.3). There was no pneumothorax on immediate post-procedural CT or on the routine chest radiograph 4 h later. She remained well and was discharged the following day.

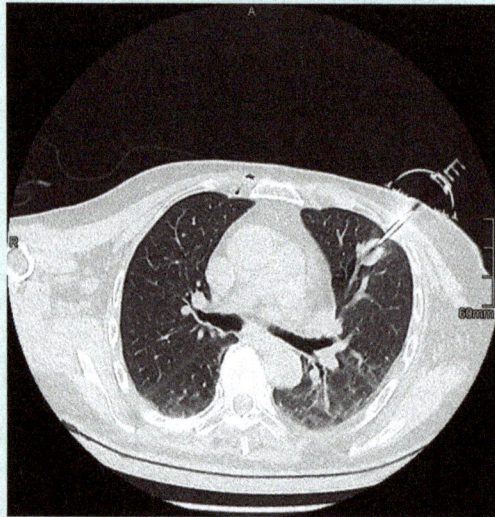

Figure 24.2 Placement of the radiofrequency ablation probe with tines open, prior to commencing treatment.

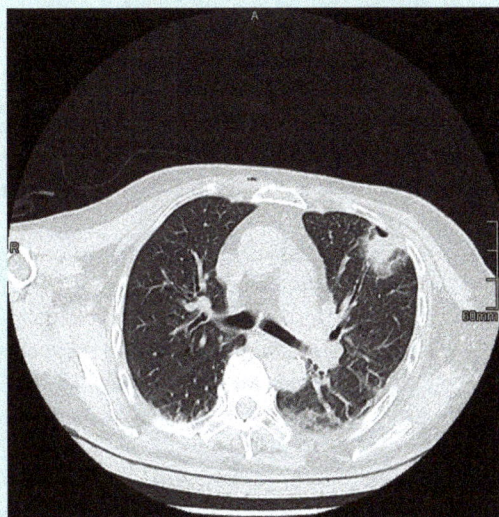

Figure 24.3 Post-ablation appearances, with a small surrounding pulmonary haemorrhage.

What was the goal of oncological treatment for this patient?

What is the rationale and evidence base for her treatment options?

What do the long-term data suggest?

How did her comorbidities influence the treatment decisions?

How did a collaborative approach help this patient achieve a good outcome?

What was the goal of oncological treatment for this patient?

Complete treatment of the lung metastasis with preservation of lung function, regardless of underlying fitness, is one of the aims of the lung cancer service. Nevertheless, the patient's wishes must be considered when planning therapies which may significantly affect quality of life, particularly if the patient has significant underlying comorbidity. Treatment in the current case aimed to balance potential gains in survival with preservation of quality of life and functional status.

What is the rationale and evidence base for her treatment options?

Lung metastases develop in up to 15% of patients with colorectal cancer. Thermal ablation preserves the lung parenchyma with minimal collateral damage. The main risks of surgical resection are preoperative toxicity and impaired lung reserve in a patient with known metastatic disease and comorbidity. Recurrence after pulmonary metastasectomy has been reported to be as high as 68%, with subsequent surgeries limited owing to decreased pulmonary reserve.[1] No randomized studies have directly compared surgery with thermal ablation. Percutaneous thermal ablation is a valuable option, as it achieves control of disease progression comparable to that found with surgery, while, importantly, avoiding the morbidity associated with surgical intervention.[2]

Radiofrequency ablation is the most widely studied modality in the literature and several studies have demonstrated favourable outcomes.

The RAPTURE study (ClinicalTrials.gov NCT00690703) was a prospective, intention-to-treat, multicentre clinical trial from Italy, in which 106 patients with different primary tumour histology were enrolled for radiofrequency ablation.[3] Of 183 metastatic lung tumours treated, 29% were colorectal metastases. The technical success rate was 99%. Cancer-specific survival was 91% (95% CI 0.78%, 0.96%) at 1 year and 68% (95% CI 0.54%, 0.80%) at 2 years in patients with colorectal metastases.

A large systematic review comprised eight studies including 903 patients, all treated with radiofrequency ablation for lung metastases from colorectal cancer.[4] Mortality was <1%, with overall survival (OS) ranging from 31 to 67 months; 1, 3 and 5 year survival ranges were 84–95%, 35–72% and 20–54%, respectively. Local progression following ablation ranged from 9% to 21%.

In a large series, de Baère et al.[5] compared radiofrequency ablation for lung metastases from various tumour types. A total of 566 patients were treated for 1037 lung metastases, most frequently colorectal cancer (34%). Most patients had one (53%) or two (25%) lung metastases. The size of tumour was predictive of local tumour progression. Median OS was 62 months; 5 year OS was 51%, which is similar to the best results obtained by surgical metastasectomy. Radiofrequency ablation was concluded to be an option for treatment of metastatic tumours between 2 cm and 3 cm in size, in patients with fewer than three metastases.

What do the long-term data suggest?

The surgical literature focuses on 5 year survival with estimates ranging between 38% and 71%; however, these favourable survival rates may be partly attributable to patient selection criteria.[6] In a retrospective, single-centre study, 125 colorectal lung metastases were treated with image-guided radiofrequency ablation; median duration of follow-up was 45.5 months. The findings indicated comparable long-term OS and progression-free survival (PFS) following radiofrequency ablation for the treatment of histologically confirmed colorectal lung metastases vs surgery.[6] Median OS was 52 months (95% CI 0.39, 0.64) and median PFS was 19 months (95% CI 0.1, 0.28). The 1, 3, 5, 7 and 9 year PFS rates were 66.7%, 31.2%, 25.9%, 21.2% and 5.9%, respectively.

How did her comorbidities influence the treatment decisions?

Stroke is a known risk factor for adverse perioperative outcomes. A large Danish study suggested a waiting period of at least 9 months before scheduling acute ischaemic stroke patients for elective non-cardiac surgery.[7] It is also well established that, compared with non-smokers, tobacco smokers are at significantly higher risk of postsurgical complications.[8] Given that it is minimally invasive and can be performed many times, thermal ablation plays a suitable role as a first-line treatment in these patients, allowing surgery to be reserved for those who are unable to be treated by minimally invasive methods.

How did a collaborative approach help this patient achieve a good outcome?

Historically, metastatic cancer has been considered to be the end stage of the disease. Through multimodal and multidisciplinary approaches, current efforts are directed towards improving the prognosis of these patients. Appropriate management requires the MDT to make a decision based on tumour biology and local experience, but it must take patient preferences into consideration. Preserving quality of life through a low morbidity rate is a major advantage of pulmonary thermal ablation.[9,10] Fundamental to the success of this treatment was a collective approach where percutaneous image-guided thermal ablation operated as an adjunct, not a competitor, to the existing surgical oncology service.

Conclusion and learning points

- For patients with colorectal cancer lung metastases, there are demonstrated benefits to local therapy, which can be offered through various modalities.

- Image-guided percutaneous thermal ablation is a safe, reliable technique demonstrating excellent local control rates for small tumours and may be considered first-line treatment for pulmonary colorectal metastases in selected patients.

- A holistic multidisciplinary and multimodality approach is essential to inform decision making and for choosing an appropriate treatment, with careful consideration of the patient's underlying risk factors and comorbidities.

- Novel systemic agents continue to extend life expectancy in metastatic disease. Combined multimodality treatments using ablation, surgery, radiation or chemotherapy may result in improved survival when compared with these modalities alone. Through trials and multidisciplinary efforts demonstrating the best strategy for combination local therapy, we can continue to individualize the optimal therapy regimen for each patient.

References

1 Kim HK, Cho JH, Lee HY, et al. Pulmonary metastasectomy for colorectal cancer: how many nodules, how many times? World J Gastroenterol 2014; 20: 6133–45.

2 Sofocleous C, Sideras P, Petre E, Solomon SB. Ablation for the management of pulmonary malignancies. Am J Roentgenol 2011; 197: W581–9.

3 Lencioni R, Crocetti L, Cioni R, et al. Response to radiofrequency ablation of pulmonary tumours: a prospective, intention-to-treat, multicentre clinical trial (the RAPTURE study). Lancet Oncol 2008; 9: 621–8.

4 Lyons NJR, Pathak S, Daniels IR, et al. Percutaneous management of pulmonary metastases arising from colorectal cancer; a systematic review. Eur J Surg Oncol 2015; 41: 1447–55.

5 de Baère T, Aupérin A, Deschamps F, et al. Radiofrequency ablation is a valid treatment option for lung metastases: experience in 566 patients with 1037 metastases. Ann Oncol 2015; 26: 987–91.

6 Zhong J, Palkhi E, Ng H, et al. Long-term outcomes in percutaneous radiofrequency ablation for histologically proven colorectal lung metastasis. Cardiovasc Intervent Radiol 2020; 43: 1900–7.

7 Jørgensen ME, Torp-Pedersen C, Gislason GH, et al. Time elapsed after ischemic stroke and risk of adverse cardiovascular events and mortality following elective noncardiac surgery. JAMA 2014; 312: 269–77.

8 Yoong SL, Tursan d'Espaignet E, Wiggers J, et al. Tobacco and postsurgical outcomes: WHO tobacco knowledge summaries. Geneva: World Health Organization, 2020.

9 Delpla A, de Baère T, Varin E, et al. Role of thermal ablation in colorectal cancer lung metastases. Cancers (Basel) 2021; 13: 908.

10 Inoue Y, Miki C, Hiro J, et al. Improved survival using multi-modality therapy in patients with lung metastases from colorectal cancer: a preliminary study. Oncol Rep 2005; 14: 1571–6.

Further reading

- Antonoff MB, Sofocleous CT, Callstrom M, et al. The roles of surgery, stereotactic radiation, and ablation for treatment of pulmonary metastases. J Thoracic Cardiovasc Surg 2021; 163: 495–502.

- de Baère T, Tselikas L, Gravel G, et al. Lung ablation: best practice/results/response assessment/role alongside other ablative therapies. Clin Radiol 2017; 72: 657–64.

- Venturini M, Cariati M, Marra P, et al. CIRSE standards of practice on thermal ablation of primary and secondary lung tumours. Cardiovasc Intervent Radiol 2020; 43: 667–83.

- Yuan Z, Wang Y, Zhang J, et al. A meta-analysis of clinical outcomes after radiofrequency ablation and microwave ablation for lung cancer and pulmonary metastases. J Am Coll Radiol 2019; 16: 302–14.

25 An older patient with stage I non-small-cell lung cancer

Mahaz Kayani, Peter Dickinson

Case history

An 82-year-old woman presented with a worsening cough, weight loss and fatigue. Her medical history included a previous T2aN0M0 left upper lobe pulmonary adenocarcinoma (treated with a left upper lobectomy 9 years earlier), ischaemic heart disease and chronic obstructive pulmonary disease (COPD). A CT scan showed stable changes in the left hemithorax but a new spiculated 2.5 cm right upper lobe mass. A PET-CT scan found the lesion to be FDG-avid: maximum standardized uptake value (SUV_{max}) 8.7; blood pool SUV_{max} 2.6; low-grade uptake within a right hilar lymph node (SUV_{max} 2.8). There was no evidence of distant metastases.

Endobronchial ultrasound sampling of the station R10 lymph node was adequate and negative for malignancy. Bronchial brushings were reported as strips of benign bronchial epithelium with no malignant cells. The patient underwent CT-guided biopsy of the upper lobe lesion, which confirmed non-small-cell lung cancer (NSCLC); immunostaining was consistent with squamous cell carcinoma. The final clinical and radiological stage was T1cN0M0. After discussion among the multidisciplinary team, she was referred to thoracic surgery.

At the surgical review it was noted that her exercise tolerance was 200 yards and she was breathless climbing a flight of stairs. Her ECOG performance status was 1 and her clinical frailty score was 3. The surgical team referred her for lung function testing and cardiopulmonary exercise testing: forced expiratory volume 1.10 l (50% predicted); diffusing capacity for carbon monoxide 43% predicted; maximal oxygen consumption (VO_{2max}) 12 ml/kg per min. After discussing the risks associated with surgery, the woman declined an operation.

She was referred for consideration of non-surgical treatment and offered stereotactic body radiotherapy (SBRT), which she accepted. The dosage was 55 Gy in five fractions, delivered on alternate days.

What was the goal of cancer treatment in this patient?

What is the evidence base for SBRT as a treatment for primary lung cancer?

How did her comorbidities affect her cancer treatment decisions?

Can all patients with stage I–IIA lung cancer be treated with SBRT?

What was the goal of cancer treatment in this patient?

The goal of treatment was cure. The size and position of the lesion were such that surgery and SBRT were possible radical treatment options. The decision regarding the eventual treatment modality was influenced by the patient's fitness and comorbidities as well as her personal beliefs and goals.

What is the evidence base for SBRT as a treatment for primary lung cancer?

SBRT is an advanced radiotherapy technique which delivers high doses of conformal radiation to a target, in a low number of treatment sessions. The dose delivered to the tumour is much greater than that delivered with conventional radical radiotherapy.

The Radiation Therapy Oncology Group (RTOG) 0236 study (ClinicalTrials.gov NCT00087438) was a landmark phase II trial that demonstrated the potential efficacy of SBRT in the management of patients with medically inoperable early-stage NSCLC.[1] In this single-arm study, 59 patients with T1 or T2 NSCLC were treated with SBRT. Primary tumour control was 97.6% at 3 years. Three year disease-free survival and overall survival (OS) were 48.3% and 55.8%, respectively. Seven patients (12.7%) experienced a grade 3 toxicity and two patients (3.6%) experienced a grade 4 toxicity. Further phase II trials (RTOG 0618, ClinicalTrials.gov NCT00551369[2]; RTOG 0915, ClinicalTrials.gov NCT00960999[3]; JCOG0403, ClinicalTrials.gov NCT00238875[4]) support these findings.

CHISEL, a phase III trial (ClinicalTrials.gov NCT01014130), confirmed that SBRT achieves superior local control compared with conventionally fractionated radiotherapy.[5] The local failure rate after SBRT was 14% vs 31% after conventional radiotherapy. While the data were immature, median OS, a secondary endpoint, was 5 years with SBRT vs 3 years with standard radiotherapy (HR 0.53; 95% CI 0.30, 0.94; $p=0.027$).

It has been difficult to establish whether radiotherapy or surgery leads to improved outcomes in patients with operable disease. Three phase III prospective randomized controlled trials (RCTs) comparing the use of surgery against SBRT for the management of early-stage NSCLC (ROSEL, ClinicalTrials.gov NCT00687986; STARS, ClinicalTrials.gov NCT00840749; American College of Surgeons Oncology Group Z4099, ClinicalTrials.gov NCT01336894) suffered from poor accrual and did not meet their recruitment targets. In 2015, a pooled analysis of patients who were enrolled into the ROSEL and STARS trials reported a statistically significant improvement in OS in patients treated with SBRT compared with surgery (HR 0.14).[6] There was no difference in local, regional or distant metastasis or in recurrence-free survival between the two groups. These findings should, however, be interpreted with caution owing to the low patient numbers and some differences in the design of each trial.

The SABRTooth feasibility study (ClinicalTrials.gov NCT02629458), which randomized higher risk patients between SBRT and surgery, also failed to recruit as planned.[7] One reason cited for low recruitment was pre-existing patient preference for a specific treatment modality. We await the results of further RCTs (STABLE-MATES, ClinicalTrials.gov NCT02468024; VALOR, ClinicalTrials.gov NCT02984761; POSTILV, ClinicalTrials.gov NCT01753414).

How did her comorbidities affect her cancer treatment decisions?

For individuals with operable lung tumours, the risks of perioperative morbidity and mortality must be considered carefully. To this end, preoperative physiological and safety tests are performed as parts of the presurgical assessment to risk stratify each patient and inform discussions around risks and benefits. At the very least, spirometry, a transfer factor for carbon monoxide test and a functional segment count to predict postoperative lung function should be performed.[8]

Cardiopulmonary exercise testing is a physiological testing procedure that can be used to estimate cardiopulmonary fitness. VO_{2max} has prognostic value and can be used to predict the likelihood of perioperative mortality and morbidity in patients being considered for surgery.[9] A VO_{2max} <10 ml/kg per min indicates a high risk of perioperative death and cardiopulmonary complications. NICE considers the acceptable cut-off to be 15 ml/kg per min.[10]

Even when accounting for cardiorespiratory fitness, it is known that elderly patients are less likely to receive curative treatment for early-stage lung cancers owing to a combination of comorbidity, frailty and perceived futility. An observational Dutch study demonstrated that increasing use of SBRT led to a survival improvement in elderly patients, while a similar improvement was not seen in patients managed surgically.[11]

There are no absolute cut-off values for lung function below which SBRT cannot be considered; however, patients must be counselled and consented appropriately. Reports have found that SBRT can be offered safely in patients with severe COPD.[12]

Can all patients with stage I–IIA lung cancer be treated with SBRT?

Not all early-stage lung cancers are suitable for treatment with SBRT. An early study showed that patients with hilar or central tumours were more likely to experience grades 3–5 toxicities when treated with SBRT.[13] Complications included bronchial stenosis, haemoptysis and fistulation. At 2 years, 83% of patients with peripheral tumours were free of severe toxicity compared with 54% of patients with perihilar/central tumours. Four out of six deaths in this study were in patients with central tumours. This led to the convention of not treating tumours within 2 cm of the proximal bronchial tree, commonly referred to as the 'no fly zone'.

Subsequent reports suggest that it may be possible to treat lesions within the 'no fly zone' with risk-adapted schedules and acceptable rates of toxicity.[14] The RTOG 0813 trial (ClinicalTrials. gov NCT00750269) enrolled patients with tumours either touching upon or within the no fly zone, demonstrating that at the highest dose level of 60 Gy in five fractions (12 Gy per fraction), dose-limiting toxicities occurred at a rate of 7.2%[15]; however, relatively few tumours were ultracentral (variably defined, but often considered to be <1 cm from the proximal bronchial tree). The HILUS trial investigated outcomes in patients with ultracentral tumours treated with SBRT.[16] Tumours that were within 1 cm of the trachea or main bronchus were associated with higher rates of toxicity, including eight cases of grade 5 haemoptysis.

Other relative contraindications to treatment with SBRT include concurrent delivery of systemic cancer therapies (outside a clinical trial) and the presence of lung fibrosis. In a systematic review of toxicity in patients with interstitial lung disease (ILD) treated with SBRT, the risk of treatment-related mortality and ILD-specific toxicity was estimated at 15.6% and 25%, respectively.[17]

Conclusion and learning points

- For stage I–IIA NSCLC, treatment with curative intent should be considered. Surgery and radiotherapy are treatment options.
- For medically inoperable, non-central stage I–IIA NSCLC, SBRT is the recommended treatment modality.
- For non-central NSCLC, SBRT is superior to conventional radiotherapy, in terms of local disease control, and has a favourable toxicity profile.

- The role of SBRT in the treatment of central and ultracentral lung tumours has not yet been fully defined; risk-adapted dose fractionation schedules may be required. Treating such tumours with SBRT is associated with an increased risk of significant toxicity.

- Trials comparing surgery and SBRT as treatment of operable stage I–IIA NSCLC have failed to recruit and report as planned; it is still debated as to whether there is clinical equipoise. Factors which influence choice of treatment modality for any given patient include respiratory function and cardiopulmonary exercise testing results, comorbidities, patient preference, and risk of perioperative morbidity and mortality.

- Further research is ongoing comparing SBRT with surgery in operable cases, to establish the safety of SBRT for central tumours and define its role in oligometastatic disease.

References

1 Timmerman R, Paulus R, Galvin J, et al. Stereotactic body radiation therapy for inoperable early stage lung cancer. JAMA 2010; 303: 1070–6.

2 Timmerman RD, Paulus R, Pass HI, et al. Stereotactic body radiation therapy for operable early-stage lung cancer: findings from the NRG Oncology RTOG 0618 trial. JAMA Oncol 2018; 4: 1263–6.

3 Videtic GM, Paulus R, Singh AK, et al. Long-term follow-up on NRG Oncology RTOG 0915 (NCCTG N0927): a randomized phase 2 study comparing 2 stereotactic body radiation therapy schedules for medically inoperable patients with stage I peripheral non-small cell lung cancer. Int J Radiat Oncol Biol Phys 2019; 103: 1077–84.

4 Nagata Y, Hiraoka M, Shibata T, et al. Prospective trial of stereotactic body radiation therapy for both operable and inoperable T1N0M0 non-small cell lung cancer: Japan Clinical Oncology Group Study JCOG0403. Int J Radiat Oncol Biol Phys 2015; 93: 989–96.

5 Ball D, Mai GT, Vinod S, et al. Stereotactic ablative radiotherapy versus standard radiotherapy in stage 1 non-small-cell lung cancer (TROG 09.02 CHISEL): a phase 3, open-label, randomised controlled trial. Lancet Oncol 2019; 20: 494–503.

6 Chang JY, Senan S, Paul MA, et al. Stereotactic ablative radiotherapy versus lobectomy for operable stage I non-small-cell lung cancer: a pooled analysis of two randomised trials. Lancet Oncol 2015; 16: 630–7.

7 Franks KN, McParland L, Webster J, et al. SABRTooth: a randomised controlled feasibility study of stereotactic ablative radiotherapy (SABR) with surgery in patients with peripheral stage I nonsmall cell lung cancer considered to be at higher risk of complications from surgical resection. Eur Respir J 2020; 56: 2000118.

8 Brunelli A, Kim AW, Berger KI, Addrizzo-Harris DJ. Physiologic evaluation of the patient with lung cancer being considered for resectional surgery: diagnosis and management of lung cancer, 3rd ed: American College of Chest Physicians evidence-based clinical practice guidelines. Chest 2013; 143 (5 suppl): e166–90S.

9 Ha D, Mazzone PJ, Ries AL, et al. The utility of exercise testing in patients with lung cancer. J Thorac Oncol 2016; 11: 1397–410.

10 NICE (2019, updated 2022). Lung cancer: diagnosis and management. NICE guideline NG122. Available from: www.nice.org.uk/guidance/ng122 (accessed 11 March 2022).

11 Palma D, Visser O, Lagerwaard FJ, et al. Impact of introducing stereotactic lung radiotherapy for elderly patients with stage I non-small-cell lung cancer: a population-based time-trend analysis. J Clin Oncol 2010; 28: 5153–9

12 Palma D, Lagerwaard F, Rodrigues G, et al. Curative treatment of stage I non-small-cell lung cancer in patients with severe COPD: stereotactic radiotherapy outcomes and systematic review. Int J Radiat Oncol Biol Phys 2012; 82: 1149–56.

13 Timmerman R, McGarry R, Yiannoutsos C, et al. Excessive toxicity when treating central tumors in a phase II study of stereotactic body radiation therapy for medically inoperable early-stage lung cancer. J Clin Oncol 2006; 24: 4833–9.

14 Senthi S, Haasbeek CJA, Slotman BJ, Senan S. Outcomes of stereotactic ablative radiotherapy for central lung tumours: a systematic review. Radiother Oncol 2013; 106: 276–82.

15 Bezjak A, Paulus R, Gaspar LE, et al. Safety and efficacy of a five-fraction stereotactic body radiotherapy schedule for centrally located non-small-cell lung cancer: NRG Oncology/RTOG 0813 trial. J Clin Oncol 2019; 37: 1316–25.

16 Lindberg K, Grozman V, Karlsson K, et al. The HILUS trial – a prospective Nordic multicenter phase 2 study of ultracentral lung tumors treated with stereotactic body radiotherapy. J Thorac Oncol 2021; 16: 1200–10.

17 Chen H, Senan S, Nossent EJ, et al. Treatment-related toxicity in patients with early-stage non-small cell lung cancer and coexisting interstitial lung disease: a systematic review. Int J Radiat Oncol Biol Phys 2017; 98: 622–31.

Further reading

- Royal College of Radiologists (2020). Radiotherapy for lung cancer – RCR consensus statements. Available from: www.rcr.ac.uk/publication/radiotherapy-lung-cancer-rcr-consensus-statements.
- UK SABR Consortium (2019). Stereotactic ablative radiotherapy (SABR): a resource. Version 6.1. Available from: www.sabr.org.uk/wp-content/uploads/2019/04/SABRconsortium-guidelines-2019-v6.1.0.pdf.

26 Locally advanced lung cancer

Ruhi Kanani, Shyamal Saujani, Suraiya Dubash, Ewan Mark Anderson

Case history

A 78-year-old woman presented with a left breast lump on a background of previously treated left-sided breast cancer. A staging ^{18}F-FDG PET-CT scan identified a new lung mass. The woman's medical history included a left breast lumpectomy, adjuvant left breast radiotherapy, previously treated endometrial cancer and anxiety.

The PET-CT scan revealed focally increased uptake in the left breast. Uptake was also seen in a 3×3.5 cm left upper lobe mass, and ipsilateral mediastinal lymph node disease was confirmed. A CT-guided biopsy of the lung lesion confirmed a squamous cell carcinoma of primary lung origin expressing 60% programmed death–ligand 1 (PD-L1). A contrast MRI scan of the head revealed no brain metastases. Lung function tests showed a forced expiratory volume of 85% and transfer factor for carbon monoxide of 81%. The new breast lump was diagnosed as a grade 2, hormone receptor-positive breast cancer.

The patient had T4N2M0 squamous cell lung cancer and grade 2 ductal carcinoma of the breast. Her case was discussed by the lung multidisciplinary team (MDT). The recommended treatment for the lung cancer was chemoradiotherapy followed by adjuvant immunotherapy. The breast cancer was to be treated with letrozole while the patient underwent lung cancer treatment. On completion of this treatment, she was to undergo a left mastectomy and axillary staging.

The patient was commenced on carboplatin and vinorelbine chemotherapy for two cycles concurrently with daily radiotherapy (55 Gy in 20 fractions over 4 weeks). She tolerated treatment well except for grade 1 fatigue and odynophagia, which was managed conservatively with supportive medication. A CT scan of the chest, abdomen and pelvis on completion of the chemoradiotherapy demonstrated a partial response of the lung cancer. She proceeded to have 1 year of adjuvant durvalumab immunotherapy, after which the breast cancer team proceeded with completion of the left-sided mastectomy and axillary staging. She remains under active surveillance from a lung cancer perspective with 3 monthly follow-up and regular surveillance scans.

What was the goal of cancer treatment in this patient?

What key investigations are required prior to treatment?

What are the different options for treatment and what is the evidence base for these treatments?

How did her comorbidities affect her cancer treatment decisions?

What are the indications for referral for genetic screening?

What services are available to support patients with high levels of anxiety?

What was the goal of cancer treatment in this patient?

Concurrent chemoradiotherapy may be offered with curative intent for patients with locally advanced lung cancer (stages IIB and IIIA–C) that is not amenable to surgical resection but that is encompassed within a radiotherapy field. This leads to an overall survival (OS) rate of 15–25% at 5 years.[1] Additional immunotherapy can be offered as maintenance for a year to further improve progression-free survival (PFS) and OS in patients with tumours expressing PD-L1 ($\geq$1%). Suitability for this treatment is dependent on the patient's comorbidities and baseline performance status.

What key investigations are required prior to treatment?

All patients with locally advanced lung cancer should be seen and assessed in clinic to determine their performance status and suitability for treatment. A full medical history should be obtained to ascertain comorbidities and any conditions from a cardiovascular, respiratory, autoimmune or renal perspective that may impede suitability for treatment. Staging should consist of a CT scan, an ^{18}F-FDG PET-CT scan, contrast MRI scan of the head, and histopathology (including PD-L1). Prior to chemoradiotherapy (in particular with cisplatin), baseline audiometry, nuclear medicine glomerular filtration rate and full spirometry testing should be carried out.

What are the different options for treatment and what is the evidence base for these treatments?

Definitive chemoradiotherapy is the standard of care across the UK and Europe, assuming patient fitness and consideration of relevant comorbidities (performance status 0–1).

Surgery alone

Management of stage III disease varies across clinical practice and by case. For single station N2 disease, the 2010 British Thoracic Society and the Society for Cardiothoracic Surgery guidelines on radical management of lung cancer recommend surgery in the first instance if the patient is fit enough.[2] The NICE Lung Cancer Diagnosis and Management Guidelines Group compared chemoradiotherapy, chemosurgery and chemoradiotherapy plus surgery.[3] They found that patients suitable for surgery should have chemoradiotherapy followed by surgery, as this was more cost-effective and associated with fewer adverse events and longer PFS compared with chemoradiotherapy or chemosurgery alone. However, these recommendations are based on historic trial data and do not factor in modern day treatment techniques. The most common approach is therefore concurrent chemoradiotherapy for confirmed stage III N2 nodal disease. This involves platinum doublet-based chemotherapy with radical dose radiotherapy. Some of these patients may be considered for surgical resection after chemoradiotherapy, depending on the response, namely those with minimal N2 disease upfront. If there is not minimal N2 disease, patients will require a pneumonectomy, which is associated with high mortality rates. For patients with N3 (encompassable within a radiotherapy field) or stage IV disease where oligometastatic disease is identified, concurrent chemoradiotherapy would remain the treatment of choice.[4]

Chemotherapy plus radiotherapy vs radiotherapy alone

Marino et al.[5] demonstrated a reduction in mortality (by 24% in year 1 and by 30% in year 2) with the addition of cisplatin chemotherapy to concurrent radiotherapy compared with radiotherapy alone. A meta-analysis of randomized controlled trials (RCTs) demonstrated reduced overall risk of death (8%) at 2 years and improved overall survival benefit (HR 0.71; 95% CI 0.64, 0.80) (*n*=1607), as well as improvement in PFS (HR 0.69; 95% CI 0.58, 0.81; I^2=45%) (*n*=1405) with the addition of concurrent chemotherapy compared with radiotherapy alone.[6] As expected, the addition of chemotherapy increased the prevalence of side effects such as anaemia, neutropenia and oesophagitis.

Chemotherapy plus radiotherapy concurrently vs sequentially

A meta-analysis by the NSCLC Collaborative Group reviewed six trials (*N*=1205) comparing concurrent with sequential chemoradiation.[7] Concurrent radiotherapy yielded a 5.7% survival benefit at 3 years and a 4.5% survival benefit at 5 years. A trial by the Radiation Therapy Oncology Group (RTOG 9410; ClinicalTrials.gov NCT01134861) similarly demonstrated improved median OS at 5 years with concurrent chemoradiotherapy (*n*=610), although there were increased rates of grade 3 non-haematological toxicity.[8] The SOCCAR trial (ClinicalTrials.gov NCT00309972) demonstrated a 4% improvement in survival at 2 years with concurrent chemotherapy.[9] Furuse et al.[10] led a phase III randomized study demonstrating improvement in survival up to 5 years in the concurrent treatment arm. A Cochrane meta-analysis collating information from six RCTs demonstrated a 10% absolute benefit at 2 years compared with sequential chemoradiotherapy.[6] With regard to tolerance, there was no statistically significant difference in treatment-related deaths but there was an increased risk of oesophagitis.

Chemotherapy plus radiotherapy concurrently plus adjuvant durvalumab

The phase III PACIFIC study (ClinicalTrials.gov NCT02125461) compared the addition of the PD-L1 antibody durvalumab as consolidation treatment following completion of two cycles of chemoradiotherapy. A total of 713 patients with locally advanced, unresectable non-small-cell lung cancer were randomized in a 2:1 ratio to durvalumab or placebo. In April 2022, 5 year follow-up data showed improved OS with durvalumab vs placebo (47.5 months vs 29.1 months, respectively) as well as improved PFS (16.9 months vs 5.6 months, respectively). Compared with placebo, durvalumab demonstrated improved 5 year survival rates (42.9% vs 33.4%, respectively) and 5 year PFS rates (33.1% vs 19%, respectively).[11-13] Grade 3 or 4 adverse events were similar in both groups in the primary analysis.[11,12]

How did her comorbidities affect her cancer treatment decisions?

Significant personal cancer history

The patient had a history of endometrial cancer and two active cancers requiring treatment: localized breast cancer and locally advanced lung cancer. Decisions regarding treatment in these cases are often complex and require discussion in an MDT meeting because of limited evidence in the literature. Treatment approaches are mainly guided by treating the tumour, with the most significant impact on prognosis, depending on the aim of treatment (either curative or palliative), availability of common systemic treatment regimens, anticipation of potential treatment-related complications, tumour profiling and previous treatments, and risk of cumulative toxicity.[14] In this scenario, both synchronous tumours could be treated with curative intent. The lung cancer was felt to be more aggressive as it was the more advanced cancer and therefore more likely to negatively impact on prognosis. The breast cancer (hormone-sensitive) was initially treated with upfront letrozole.

Re-irradiation

The patient had received radiotherapy to the left breast 30 years earlier. The left lung and heart would have therefore received some radiation. Decisions regarding the safety of re-irradiation are made on an individual case-by-case basis depending on the field treated, the dose delivered and the recovery time. Research suggests safety and efficacy with thorax re-irradiation.[15,16] There is increasing evidence of recovery of certain organs, such as the lung, following a period of radiotherapy, allowing further radiotherapy to be delivered to overlapping fields.[17] Re-irradiation is, however, linked to an increased risk of normal tissue damage and late-onset side effects.[18] It is therefore important to carefully consider the radiobiology and factor it into decisions regarding fractionation, delivery and field size, in close collaboration with clinical oncology specialists and the medical physics team.[18] Taking this into account, in the present case it was felt safe to deliver full treatment dose radiotherapy as per standard of care.

What are the indications for referral for genetic screening?

The patient had a history of endometrial cancer, previously treated breast cancer, a locally re-current breast cancer and lung cancer. All patients with a history of multiple cancers should be referred for genetic screening. Risk factors for multiple primaries can be due to genetic predisposition or lifestyle factors such as smoking. Previous treatment (endocrine treatment for breast cancer and risk of consequent endometrial cancer) may also play a role, as can long-term surveillance of these patients (picking up incidental primaries or increased radiation risk with imaging). Obtaining a clear family history is vital. Genetic screening can highlight underlying mutations that can be targeted directly and allow treatment of more than one tumour at any one time. It can also highlight any preventative and surveillance measures following completion of treatment. Many UK oncology centres have a linked genetic referral service for patients who are considered high risk, based on centre-specific referral criteria, and also for patients who demonstrate high levels of clinical suspicion that do not specifically meet the pre-set referral criteria.

What services are available to support patients with high levels of anxiety?

Anxiety levels are high in cancer patients: 19% are reported to have clinical levels of anxiety, with more demonstrating subclinical levels.[19] Depression and anxiety are linked to poorer quality of life, poorer compliance and tolerance of treatment, as well as poorer survival.[20,21] It is important to consider pharmaceutical support and referral for psychological support as appropriate.

Conclusion and learning points

- Stage III lung cancer can be treated with curative intent with concurrent chemoradiotherapy or surgery depending on resectability and fitness of the patient.
- Concurrent chemoradiotherapy is superior to sequential chemoradiotherapy and radiotherapy alone.
- It is important to take a full clinical history, including a medical history, and clearly assess fitness and performance status to help guide the most appropriate management plan.
- It is important to consider previous radiation and chemotherapy exposure and factor this into patient care plans.

- Careful consideration of family history and medical history of cancer are key to help identify any genetic component that may alter management or guide further surveillance.

- In addition to treating the physical health of a patient, a focus on psychological and mental well-being and rehabilitation is important in providing holistic care to cancer patients.

References

1 Vrankar M, Stanic K. Long-term survival of locally advanced stage III non-small cell lung cancer patients treated with chemoradiotherapy and perspectives for the treatment with immunotherapy. Radiol Oncol 2018; 52: 281–8.

2 Lim E, Baldwin D, Beckles M, et al. Guidelines on the radical management of patients with lung cancer. Thorax 2010; 65 (suppl 3): iii1–27.

3 NICE (2019, updated 2022). Lung cancer: diagnosis and management. NICE guideline NG122. Available from: www.nice.org.uk/guidance/NG122 (accessed 2 January 2023).

4 Conibear J. Rationale for concurrent chemoradiotherapy for patients with stage III non-small-cell lung cancer. Br J Cancer 2020; 123: 10–17.

5 Marino P, Preatoni A, Cantoni A. Randomized trials of radiotherapy alone versus combined chemotherapy and radiotherapy in stages IIIa and IIIb nonsmall cell lung cancer. A meta-analysis. Cancer 1995; 76: 593–601.

6 O'Rourke N, Roqué I Figuls M, Farré Bernadó N, Macbeth F. Concurrent chemoradiotherapy in non-small cell lung cancer. Cochrane Database Syst Rev 2010; 6: CD002140.

7 Aupérin A, Le Péchoux C, Rolland E, et al. Meta-analysis of concomitant versus sequential radiochemotherapy in locally advanced non-small-cell lung cancer. J Clin Oncol 2010; 28: 2181–90.

8 Curran WJ Jr, Paulus R, Langer CJ, et al. Sequential vs concurrent chemoradiation for stage III non-small cell lung cancer: randomized phase III trial RTOG 9410. J Natl Cancer Inst 2011; 103: 1452–60.

9 Maguire J, Khan I, McMenemin R, et al. SOCCAR: a randomised phase II trial comparing sequential versus concurrent chemotherapy and radical hypofractionated radiotherapy in patients with inoperable stage III non-small cell lung cancer and good performance status. Eur J Cancer 2014; 50: 2939–49.

10 Furuse K, Fukuoka M, Kawahara M, et al. Phase III study of concurrent versus sequential thoracic radiotherapy in combination with mitomycin, vindesine, and cisplatin in unresectable stage III non-small-cell lung cancer. J Clin Oncol 1999; 17: 2692–9.

11 Antonia SJ, Villegas A, Daniel D, et al. Overall survival with durvalumab after chemoradiotherapy in stage III NSCLC. N Engl J Med 2018; 379: 2342–50.

12 Hui R, Özgüroğlu M, Villegas A, et al. Patient-reported outcomes with durvalumab after chemoradiotherapy in stage III, unresectable non-small-cell lung cancer (PACIFIC): a randomised, controlled, phase 3 study. Lancet Oncol 2019; 20: 1670–80.

13 Spigel DR, Faivre-Finn C, Gray JE, et al. Five-year survival outcomes from the PACIFIC trial: durvalumab after chemoradiotherapy in stage III non-small-cell lung cancer. J Clin Oncol 2022; 40: 1301.

14 Vogt A, Schmid S, Heinimann K, et al. Multiple primary tumours: challenges and approaches, a review. ESMO Open 2017; 2: e000172.

15 Schröder C, Stiefel I, Tanadini-Lang S, et al. Re-irradiation in the thorax – an analysis of efficacy and safety based on accumulated EQD2 doses. Radiother Oncol 2020; 152: 56–62.

16 Sumita K, Harada H, Asakura H, et al. Re-irradiation for locoregionally recurrent tumors of the thorax: a single-institution, retrospective study. Radiat Oncol 2016; 11: 1–8.

17 Nieder C. Second re-irradiation: a delicate balance between safety and efficacy. Phys Med 2019; 58: 155–8.

18 Dörr W, Gabryś D. The principles and practice of re-irradiation in clinical oncology: an overview. Clin Oncol 2018; 30: 67–72.

19 Linden W, Vodermaier A, MacKenzie R, Greig D. Anxiety and depression after cancer diagnosis: prevalence rates by cancer type, gender, and age. J Affect Disord 2012; 141: 343–51.

20 Brintzenhofe-Szoc KM, Levin TT, Li Y, et al. Mixed anxiety/depression symptoms in a large cancer cohort: prevalence by cancer type. Psychosomatics 2009; 50: 383–91.

21 Wang YH, Li JQ, Shi JF, et al. Depression and anxiety in relation to cancer incidence and mortality: a systematic review and meta-analysis of cohort studies. Mol Psychiatry 2020; 25: 1487–99.

Further reading

- Cox JD, Le Chevalier T, Arriagada R, et al. Management of unresectable non-small cell carcinoma of the lung (NSCLC). Lung Cancer 2003; 42: 15–16.

- Dillman RO, Herndon J, Seagren SL, et al. Improved survival in stage III non-small-cell lung cancer: seven-year follow-up of Cancer and Leukemia Group B (CALGB) 8433 trial. J Natl Cancer Inst 1996; 88: 1210–15.

- Evison M. The current treatment landscape in the UK for stage III NSCLC. Br J Cancer 2020; 123: 3 9.

- Gridelli C, Aapro M, Ardizzoni A, et al. Treatment of advanced non-small-cell lung cancer in the elderly: results of an international expert panel. J Clin Oncol 2005; 23: 3125–37.

- Maconachie R, Mercer T, Navani N, McVeigh G. Lung cancer: diagnosis and management: summary of updated NICE guidance. BMJ 2019; 364: 1049.

- Rolland E, Le Pechoux C, Curran WJ, et al. Concomitant radio-chemotherapy (CT-RT) versus sequential CT-RT In locally advanced non-small-cell lung cancer (NSCLC): a meta-analysis using individual patient data (IPD) from randomised clinical trials (RCTs). Int J Radiat Oncol Biol Phys 2007; 69 (suppl 5).

27 Use of fiducial markers in navigational bronchoscopy for lung cancer resection

Arvind Muthirevula, Nilanjan Chaudhuri

Case histories

Case A

A 65-year-old man with a ypT3pN2R0 Dukes' C1 moderately differentiated adenocarcinoma of the rectum was diagnosed on surveillance imaging with a slow-growing subcentimetre (<1 cm) lung nodule in the right upper lobe. The multidisciplinary team thought it could be either a primary lung tumour or a metastatic tumour. Owing to the small size of the lesion, neither percutaneous CT-guided biopsy nor standard diagnostic navigational bronchoscopy was an ideal modality to obtain a tissue sample. It was therefore decided to localize the pulmonary nodule using fiducial marker placement with the help of navigational bronchoscopy. This was followed by a fluoroscopy-guided uniportal thoracoscopic wedge resection of the lung. Histopathology examination confirmed the nodule to be a metastatic colorectal deposit. The lesion could not be palpated intraoperatively, but the prior fiducial marker placement allowed it to be easily localized with fluoroscopy (Figure 27.1), thus avoiding the morbidity of a larger incision and further uncertainty of being able to reliably palpate such a small pulmonary nodule.

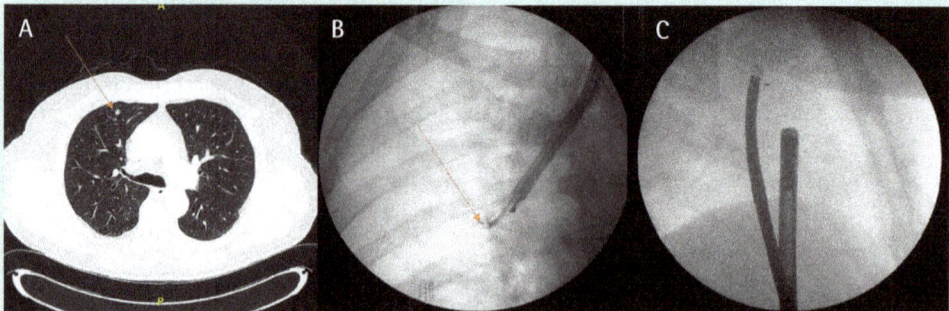

Figure 27.1 (A) CT image representing the subcentimetric nodule (arrow). (B) Locating guidewire with deployed fiducial marker (arrow) on fluoroscopy. (C) Localization of the fiducial marker with an instrument.

Case B

A 74-year-old man had a previous right upper lobectomy for a pT1bpN2R0 adenocarcinoma of the lung and had declined adjuvant chemotherapy. He was referred for biopsy of one of the multiple right-sided lung lesions found on surveillance imaging, to rule out whether the lesions were recurrent or a new primary with metastases. Comorbidities included ischaemic heart disease with prior angioplasty, hypertension and prediabetes. We performed a navigational bronchoscopy and placed a fiducial marker for localization, as we anticipated that dense pleural adhesions from the previous operation might make it difficult for us to approach and identify the pulmonary nodule/s. A mini-thoracotomy and rib resection were carried out directly over the lesion because of the expected adhesions since it was a redo operation. We encountered dense adhesions, but the fluoroscopy helped to localize the site (Figure 27.2). A limited dissection and wedge resection were performed with blood loss of only 50 ml; otherwise, the dissection would have been extensive and with much greater blood loss. Histology suggested recurrent lung cancer in the lung. The patient was commenced on systemic treatment with chemotherapeutic drugs based on the diagnosis.

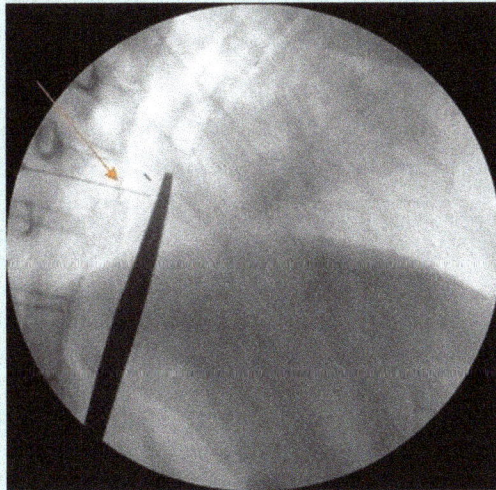

Figure 27.2 Deployed fiducial marker localization. Note the needle (arrow) which directed the incision.

Why do we need to use image-guided techniques to localize lesions?

What are the prerequisites for this procedure?

How should the procedure be performed?

When have we found the procedure to be most useful?

What modalities currently exist in localization?

Where else could the placement of markers be beneficial?

Why do we need to use image-guided techniques to localize lesions?

The advent of low-dose CT screening for lung cancer has increased the detection rate of small pulmonary nodules.[1] In light of the lesions' small size or ground-glass nature, a regular biopsy would be difficult to perform and would carry a low yield, thus requiring a surgical biopsy. Either an open or a thoracoscopic procedure can be used for carrying out a surgical biopsy. Since thoracoscopic procedures have comparable long-term outcomes, better cosmesis, less pain and a reduced inflammatory process compared with open procedures, they have become the procedure of choice for biopsy. If, however, the lesions are deeper or have a less solid component, digital or instrument-assisted palpation is difficult or unhelpful; therefore, different techniques have been developed to help localize these lesions and aid their resection with smaller incisions.

What are the prerequisites for this procedure?

In addition to the standard requirements for a routine thoracoscopic surgical procedure, there are several other factors that need to be considered.

- A surgical team familiar with all aspects of the procedure.
- A CT scan of the chest with a slice thickness of 1 mm at an overlapping interval of 0.8 mm.[2]
- Digital Imaging and Communications in Medicine information from the scan needs to be uploaded into the i-Logic Software system which helps in reconstructing a three-dimensional airway tree.[2]
- Prior planning of an airway path to the target based on the reconstruction.
- Sufficient radiation protective gear.
- Effective communication with the radiographers for fluoroscopy availability to reduce time delays.
- Theatre set up to accommodate the equipment.

How should the procedure be performed?

After obtaining their informed consent, the patient will initially be placed in a supine position and ventilated with a single-lumen endotracheal tube, followed by navigational bronchoscopy. The operator steers the locator guidewire to about a centimetre or so proximal to the target. The team then uses fluoroscopy to locate the guidewire in the lung and deploy the fiducial marker. Following this, the patient is intubated with a double-lumen tube to facilitate single lung isolation for a thoracoscopic procedure and changed to a lateral decubitus position. The surgeon then uses a thoracoscopic or open surgical approach, as appropriate, using fluoroscopy to locate the fiducial marker in the lung as well as resect the lesion with an adequate surgical margin. The operator then uses X-ray to confirm the location of the nodule along with the fiducial marker in the resected specimen. Ideally, this would require a hybrid theatre with a cone beam CT scanner, but we employ fluoroscopy as a cheaper alternative.

When have we found the procedure to be most useful?

We have found the procedure most useful for:

- small lesions that are difficult to palpate;
- lesions that are not superficial;
- redo operations, to guide the incision and limit dissection by pinpointing the location of the lesion;
- emphysema or fibrosis of the lungs where it is difficult to palpate.

In our experience with 33 cases, we found the fiducial marker to be very useful. In most cases, we could not palpate the lesions by thoracoscopy, as most were subcentimetric in size. However, we did experience some difficulties, especially in our initial learning curve with the procedure. In one of the patients, we had to perform a reoperation in a short time as the histopathology revealed that we had missed the lesion. We had left the fiducial marker during the first procedure as the fibrosis of the lung made lesion palpation difficult and we felt we had the lesion resected (Figure 27.3). A postoperative CT scan revealed, however, that the lesion had been missed in the initial procedure and it was adjacent to the fiducial marker. We had to reoperate and excise the lesion with the help of fluoroscopy again.

In another of our cases, our patient had had a right upper lobectomy and later a left upper lobectomy, and now presented with a nodule in the left lower lobe without a prior diagnosis. We planned for resection to obtain a biopsy and a possible attempt at cure. The patient, however, was not fit for a lower lobectomy, which meant we were limited to a wedge resection or a segmentectomy. Since this was a redo procedure, the lung was densely adherent to the chest wall and mediastinum. During the fluoroscopic evaluation, we realized the fiducial marker was close to the lower lobe's pulmonary artery. The lobectomy procedure had to be abandoned because it was too risky: given his prior resections, he would be at higher risk in terms of his respiratory function. In this particular case, the fiducial marker was crucial in averting a complication.

What modalities currently exist in localization?

A variety of options are currently available to localize the nodules, each having pros and cons (Table 27.1).[3]

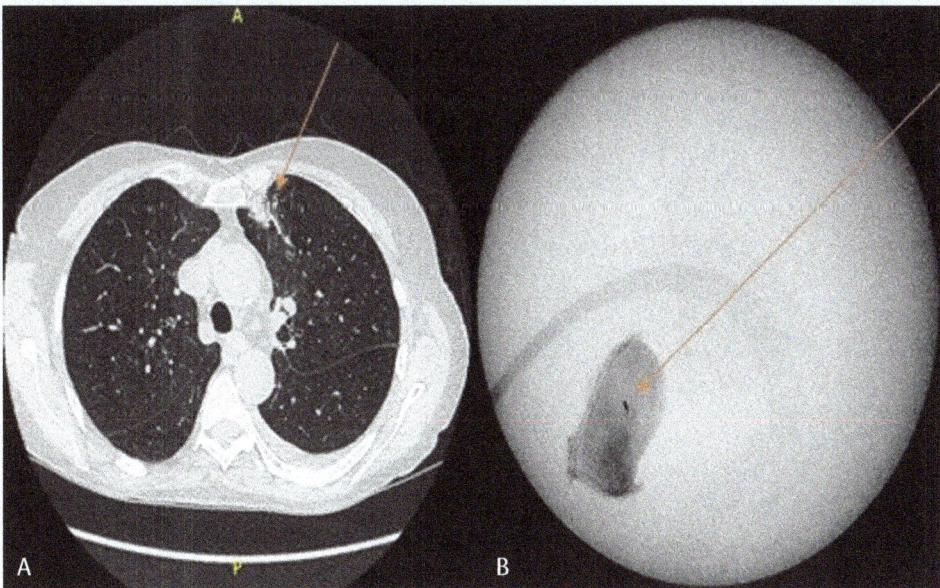

Figure 27.3 (A) Imaging following prior surgery showing lesion adjacent to the previously deployed fiducial marker (arrow). (B) Fiducial marker (arrow) in the lesion once the specimen is retrieved.

Table 27.1 Techniques of localization of pulmonary nodules in thoracoscopic surgery.

	Advantages	Disadvantages
CT-guided		
Hook wire localization (oldest and probably most used technique)	Acceptable successful localization rate (95%)[4] Short localization duration Intraoperatively, no need for fluoroscopy and, hence, no radiation exposure	Dislodgement Pneumothorax Focal parenchymal haemorrhage Subcutaneous emphysema Massive air embolism Not useful for some locations (diaphragm, apex, near cardiac/great vessels)
Dye localization (methylene blue)	High success rate Short localization duration No radiation exposure No limitation based on location of lesions	Diffusion into adjacent parenchyma Pneumothorax Focal parenchymal haemorrhage Anaphylaxis to dye (rare)
Micro coil (platinum) and fiducial (gold) marker placement	Acceptable success rate (97%)[5] No extracorporeal wire	Requires fluoroscopy, so radiation exposure is present Migration (3%)[5] Air embolism Fiducial marker embolism Pneumothorax Haemothorax Focal parenchymal haemorrhage
Contrast medium injection (water-insoluble barium, Lipiodol)	Will be retained for a long time with limited diffusion, so the procedure can be done in a later setting A reported success rate of 100%[6]	Requires fluoroscopy, so radiation exposure is present Barium may mimic lesions and also elicit inflammatory reactions affecting diagnosis Pneumothorax Minimal haemothorax Air embolism Contrast embolism
Radiotracer-guided localization (^{99}Tc gamma-emitting radioisotopes attached to large albumin molecules)	High success rate (100%)[7] Isotopes can remain stable for 24 h, so surgery can be done leisurely	Highly facility-dependent Radiation exposure Pneumothorax Haemothorax Focal parenchymal haemorrhage
Dual localization (using a hook wire and radiotracer/ Lipiodol)	Higher success rate as it combines both techniques[8]	Highly facility-dependent Radiation exposure Pneumothorax May be time-consuming

	Advantages	Disadvantages
CT-guided localization in hybrid theatres	Invasive localization can be done under anaesthesia Salvage CT scan available if first localization fails Less possibility of complications like pneumothorax or haemothorax Provides information on resection margin	Availability of facility Radiation exposure
Bronchoscopic-guided		
Electromagnetic navigational bronchoscopy	Multiple lesions can be targeted in one setting Done under anaesthesia, so less discomfort for patients Complications like pneumothorax or haemothorax are not of much concern	Availability of facility Radiation exposure
Other		
Intraoperative ultrasound	No radiation exposure Can be applied to any pleural surface	Requires experienced sonographers Requires complete collapse of lungs, so emphysema makes it difficult to localize Ground-glass lesions are difficult to localize
Intraoperative near-infrared imaging (indocyanine green injection 4 h before surgery)	Can detect impalpable lesions and resect with good margins Can facilitate small, invisible, multiple lung malignancies intraoperatively	False-positive and -negative fluorescence Tissue penetration limitations

- CT-guided techniques:
  - hook wire localization;
  - dye localization;
  - micro coil and fiducial marker placement;
  - contrast medium injection;
  - radiotracer-guided localization;
  - dual localization;
  - CT-guided localization in hybrid theatres.

- Bronchoscopic-guided techniques:
  - electromagnetic navigational bronchoscopy.
- Other techniques:
  - intraoperative ultrasound;
  - intraoperative near-infrared imaging.

Where else could the placement of markers be beneficial?

Navigational bronchoscopy with fiducial marker deployment is also useful to direct stereotactic body radiotherapy in lung cancer treatment.[9]

Conclusion and learning points

- Lung screening results in increased detection of small-sized or ground-glass nodules.
- Thoracoscopic procedures are the current way ahead for biopsy of these otherwise impalpable nodules.
- Various modalities currently exist to aid the surgeon to perform these procedures with a minimally invasive approach; bronchoscopic localization with placement of a radiopaque marker is one of these options.
- A hybrid operating room for intraoperative localization of these indeterminate lung nodules could be a future trend as it could both reduce patient discomfort and be more cost-effective.
- The use of fluoroscopy as an alternative to equipping a hybrid theatre means this procedure can be performed on a smaller budget and at smaller centres. The therapeutic effectiveness looks reasonable in our experience.

References

1 National Lung Screening Trial Research Team, Aberle DR, Adams AM, et al. Reduced lung-cancer mortality with low-dose computed tomographic screening. N Engl J Med 2011; 365: 395–409.

2 Nabavizadeh N, Zhang J, Elliott DA, et al. Electromagnetic navigational bronchoscopy-guided fiducial markers for lung stereotactic body radiation therapy: analysis of safety, feasibility, and interfraction stability. J Bronchology Interv Pulmonol 2014; 21: 123–30.

3 Lin MW, Chen JS. Image-guided techniques for localizing pulmonary nodules in thoracoscopic surgery. J Thorac Dis 2016; 8 (suppl 9): S749–55.

4 Chen YR, Yeow KM, Lee JY, et al. CT-guided hook wire localization of subpleural lung lesions for video-assisted thoracoscopic surgery (VATS). J Formos Med Assoc 2007; 106: 911–18.

5 Mayo JR, Clifton JC, Powell TI, et al. Lung nodules: CT-guided placement of microcoils to direct video-assisted thoracoscopic surgical resection. Radiology 2009; 250: 576–85.

6 Watanabe K, Nomori H, Ohtsuka T, et al. Usefulness and complications of computed tomography-guided Lipiodol marking for fluoroscopy-assisted thoracoscopic resection of small pulmonary nodules: experience with 174 nodules. J Thorac Cardiovasc Surg 2006; 132: 320–4.

7 Chella A, Lucchi M, Ambrogi MC, et al. A pilot study of the role of Tc-99 radionuclide in localization of pulmonary nodular lesions for thoracoscopic resection. Eur J Cardiothorac Surg 2000; 18: 17–21.

8 Kang DY, Kim HK, Kim YK, et al. Needlescopy-assisted resection of pulmonary nodule after dual localisation. Eur Respir J 2011; 37: 13–17.

9 Bowling MR, Folch EE, Khandhar SJ, et al. Fiducial marker placement with electromagnetic navigation bronchoscopy: a subgroup analysis of the prospective, multicenter NAVIGATE study. Ther Adv Respir Dis 2019; 13: 1753466619841234.

Further reading

- Chan JWY, Lau RWH, Ng CSH. Electromagnetic navigation bronchoscopy fiducial marker margin identification plus triple dye for complete lung nodule resection. JTCVS Tech 2020; 3: 329–33.

28 Surgical management of pancreatic ductal adenocarcinoma

Zaed Hamady

Case history

A 70-year-old man with a history of hypertension and Barrett's oesophagus underwent a CT scan because of persistent epigastric pain, unintentional weight loss and new-onset diabetes (HbA$_{1c}$ 57 mmol/mol). He also had a 30 pack-year smoking history. Routine blood tests and tumour markers revealed a raised CA 19-9 level of 93 U/ml (normal range 0–35 U/ml). Cross-sectional CT imaging showed heterogeneity in the pancreatic neck with upstream pancreatic ductal dilation and a trace of peri-pancreatic free fluid. A subsequent MRI scan showed a 21 mm area of hyperenhancement, without the presence of a definitive mass lesion. A further endoscopic ultrasound (EUS) scan showed the presence of a coarse lobular pancreatic parenchyma with microcalcification and pancreatic duct dilation to 4 mm. The cytology report following EUS-guided fine needle aspiration biopsy described findings consistent with chronic pancreatitis.

Owing to the presence of new-onset diabetes, marked weight loss and elevated CA 19-9, there was some hesitancy in considering chronic pancreatitis as a definitive diagnosis; consequently, the decision was taken to follow up with a repeat MRI scan after 6 months. The follow-up MRI scan revealed the presence of a definitive mass in the pancreatic neck, worsening pancreatic duct dilation (8 mm) and tumour abutment of the portal vein. Repeat EUS confirmed the presence of a hypoechoic mass in the neck of the pancreas causing stricturing of the pancreatic duct. Fine needle aspiration biopsy was repeated and the cytology demonstrated atypical cells suggestive of an adenocarcinoma.

Owing to the presence of the tumour in the pancreatic neck, an open subtotal pancreatectomy was initially planned. However, on intraoperative assessment a bulky mass with tumour abutment of the portal vein was seen. After careful assessment the decision was made to undertake a total pancreatectomy and splenectomy with portal vein resection and reconstruction. The portal vein reconstruction was intraoperatively complicated by loss of flow due to thrombus formation in a branch of the superior mesenteric vein. The anastomosis was therefore reconstructed and a Doppler ultrasound scan confirmed portal venous flow.

Postoperatively the patient was closely monitored in a high-dependency unit. Once oral intake was established, CREON (oral pancreatic enzymes) was restarted to optimize his nutritional status and he was advised to continue on this for the rest of his life. Additionally, he was started on insulin and closely managed to optimize his glycaemic control. Prior to discharge, post-splenectomy vaccinations were given and he was prescribed oral phenoxymethylpenicillin to reduce the risk of overwhelming post-splenectomy infection.

The final histology report described a 19 mm tumour with chronic inflammatory changes in the pancreas. As none of the 33 sampled lymph nodes demonstrated any evidence of metastasis, the final TNM classification was T1cN0M0 (stage IA). The patient was seen in clinic 2 weeks after the procedure to ensure optimal healing of the surgical wound and referred to the oncology team for consideration of adjuvant chemotherapy.

What is the significance of new-onset diabetes in the diagnosis of pancreatic ductal adenocarcinoma (PDAC)?

How useful is CA 19-9 in the detection of PDAC?

What is the relationship between chronic pancreatitis and PDAC?

How did the location of the tumour dictate the operative approach?

How does the postoperative management differ between those who have undergone a Whipple's procedure or distal pancreatectomy compared with a total pancreatectomy?

What is the significance of new-onset diabetes in the diagnosis of PDAC?

In a US population-based study (N=2122), Chari et al.[1] found that almost 1% of individuals aged 50 and over with new-onset diabetes were diagnosed with PDAC within 36 months of first meeting the criteria for diabetes diagnosis. This is thought to be due to a paraneoplastic phenomenon, the exact pathophysiology of which is poorly understood. Sharma et al.[2] recently reported a 5.4-fold increase in the relative risk of developing PDAC in individuals over the age of 50 diagnosed with new-onset diabetes (within 12 months). A diagnosis of new-onset diabetes is an important consideration when assessing a patient, as recognition of such risk factors will help to identify those who may benefit from additional investigation by cross-sectional imaging.

How useful is CA 19-9 in the detection of PDAC?

CA 19-9 is a well-documented serum biomarker associated with PDAC; it has a sensitivity of 79–81% and a specificity of 82–90%.[3] It is not routinely used as a diagnostic biomarker but is used to monitor response to systemic treatment, as a markedly elevated CA 19-9 level is associated with a poor prognosis.[4] It may be elevated in other obstructive biliary conditions, limiting its utility as a screening test to diagnose PDAC.[5]

What is the relationship between chronic pancreatitis and PDAC?

Chronic pancreatitis increases the risk of developing PDAC; some studies have reported an eight-fold increased risk of PDAC within 5 years of a diagnosis of chronic pancreatitis.[6] In one study, over 30% of those who underwent surgery for chronic pancreatitis were found to have a synchronous PDAC.[7]

Owing to the inflammatory nature of chronic pancreatitis, a mass lesion can be found on imaging in approximately 10–20% of patients.[8] These mass-forming lesions can appear identical to PDAC on cross-sectional imaging, thus making a definitive diagnosis challenging. Subtle radiological features such as reduced calcification and abutment/invasion of blood vessels may provide valuable clues in making the diagnosis.

How did the location of the tumour dictate the operative approach?

The pancreas has five anatomical parts: the uncinate process, head, neck, body and tail. The neck is the region superior to the portal vein and superior mesenteric artery. A distal pancreatectomy describes resection of the body and tail, while a subtotal pancreatectomy refers to excision of the neck, body and tail. Usually, tumours of the neck of the pancreas are resected by a subtotal pancreatectomy and splenectomy owing to the neck of the pancreas being derived from the dorsal bud during embryological development.[9–11] The embryological derivation dictates that the lymphatics flow from peri-pancreatic lymph node stations towards the tail of the pancreas and splenic hilum. Thus a subtotal pancreatectomy will ensure that an optimal lymph node harvest is obtained. Although located in the neck of the pancreas, our patient's tumour was partially encasing the portal vein, making it borderline resectable. A portal vein resection was thus required and could not have been undertaken safely with the pancreatic head and uncinate process *in situ*. Undertaking a total pancreatectomy also abrogates the possibility of a postoperative anastomotic leak/pancreatic fistula, which may result in significant complications and morbidity. The decision, however, comes at the cost of rendering the patient diabetic, nutritionally dependent on oral exocrine pancreatic enzymes and immune-compromised from the splenectomy.

How does the postoperative management differ between those who have undergone a Whipple's procedure or distal pancreatectomy compared with a total pancreatectomy?

Studies comparing morbidity and mortality after total pancreatectomy and splenectomy have not reported inferiority when compared with a pancreatico-duodenectomy.[12] The primary advantage of undertaking a total pancreatectomy is that it removes the potential for a postoperative anastomotic leak from the pancreatico-jejunostomy and removes the possibility of involved margins on pathological analysis. However, this comes at the cost of development of insulin-dependent diabetes in all patients who undergo a total pancreatectomy. Only 15% of non-diabetic patients who undergo a Whipple's procedure for malignancy develop diabetes 6 months after the procedure.[13] Interestingly, resolution of preoperative diabetes was observed in a subgroup of patients who underwent pancreatic resection.[14] Both groups of patients will require supplemental enzyme therapy for pancreatic exocrine insufficiency. Total pancreatectomy is almost always associated with a splenectomy and these patients are susceptible to overwhelming sepsis from encapsulated organisms (*Escherichia coli, Haemophilus influenzae, Neisseria meningitidis* and *Streptococcus pneumoniae*) and must be vaccinated prophylactically 2 weeks before or after the procedure. These patients also need to be started on phenoxymethylpenicillin to reduce the risk of overwhelming post-splenectomy infection.

Conclusion and learning points

- Diabetes and PDAC have a strong association.
- Chronic pancreatitis and PDAC may coexist; one should consider the possibility of the latter, depending on other signs and symptoms.
- All patients should be counselled for the possibility of undergoing total pancreatectomy if the tumour margin is involved, particularly when the surgery involves the neck of the pancreas.

References

1　Chari ST, Leibson CL, Rabe KG, et al. Probability of pancreatic cancer following diabetes: a population-based study. Gastroenterology 2005; 129: 504–11.

2　Sharma S, Tapper WJ, Collins A, Hamady ZZR. Predicting pancreatic cancer in the UK Biobank cohort using polygenic risk scores and diabetes mellitus. Gastroenterology 2022; 162: 1665–74.e2.

3　Ballehaninna UK, Chamberlain RS. The clinical utility of serum CA 19-9 in the diagnosis, prognosis and management of pancreatic adenocarcinoma: an evidence based appraisal. J Gastrointest Oncol 2012; 3: 105–19.

4　Hartwig W, Strobel O, Hinz U, et al. CA 19-9 in potentially resectable pancreatic cancer: perspective to adjust surgical and perioperative therapy. Ann Surg Oncol 2013; 20: 2188–96.

5　Mann DV, Edwards R, Ho S, et al. Elevated tumour marker CA 19-9: clinical interpretation and influence of obstructive jaundice. Eur J Surg Oncol 2000; 26: 474–9.

6　Kirkegård J, Mortensen FV, Cronin-Fenton D. Chronic pancreatitis and pancreatic cancer risk: a systematic review and meta-analysis. Am J Gastroenterol 2017; 112: 1366–72.

7　Birgin E, Hablawetz P, Téoule P, et al. Chronic pancreatitis and resectable synchronous pancreatic carcinoma: a survival analysis. Pancreatology 2018; 18: 394–8.

8　Schima W, Böhm G, Rösch CS, et al. Mass-forming pancreatitis versus pancreatic ductal adenocarcinoma: CT and MR imaging for differentiation. Cancer Imaging 2020; 20: 52.

9　Kozu T, Suda K, Toki F. Pancreatic development and anatomical variation. Gastrointest Endosc Clin N Am 1995; 5: 1–30.

10　Henry BM, Skinningsrud B, Saganiak K, et al. Development of the human pancreas and its vasculature – an integrated review covering anatomical, embryological, histological, and molecular aspects. Ann Anat 2019; 221: 115–24.

11　Tadokoro H, Takase M, Nobukawa B. Development and congenital anomalies of the pancreas. Anat Res Int 2011; 2011: 351217.

12　Müller MW, Friess H, Kleeff J, et al. Is there still a role for total pancreatectomy? Ann Surg 2007; 246: 966–74; discussion 974–5.

13　Beger HG, Poch B, Mayer B, Siech M. New onset of diabetes and pancreatic exocrine insufficiency after pancreaticoduodenectomy for benign and malignant tumors: a systematic review and meta-analysis of long-term results. Ann Surg 2018; 267: 259–70.

14　Kang MJ, Jung HS, Jang JY, et al. Metabolic effect of pancreatoduodenectomy: resolution of diabetes mellitus after surgery. Pancreatology 2016; 16: 272–7.

Further reading

• Almond M, Roberts KJ, Hodson J, et al. Changing indications for a total pancreatectomy: perspectives over a quarter of a century. HPB (Oxford) 2015; 17: 416–21.

• Petrucciani N, Nigri G, Giannini G, et al. Total pancreatectomy for pancreatic carcinoma: when, why, and what are the outcomes? Results of a systematic review. Pancreas 2020; 49: 175–80.

• Schmidt CM, Glant J, Winter JM, et al. Total pancreatectomy (R0 resection) improves survival over subtotal pancreatectomy in isolated neck margin positive pancreatic adenocarcinoma. Surgery 2007; 142: 572–8.

29 Interventional radiology approaches for diagnosis and palliation/symptom control

Pavan Najran

Case history

A 76-year-old man presented with weight loss, jaundice and pale stools. A diagnostic CT scan revealed locally advanced pancreatic cancer with soft tissue involvement of the superior mesenteric artery (Figure 29.1). As the cancer was deemed unresectable, systemic treatment was recommended. The distal common bile duct was obstructed owing to the extent of local primary disease (Figure 29.2), requiring common bile duct stent insertion to enable systemic treatment.

After six cycles of systemic chemotherapy the patient presented with non-specific central abdominal pain and an associated mild rise in bilirubin level. Cross-sectional imaging showed migration of the previously placed common bile duct stent and associated mild intrahepatic biliary ductal dilation. Percutaneous transhepatic cholangiography (PTC) showed residual distal common bile duct narrowing (Figure 29.3), requiring insertion of a further common bile duct stent (Figure 29.4).

Further imaging showed disease progression extending into the uncinate process of the pancreas (Figure 29.5) and encroaching on the adjacent duodenum, resulting in

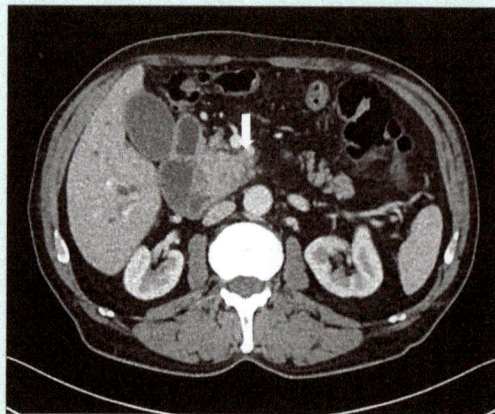

Figure 29.1 Locally advanced pancreatic cancer with disease encasing the superior mesenteric artery (arrow).

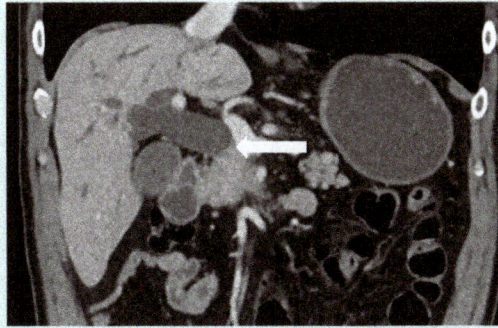

Figure 29.2 Distal common bile duct obstruction secondary to locally advanced pancreatic malignancy (arrow showing transition point).

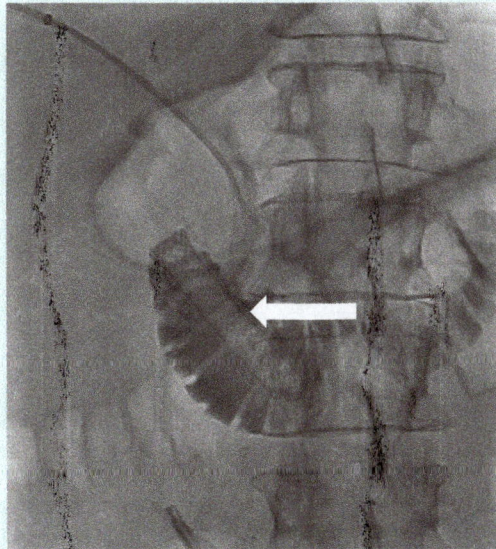

Figure 29.3 PTC imaging showing migrated common bile duct stent located in the duodenum (arrow).

bowel obstruction requiring stent insertion (Figure 29.6). The patient re-presented with progressive vomiting and symptoms suggestive of gastric outlet obstruction. A water-soluble contrast swallow showed stenosis of the intraluminal stent suggestive of tumour ingrowth (Figure 29.7).

Endoscopy, performed with a view to examining the stent, showed stagnant material and sludge with little tumour ingrowth (Figure 29.8). An intraluminal stent trawling was performed with good post-procedural appearances and adequate intraluminal volume.

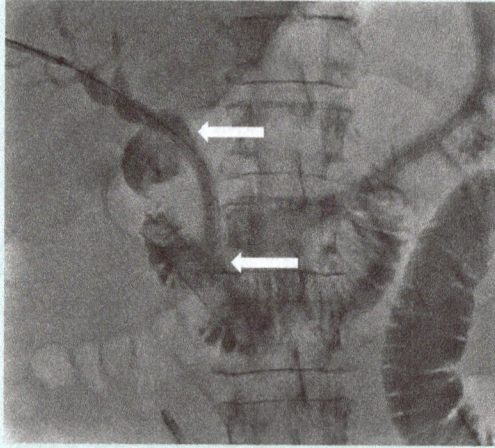

Figure 29.4 Subsequent bile duct stent inserted (arrows).

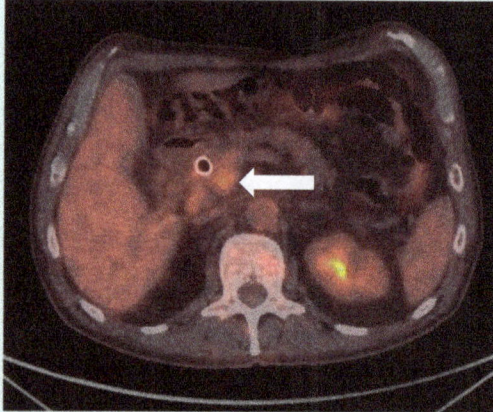

Figure 29.5 Progressive disease extending into the uncinate process of the pancreas (arrow).

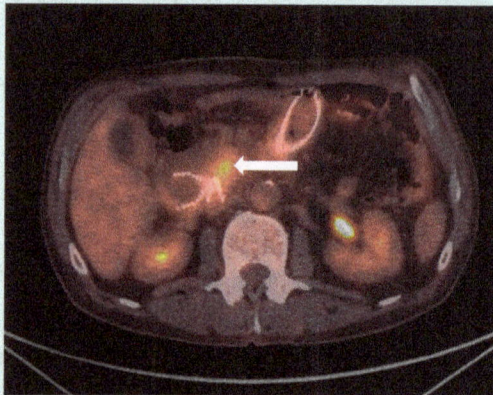

Figure 29.6 Metabolically active disease extending medially to involve the adjacent duodenum requiring duodenal stent insertion (arrow).

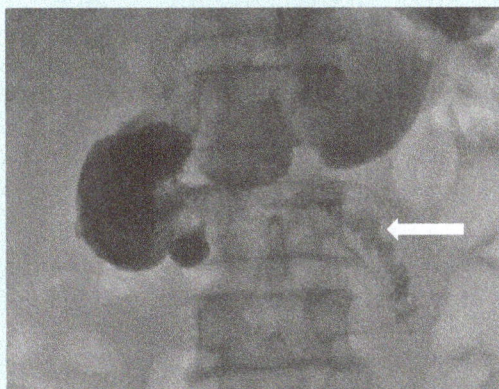

Figure 29.7 Water-soluble contrast swallow showing little contrast passing through the duodenal stent (arrow) suggestive of tumour ingrowth.

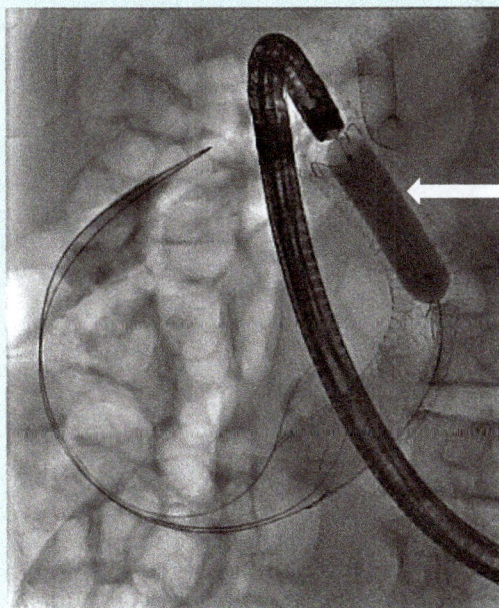

Figure 29.8 Stent trawling performed (arrow).

What are the imaging modalities for pancreatic cancer diagnosis?

What was the goal of cancer treatment in this patient?

What are the management options for biliary duct obstruction?

What is the role of the endoscopic approach in luminal obstruction?

What are the imaging modalities for pancreatic cancer diagnosis?

Initial imaging, in the form of a CT scan of the thorax, abdomen and pelvis, should be performed to fully stage the malignancy.[1] An arterial phase CT covering the pancreatic region is required to ascertain local vascular involvement, which will dictate the extent of local disease and resectability. Imaging of the thorax and remaining portions of the abdomen/pelvis will ascertain distant disease status. A histological diagnosis can be obtained by endoscopic sampling[2] or via sampling of a metastatic site percutaneously.

What was the goal of cancer treatment in this patient?

Surgical resection was not possible because of local disease. Systemic treatment was begun with a view to downstaging the local disease. Biliary drainage was required before the patient could start systemic chemotherapy. Unfortunately, as his disease progressed through systemic treatment, subsequent procedures were for symptom control.

What are the management options for biliary duct obstruction?

Depending on the location, distal common bile duct obstruction can be managed via endoscopic stent insertion. This is limited by service availability and anatomy; for example, patients who have had a Whipple's procedure cannot have a stent inserted endoscopically owing to the surgical diversion. Where this is the case, a stent can be inserted using PTC. In patients with a duodenal stent *in situ*, PTC is a preferable method for biliary stent insertion as endoscopic cannulation of the common bile duct would not be possible.

Although self-expandable metallic stents are commonly used to relieve biliary obstruction, their use may make future surgical resection challenging. In patients with progressive disease involving the liver and proximal biliary obstruction, PTC and metallic stenting are favourable.[3] Plastic stents provide a temporary method of relieving biliary obstruction with the option of removing the stent endoscopically. Plastic stents are more commonly used in the benign setting where there is a higher incidence of obstruction.

What is the role of the endoscopic approach in luminal obstruction?

Because of the location of the patient's duodenal stent it was difficult to further characterize the intraluminal pathology. A water-soluble contrast swallow can identify functional intraluminal compromise, but, as demonstrated in this case, intraluminal compromise may be due to a range of causes. An endoscopic evaluation is not only diagnostic but will allow for a therapeutic option; in this case a balloon was inserted to trawl out the obstructing stagnant content within the stent.

This case demonstrates a multimodal approach in managing pancreatic cancer in a palliative setting. Common bile duct metallic stent insertion is frequently performed to optimize liver function before instigation of systemic treatment.[4]

As the insertion of a common bile duct stent can increase the risk of pancreatitis and recurrent biliary obstruction, the initial choice and placement of the stent need to be accurate to minimize the likelihood of re-intervention.[5] There is debate as to whether a plastic stent or a self-expandable metallic stent should be used in borderline resectable cases. Plastic stents can be retrieved endoscopically and as such are desirable in the benign setting, but they are associated with a higher rate of obstruction compared with self-expandable metal stents.[6]

This case highlights the importance of collaboration, as disease progression can result in clinically challenging scenarios. In this case the patient progressed, resulting in disease compromising the duodenum. A surgical gastro-jejunostomy is a significant undertaking for patients, particularly those who are exposed to systemic treatments. Endoscopic placement of a duodenal stent will avoid significant surgery and provide symptomatic relief.[7] Care needs to be taken when placing a duodenal stent with a biliary stent *in situ* as the procedure may compromise biliary drainage. A combined approach is ideal with coaxial placements of biliary and duodenal stents or endoscopic placement of both stents.[8]

Conclusion and learning points

- Accurate initial staging is essential for appropriate patient management, which should include an arterial phase CT scan to assess local vessel involvement.

- Prompt intervention is required as adequate biliary decompression is important to allow for systemic chemotherapy.

- Distal common bile duct obstruction can be managed with a stent insertion placed via endoscopic retrograde cholangiopancreatography as it will also provide the opportunity for diagnostic sampling of the primary disease.

- PTC provides the opportunity to perform intervention in patients who have had a previous Whipple's procedure.

- Local disease progression provides a challenging environment for symptomatic control; a combined endoscopic and percutaneous approach is an effective method of managing duodenal involvement and biliary disease.

References

1 Zhang L, Sanagapalli S, Stoita A. Challenges in diagnosis of pancreatic cancer. World J Gastroenterol 2018; 24: 2047–60.

2 Hanada K, Okazaki A, Hirano N, et al. Effective screening for early diagnosis of pancreatic cancer. Best Pract Res Clin Gastroenterol 2015; 29: 929–39.

3 Lee BH, Choe DH, Lee JH, et al. Metallic stents in malignant biliary obstruction: prospective long-term clinical results. Am J Roentgenol 1997; 168: 741–5.

4 Hasegawa S, Kubota K, Yagi S, et al. Covered metallic stent placement for biliary drainage could be promising in the coming era of neoadjuvant chemo-radiation therapy for all pancreatic cancer. J Hepatobiliary Pancreat Sci 2021; 28: 617–24.

5 Takeda T, Sasaki T, Mie T, et al. Novel risk factors for recurrent biliary obstruction and pancreatitis after metallic stent placement in pancreatic cancer. Endosc Int Open 2020; 8: E1603–10.

6 Lee HW, Moon JH, Lee YN, et al. Modified non-flared fully covered self-expandable metal stent vs plastic stent for preoperative biliary drainage in patients with resectable malignant biliary obstruction. J Gastroenterol Hepatol 2019; 34: 1590–6.

7 Kobayashi S, Ueno M, Kameda R, et al. Duodenal stenting followed by systemic chemotherapy for patients with pancreatic cancer and gastric outlet obstruction. Pancreatology 2016; 16: 1085–91.

8 Moon JH, Choi HJ. Endoscopic double-metallic stenting for malignant biliary and duodenal obstructions. J Hepatobiliary Pancreat Sci 2011; 18: 658–63.

30 Inoperable locally advanced pancreatic head tumour

Praveen Peddu

Case history

A 54-year-old woman presented with jaundice, weight loss and fatigue. She was previously fit and well and had no significant medical history. Her blood tests showed hyperbilirubinaemia and elevated liver enzymes with a cholestatic picture. An ultrasound scan of the abdomen demonstrated dilated bile ducts and no gallstones. A CT scan revealed a 3 cm mass in the head of pancreas causing biliary and pancreatic ductal obstruction. The mass was circumferentially encasing the portal vein and superior mesenteric vein confluence. The scan also showed small lymph nodes around the pancreatic head but no evidence of distant metastases. The case was reviewed in the hepatobiliary multidisciplinary team (MDT) cancer meeting. The woman was diagnosed radiologically as having an inoperable locally advanced pancreatic head cancer. It was staged as T4N1M0.

Endoscopic ultrasound sampling of the mass confirmed pancreatic ductal adenocarcinoma. Endoscopic retrograde cholangiopancreatography was used to place a plastic biliary stent in the distal bile duct. Her jaundice slowly resolved and she was referred to oncology for chemotherapy.

The patient was treated with folinic acid, fluorouracil, irinotecan and oxaliplatin (FOLFIRINOX), in six cycles initially over a 3 month period, after which a restaging CT scan was carried out. The scan showed stable disease with no significant reduction in the size of tumour or improvement in vascular encasement of the portal vein and superior mesenteric vein confluence. She received three further cycles of chemotherapy but developed significant side effects which included nausea, haematological toxicity and peripheral neuropathy. She discontinued chemotherapy and was referred to the hepatobiliary MDT for consideration of alternative loco-regional therapies. A further staging CT confirmed a 3 cm locally advanced pancreatic head tumour without distant metastases. She was offered percutaneous irreversible electroporation (IRE) for local tumour control.

The patient was admitted to the hospital and underwent percutaneous IRE under CT guidance and general anaesthesia. She made an uneventful recovery and was discharged after 48 h. A follow-up CT scan performed 6 weeks after treatment demonstrated a slight reduction in the size of tumour to 2.6 cm. The tumour remained inoperable. She declined further chemotherapy and opted for follow-up. Four months after IRE, a follow-up CT scan showed a stable local tumour but development of liver metastases. She was referred for further chemotherapy and

Case 30: Inoperable locally advanced
pancreatic head tumour
205

treated with gemcitabine but developed progressive liver metastases and passed
away 3 months after recommencement of chemotherapy.

What are the treatment options for locally advanced inoperable pancreatic
cancers?

What is IRE?

How is IRE performed?

Are there any complications from IRE?

What is the evidence base for IRE in treating locally advanced pancreatic cancer?

What are the future prospects of IRE?

What are the treatment options for locally advanced inoperable pancreatic cancers?

Approximately 80% of pancreatic cancer patients have locally advanced disease or distant metastases at presentation. Pancreatic cancer is termed locally advanced and inoperable when it is seen to circumferentially encase the superior mesenteric artery, superior mesenteric vein and/or portal vein. The presence of extrapancreatic disease is also an absolute contraindication for surgery. The treatment options for inoperable pancreatic cancer include palliative chemotherapy, stereotactic body radiotherapy (SBRT) and IRE.

What is IRE?

IRE is a novel non-thermal local ablative treatment for locally advanced pancreatic adenocarcinoma. It achieves soft tissue ablation with short (70–90 µs), high-voltage (3000 V) electric pulses causing cell membrane perforation, electrolyte instability, disruption of cellular homeostasis, and cell death by apoptosis. A major advantage is that surrounding structures such as ducts and vasculature are not injured. Although it is not standard-of-care practice at this time, with further research IRE may serve as a useful adjunct in the optimal treatment of inoperable pancreatic cancer.

How is IRE performed?

IRE is performed by interventional radiologists under CT scan guidance and general anaesthesia. Under CT guidance, between three and six monopolar electrodes are carefully placed in the tumour percutaneously. The needles should be placed parallel to each other and the distance between each needle should be 1.5–2.2 cm. The needles are then connected to a computerized generator which sends high-voltage electric impulses between the needles and creates a high-power electric field within the confined area causing damage to the cellular structure of the tumour and resulting in cellular death by apoptosis. The entire procedure lasts for up to 2 h. The treatment is also ECG-gated to avoid disturbing cardiac rhythm. Therefore, patients with uncontrolled cardiac arrhythmias are not suitable for the procedure. The presence of metal in the treatment field (e.g. a metal bile duct stent) can disturb the electric field and is a relative contraindication to the procedure.

Are there any complications from IRE?

IRE is a relatively safe procedure. Needle placement in the tumour can result in bleeding and injury to nearby viscera such as bowel, for example. There is also a risk of causing pancreatitis.

Application of a high-strength electric field can also cause cardiac arrhythmias, although these are rare.

What is the evidence base for IRE in treating locally advanced pancreatic cancer?

There have been no randomized controlled trials evaluating the efficacy of IRE in treating locally advanced pancreatic cancer. There have, however, been several retrospective and prospective multicentre studies that have demonstrated improved survival rates when IRE was used in combination with chemotherapy compared with standard chemotherapy alone. Holland et al.[1] reported a multicentre study of 152 patients with locally advanced pancreatic cancer treated with open IRE followed by chemotherapy. The median time to progression and median progression-free survival (PFS) and overall survival (OS) from diagnosis were 27.3 months, 22.8 months and 30.7 months, respectively; morbidity and mortality rates were 18% and 2%, respectively. Leen et al.[2] treated 75 patients with unresectable pancreatic cancer with percutaneous IRE under CT guidance after chemotherapy and reported median OS and PFS of 27 months and 15 months, respectively. Narayanan et al.[3] treated 50 patients with locally advanced pancreatic cancer with percutaneous IRE after completion of chemotherapy; 60% of patients also had prior radiation therapy. The median OS was 27 months from time of diagnosis and 14.2 months from time of IRE. These authors also reported a longer median OS in patients with tumours ≤3 cm than in patients with tumours >3 cm (33.8 months vs 22.7 months, respectively).

What are the future prospects of IRE?

IRE is currently offered in combination with chemotherapy, but although there has been proven improvement in OS the prognosis in patients with locally advanced pancreatic cancer remains poor. One potential advancement in combination therapy integrates immunotherapy with IRE, referred to as 'electroimmunotherapy'. Scheffer et al.[4] found that IRE induced a systemic immune response that resulted in the release of antigens and the formation of antigen-presenting cells causing systemic activation of the immune system. The activation of lymph nodal T-cells by these antigen-presenting cells could potentially induce a durable anti-tumour T-cell response. To boost the patient's own activated immune system through the IRE procedure, a combination with immunotherapy in the form of checkpoint inhibitors or other active immune-enhancing drugs may be able to create a synergistic effect. A recent preclinical study involving immunocompetent mice with pancreatic cancer that received combined treatment with IRE and an anti-programmed cell death protein 1 (PD-1) checkpoint inhibitor demonstrated significant survival benefit.[5] Furthermore, in a clinical study for unresectable locally advanced pancreatic cancer, a combination of IRE and allogeneic natural killer cells achieved significant improvement in OS compared with IRE alone.[6,7] These are preliminary results and more studies in future will determine the clinical safety and efficacy of such combination treatments.

Conclusion and learning points

- Pancreatic cancer remains a deadly disease with poor survival rates. The majority of pancreatic cancers are inoperable at presentation.
- Chemotherapy, IRE and SBRT are the currently available treatments for locally advanced pancreatic cancer.

- IRE when combined with chemotherapy or chemoradiotherapy improves survival rates in patients with locally advanced pancreatic cancer; however, larger controlled studies are needed.

- IRE was found to induce an immune response, suggesting that in combination with immunotherapy IRE may have a significant impact on tumour response rates and OS.[4]

References

1 Holland MM, Bhutiani N, Kruse EJ, et al. A prospective, multi-institution assessment of irreversible electroporation for treatment of locally advanced pancreatic adenocarcinoma: initial outcomes from the AHPBA pancreatic registry. HPB (Oxford) 2019; 21: 1024–31.

2 Leen E, Picard J, Stebbing J, et al. Percutaneous irreversible electroporation with systemic treatment for locally advanced pancreatic adenocarcinoma. J Gastrointest Oncol 2018; 9: 275–81.

3 Narayanan G, Hosein PJ, Beulaygue IC, et al. Percutaneous image-guided irreversible electroporation for the treatment of unresectable, locally advanced pancreatic adenocarcinoma. J Vasc Interv Radiol 2017; 28: 342–8.

4 Scheffer HJ, Stam AGM, Geboers B, et al. Irreversible electroporation of locally advanced pancreatic cancer transiently alleviates immune suppression and creates a window for antitumor T cell activation. Oncoimmunology 2019; 8: 1652532.

5 Zhao J, Wen X, Tian L, et al. Irreversible electroporation reverses resistance to immune checkpoint blockade in pancreatic cancer. Nat Commun 2019; 10: 899.

6 Lin M, Liang S, Wang X, et al. Percutaneous irreversible electroporation combined with allogeneic natural killer cell immunotherapy for patients with unresectable (stage III/IV) pancreatic cancer: a promising treatment. J Cancer Res Clin Oncol 2017; 143: 2607–18.

7 Lin M, Alnaggar M, Liang S, et al. An important discovery on combination of irreversible electroporation and allogeneic natural killer cell immunotherapy for unresectable pancreatic cancer. Oncotarget 2017; 8: 101795–807.

31 Borderline resectable pancreatic cancer and the role of intraoperative electron beam radiotherapy

Dharmadev Trivedi, Arjun Takhar

Case history

The case of a 71-year-old man was referred to the pancreatic multidisciplinary team (MDT). He had a 3 month history of weight loss, a feeling of fullness in the upper abdomen and gradually worsening jaundice. An initial CT scan suggested a mass lesion in the head of the pancreas with involvement of the superior mesenteric vein and encasement (<180°) of the superior mesenteric artery (Figure 31.1). No distal metastatic disease was seen. Radiological staging according to the criteria of the American Joint Committee on Cancer was T4N1M0.[1] The pancreatic MDT considered the cancer to be borderline resectable.

Endoscopic retrograde cholangiopancreatography was used to place a fully covered self-expandable metal biliary stent in the common bile duct. The biliary brushings obtained at the time of the procedure, and an endoscopic ultrasound-guided biopsy of the lesion, confirmed a moderately differentiated pancreatic ductal adenocarcinoma (PDAC).

The patient was reviewed by the local oncology team and neoadjuvant folinic acid, fluorouracil, irinotecan and oxaliplatin (FOLFIRINOX) was commenced. After 12 cycles, a moderate local response was noted (Figure 31.2). No distal metastasis was seen on imaging.

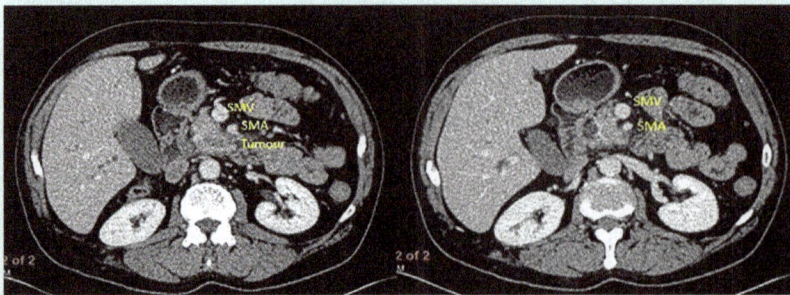

Figure 31.1 CT scan images at presentation showing pancreatic mass with vascular involvement. SMA, superior mesenteric artery; SMV, superior mesenteric vein.

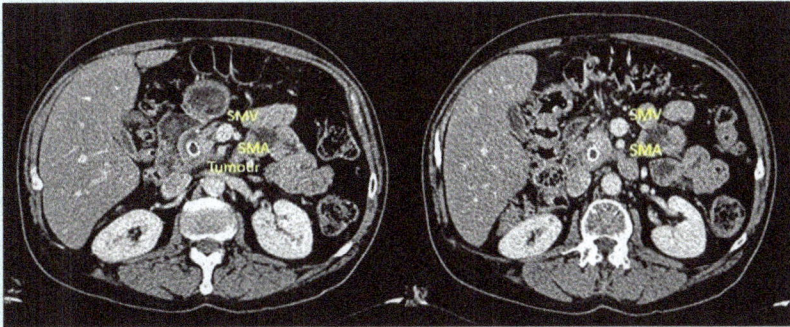

Figure 31.2 CT scan images after 12 cycles of neoadjuvant chemotherapy showing partial response. SMA, superior mesenteric artery; SMV, superior mesenteric vein.

The patient underwent a classic Whipple's procedure. After resection was completed, a 15 Gy dose of intraoperative electron beam radiotherapy (IOERT) was delivered to the tumour bed (cone applicator 6 cm in diameter, 12 MeV energy, depth 1 cm bolus) (Figures 31.3 and 31.4). The patient's recovery was uneventful. The drain amylase level at day 3 was <10 U/l. The patient was discharged home on postoperative day 8. The final histology was T1N0M0.[1]

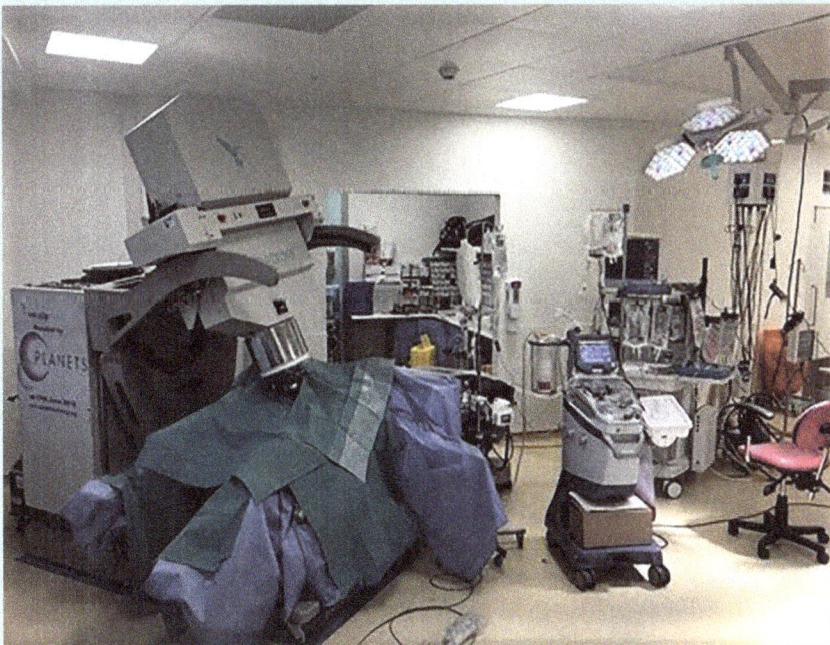

Figure 31.3 Standard patient and equipment set-up for IOERT.

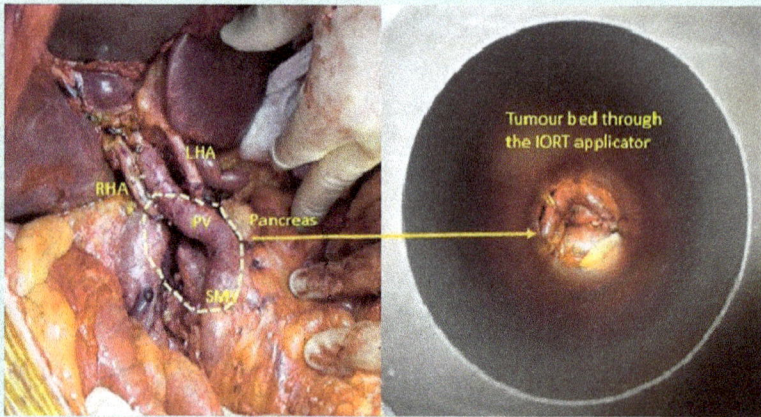

Figure 31.4 Intraoperative radiotherapy (IORT) to the tumour bed after resection stage of Whipple's procedure (reproduced with permission from Bhome et al.[6]). LHA, left hepatic artery; PV, portal vein; RHA, right hepatic artery; SMV, superior mesenteric vein.

What is the definition of resectable, borderline resectable and unresectable pancreatic cancer?

What is the evidence for neoadjuvant chemotherapy for locally advanced pancreatic cancers?

What is the rationale for IOERT in pancreatic cancers?

What are the selection criteria for IOERT for pancreatico-biliary cancers?

What is the future of IOERT for pancreatico-biliary cancers?

What is the definition of resectable, borderline resectable and unresectable pancreatic cancer?

The International Association of Pancreatology classifies PDAC into resectable, borderline resectable and unresectable.[2] The classification takes into account the anatomical (on cross-sectional imaging) and biological (regional lymph node metastasis on PET-CT or biopsy; CA 19-9 levels >500 U/l) characteristics of the tumour (Table 31.1). Patient factors, such as ECOG performance status ≥2, are also considered under the domain of 'conditional' when deciding whether an upfront surgery (surgery-first) approach and achieving R0 resection status may or may not be possible.[2]

What is the evidence for neoadjuvant chemotherapy for locally advanced pancreatic cancers?

Neoadjuvant chemotherapy and chemoradiation have been shown to improve resectability and overall survival (OS) in patients with borderline resectable PDAC.[2] A recent meta-analysis of seven randomized controlled trials comprising 938 patients concluded that OS was better in patients receiving neoadjuvant chemotherapy with or without radiotherapy compared with those having upfront surgery.[3] Median OS increased from 19 to 29 months with neoadjuvant chemotherapy (HR 0.66; 95% CI 0.52, 0.85; p=0.001). Patients with borderline resectable cancers

Table 31.1 International consensus guidance on definition of borderline pancreatic cancer based on anatomical characteristics (adapted from Isaji et al.[3]).

Resectable (R)	No tumour contact or unilateral narrowing of SMV or PV
	No tumour contact with SMA or CA or CHA
Borderline resectable (BR)	
BR-PV (SMV/PV involvement)	Tumour contact ≥180° or bilateral narrowing or occlusion, not exceeding the inferior border of the duodenum
	No contact with SMA or CA or CHA
BR-A (arterial involvement)	Tumour contact <180° with SMA or CA without arterial deformity
	Tumour contact with CHA without contact with hepatic artery proper or CA
Unresectable (UR)	
UR-LA (locally advanced)	Narrowing/occlusion of SMV or PV exceeding the inferior border of the duodenum and ≥180° contact of tumour with SMA or CA
	Tumour contact of CHA with contact/invasion of the hepatic artery proper and/or CA
	Tumour contact or invasion of aorta
UR-M (metastatic)	Presence of distal metastasis

CA, coeliac artery; CHA, common hepatic artery; PV, portal vein; SMA, superior mesenteric artery; SMV, superior mesenteric vein.

had better OS after neoadjuvant chemotherapy compared with patients who had upfront surgery (HR 0.61; 95% CI 0.44, 0.85; p=0.004).

What is the rationale for IOERT in pancreatic cancers?

IOERT for pancreatic cancers is used mainly in two broad contexts.

Resectable tumours (to achieve additional local clearance) and borderline resectable tumours (to achieve R0 resection)

Local recurrence even after curative surgery in patients with PDAC is common. A 2017 review found that IOERT to achieve local control as an adjunct to surgery was feasible and safe.[4] Additionally, IOERT facilitates provision of a higher radiation dose without causing collateral radiation damage to vital structures in the vicinity of the pancreatico-duodenectomy bed, thus reducing local recurrence. Drawbacks of IOERT are the inability to obtain further margin to confirm tumour clearance after the procedure, the initial set-up cost, operational logistics, delayed radiation side effects, and the inability to plan three-dimensional treatment preoperatively.[4]

Nevertheless, delivering IOERT after curative resection has been shown to improve survival in patients with borderline resectable tumours who have had contemporary (FOLFIRINOX) neoadjuvant chemotherapy. Harrison et al.[5] reported a median progression-free survival and OS of 21.5 and 46.7 months, respectively, in a series of 86 patients receiving 10 Gy of IOERT at the time of curative surgery; 55 of 86 patients had a pancreatico-duodenectomy and 31 a distal or left pancreatectomy. The authors reported significant complication rates of 13% (Clavien–Dindo grade 3 or more). This patient profile differs from that in the study of Bhome et al.,[6] where all 19 patients underwent pancreatico-duodenectomy with curative intent. The median IOERT dose was 15 Gy (10–15 Gy). Six of 19 patients had minor (C–D I or II) complications; no deaths were reported.

A recent and so far the only prospective phase II trial comprising 41 patients with resectable pancreatic cancers reported a local control rate of 76.1% at 1 year after IOERT of 10 Gy delivered at the time of curative surgery.[7] One patient in this cohort required surgery for a complication. Four patients developed local recurrence at 9 months' follow-up, nine patients developed distal metastases, and two had both local and distal recurrence. The authors concluded that IOERT was feasible and had an acceptable safety profile.

Locally advanced pancreatic cancers when curative resection is not possible

IOERT has been shown to provide survival benefit in patients with unresectable tumours with or without additional external beam radiotherapy (EBRT).[4,5,8] Cai et al.[8] reported long-term outcomes in 183 patients with unresectable pancreatic cancers receiving IOERT. The authors identified the size of the tumours (applicator diameter ≤8 cm), good performance status and additional chemotherapy as favourable prognostic indicators. In the cohort of patients with all three indicators, a median OS was noted of 21.2 months. Importantly, most of the patients in this study had received EBRT before IOERT.

What are the selection criteria for IOERT for pancreatico–biliary cancers?

Patient selection criteria for administering IOERT have been explicitly documented by Bhome et al.[6] as:

- initially unresectable or borderline resectable tumours:
  - arterial encasement or superior mesenteric vein/portal vein contact (180–270°);
- WHO performance status 0–1;
- no evidence of distant metastasis or disease progression on CT scan (2–4 weeks before the procedure).

What is the future of IOERT for pancreatico–biliary cancers?

IOERT is currently not the gold standard; therefore, randomized prospective studies before widespread implementation are required.[4–6,8] PACER (ClinicalTrials.gov NCT03716531) is a phase II study evaluating IOERT after chemoradiation in patients with pancreatic cancers with vascular involvement. The trial aims to recruit 200 patients before November 2023. The inclusion criteria are age ≥18 years, previous EBRT or stereotactic body radiotherapy with neoadjuvant chemotherapy, and performance status of 0 or 1.

Conclusion and learning points

- IOERT is safe and appears to have a role in a subset of the population with borderline resectable pancreatic cancers.[4–7]
- The provision of IOERT is labour-intensive and requires MDT effort.[5,6]
- The current selection criteria for patients suitable for IOERT are well defined.[6]

- Despite a lack of high-quality evidence, emerging data suggest a survival benefit of IOERT in selected patient cohorts with borderline and unresectable pancreatic cancers.[5,8]

- Future prospective trials will strengthen the evidence for wider implementation of IOERT for pancreatic cancers.

References

1 Allen PJ, Kuk D, Castillo CF, et al. Multi-institutional validation study of the American Joint Commission on Cancer (8th edition) changes for T and N staging in patients with pancreatic adenocarcinoma. Ann Surg 2017; 265: 185–91.

2 Isaji S, Mizuno S, Windsor JA, et al. International consensus on definition and criteria of borderline resectable pancreatic ductal adenocarcinoma 2017. Pancreatology 2018; 18: 2–11.

3 van Dam JL, Janssen QP, Besselink MG, et al. Neoadjuvant therapy or upfront surgery for resectable and borderline resectable pancreatic cancer: a meta-analysis of randomised controlled trials. Eur J Cancer 2022; 160: 140–9.

4 Krempien R, Roeder F. Intraoperative radiation therapy (IORT) in pancreatic cancer. Radiat Oncol 2017; 12: 1–8.

5 Harrison JM, Wo JY, Ferrone CR, et al. Intraoperative radiation therapy (IORT) for borderline resectable and locally advanced pancreatic ductal adenocarcinoma (BR/LA PDAC) in the era of modern neoadjuvant treatment: short-term and long-term outcomes. Ann Surg Oncol 2020; 27: 1400–6.

6 Bhome R, Karavias D, Armstrong T, et al. Intraoperative radiotherapy for pancreatic cancer: implementation and initial experience. Br J Surg 2021; 108: e400–1.

7 Cho Y, Kim JW, Kim HS, et al. Intraoperative radiotherapy for resectable pancreatic cancer using a low-energy X-ray source: postoperative complications and early outcomes. Yonsei Med J 2022; 63: 405–12.

8 Cai S, Hong TS, Goldberg SI, et al. Updated long-term outcomes and prognostic factors for patients with unresectable locally advanced pancreatic cancer treated with intraoperative radiotherapy at the Massachusetts General Hospital, 1978 to 2010. Cancer 2013; 119: 4196–204.

Further reading

- Cloyd JM, Heh V, Pawlik TM, et al. Neoadjuvant therapy for resectable and borderline resectable pancreatic cancer: a meta-analysis of randomized controlled trials. J Clin Med 2020; 9: 1129.

- Goodman KA, Hajj C. Role of radiation therapy in the management of pancreatic cancer. J Surg Oncol 2013; 107: 86–96.

- Rangarajan K, Pucher PH, Armstrong T, et al. Systemic neoadjuvant chemotherapy in modern pancreatic cancer treatment: a systematic review and meta-analysis. Ann R Coll Surg Engl 2019; 101: 453–62.

32 Pancreatic and biliary tract cancers: post-ablation response monitoring

Govindarajan Narayanan, Jacklyn Garcia, Ashwin Mahendra, Jonathan Eyshi

Case history

A 55-year-old woman with type 2 diabetes presented with epigastric pain, pruritus and 18 kg unintentional weight loss. Abdominal MRI showed intra- and extrahepatic and pancreatic ductal dilations and a hypo-enhancing pancreatic mass (3.3×1.9×3.5 cm) with restricted diffusion encasing the junction of the superior mesenteric and portal veins; there was no evidence of metastatic liver disease (Figure 32.1).

The woman underwent an endoscopic ultrasound-guided fine needle aspiration of the pancreatic mass, sphincterotomy and metallic stent placement. Imaging demonstrated stable pulmonary nodules and no osseous metastatic lesions. Biopsy confirmed a TNM stage II (cT2cNXcM0) pancreatic ductal adenocarcinoma (PDAC); the CA 19-9 tumour marker was elevated (1665 U/ml).

The patient completed neoadjuvant chemotherapy with 12 cycles of folinic acid, fluorouracil, irinotecan and oxaliplatin (FOLFIRINOX) and three cycles of a modified (75% of the standard dose) FOLFIRINOX regimen. Scans showed a decrease in

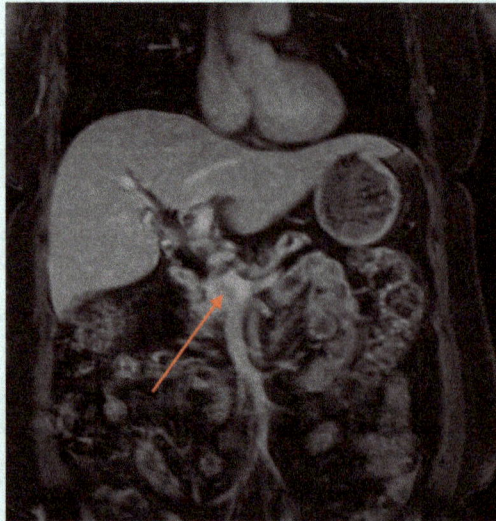

Figure 32.1 Pre-ablation MRI coronal view showing pancreatic head mass.

pancreatic mass size (1.2×1.6 cm), persistent vessel encasement and no hepatic metastases. The tumour board recommended irreversible electroporation (IRE) as an interval bridge to surgery.

A pre-procedural CT scan showed a 1.6×1.5 cm pancreatic lesion. Under CT guidance two 19-gauge IRE needles were advanced into the lesion, one in the cranial and the other in the caudal part of the lesion (Figure 32.2). IRE was delivered in 100 pulses. The probes were retracted 1 cm and IRE was repeated. The cranial needle was repositioned more medially away from the stent and the treatment was performed once more. A post-procedural CT scan showed that the IRE had been successful, with a lack of enhancement of the pancreatic lesion (Figure 32.3).

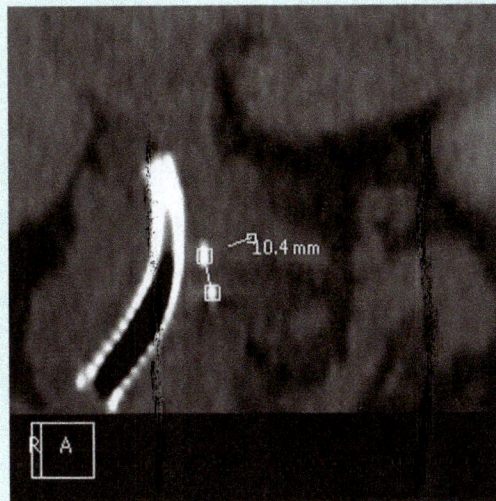

Figure 32.2 Pre-ablation CT-guided IRE probes.

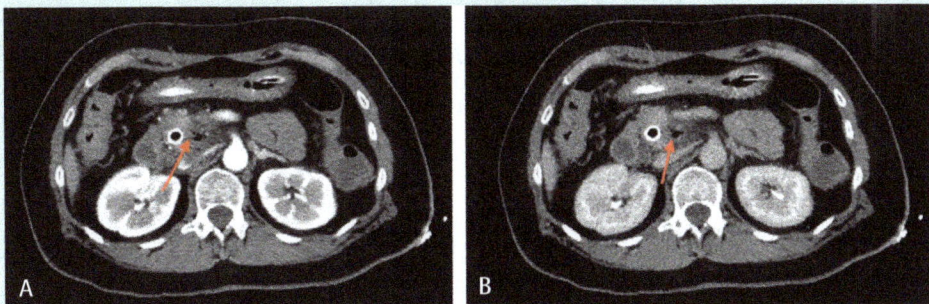

Figure 32.3 (A) Post-ablation arterial phase axial CT image showing tumour and ablation zone. (B) Post-ablation venous phase axial CT image showing tumour and ablation zone.

Following IRE, the patient's abdominal pain was controlled and there was no elevation in amylase and lipase levels. She was discharged 2 days later. Three weeks after IRE, she reported intermittent abdominal pain that worsened with constipation. MRI demonstrated IRE-related changes: a pancreatic soft tissue mass (1.3×1.2 cm), improvement in main pancreatic ductal dilation, a well-positioned stent and no metastatic lesions.

Two months after IRE, she presented with sharp abdominal pain in the right upper quadrant, fever (38.6°C) and transient transaminitis. Imaging showed no acute abdominopelvic inflammatory process and a decrease in the size of the pancreatic head mass (1.1×1.2 cm). The woman is currently on maintenance chemotherapy; a follow-up scan is scheduled and a Whipple's procedure is planned. Her CA 19-9 level has decreased since the IRE (from 179 U/ml before IRE to 60 U/ml in her latest reading). At 3 months' follow-up she continues to show a complete response to treatment (Figure 32.4).

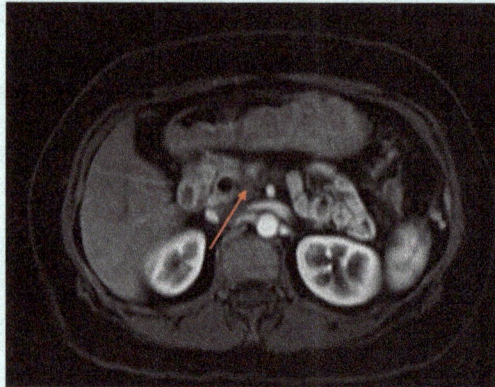

Figure 32.4 Post-ablation MRI axial view showing tumour and ablation zone at 3 months' follow-up.

What was the goal of cancer treatment in this patient?

How did the patient's comorbidities affect her cancer treatment?

What is the evidence base for her treatment?

What is the protocol for percutaneous IRE of the pancreas?

What was the goal of cancer treatment in this patient?

The lesion was considered to be borderline resectable owing to the encasement of the vascular structures. The goal of cancer treatment in this patient was to potentially downstage the tumour prior to surgery. IRE was carried out to treat the PDAC locally while preserving the vasculature[1] and downstage the tumour from borderline resectable to resectable status.

How did the patient's comorbidities affect her cancer treatment?

The patient had experienced some palpitations during chemotherapy and needed evaluation by a cardiologist. The cardiologist cleared her to continue receiving chemotherapy, which delayed her care by a few weeks. A febrile neutropenic event during a chemotherapy cycle delayed her treatments further. In addition, after cycle 12 her chemotherapy regimen was changed to fluorouracil, folinic acid and irinotecan (FOLFIRI) because of neuropathy.

What is the evidence base for her treatment?

Integration of IRE ablation with systemic chemotherapy has been proven to be a safe and potentially effective option for patients with inoperable pancreatic carcinoma.[1] IRE has been identified as an effective modality for locally advanced pancreatic cancer to optimize the margin status or as a primary tumour treatment.[2] IRE may be used in lesions that are close to peri-pancreatic vessels without the risk of vascular trauma.

Fourteen single-arm studies were published on the use of IRE in locally advanced pancreatic cancer, either to accentuate the margin or treat the primary tumour. Participants were treated percutaneously, laparoscopically or with laparotomy.[3–6] In 75 patients, Leen et al.[7] reported a median overall survival (OS) after IRE of 27 months and a median progression-free survival of 15 months, with a median follow-up of 11.7 months. The study by Rai et al.[8] found no statistical significance between median OS in patients in whom treatment was for primary tumour control (23.2 months) vs margin accentuation after resection (28.3 months). The ability to resect the lesion after IRE ranged from 6% to 10.3%, which was investigated in three studies.[9]

What is the protocol for percutaneous IRE of the pancreas?

The protocol for percutaneous IRE in pancreatic cancer requires the procedure to be performed under general anaesthesia with placement of a nasogastric tube, Foley catheter and defibrillator pads. The patient is administered ciprofloxacin 400 mg and metronidazole 500 mg preoperatively. IRE is performed under CT guidance using a NanoKnife to deliver 70 ms high-voltage (1500–3000 V) direct current (25–45 A) electric pulses.[10]

Conclusion and learning points

- For borderline resectable pancreatic cancer, treatment with curative intent may be considered. Chemotherapy with IRE and radiotherapy are treatment options for downstaging the tumour with a view to obtaining resection with a clear margin.
- IRE is a well-tolerated and safe modality of treatment for pancreatic carcinoma with few major or minor complications.
- Further research is needed to determine OS and efficacy of IRE in borderline resectable and locally advanced PDAC.

References

1 Narayanan G, Daye D, Wilson NM, et al. Ablation in pancreatic cancer: past, present and future. Cancers (Basel) 2021; 13: 2511.

2 Bower M, Sherwood L, Li Y, Martin R. Irreversible electroporation of the pancreas: definitive local therapy without systemic effects. J Surg Oncol 2011; 104: 22–8.

3 Kluger MD, Epelboym I, Schrope BA, et al. Single-institution experience with irreversible electroporation for T4 pancreatic cancer: first 50 patients. Ann Surg Oncol 2016; 23: 1736–43.

4 Martin RC 2nd, Kwon D, Chalikonda S, et al. Treatment of 200 locally advanced (stage III) pancreatic adenocarcinoma patients with irreversible electroporation: safety and efficacy. Ann Surg 2015; 262: 486–94; discussion 492–4.

5 Martin RC 2nd, McFarland K, Ellis S, Velanovich V. Irreversible electroporation therapy in the management of locally advanced pancreatic adenocarcinoma. J Am Coll Surg 2012; 215: 361–9.

6 Martin RC 2nd, McFarland K, Ellis S, Velanovich V. Irreversible electroporation in locally advanced pancreatic cancer: potential improved overall survival. Ann Surg Oncol 2013; 20 (suppl 3): S443–9.

7 Leen E, Picard J, Stebbing J, et al. Percutaneous irreversible electroporation with systemic treatment for locally advanced pancreatic adenocarcinoma. J Gastrointest Oncol 2018; 9: 275–81.

8 Rai ZL, Feakins R, Pallett LJ, et al. Irreversible electroporation (IRE) in locally advanced pancreatic cancer: a review of current clinical outcomes, mechanism of action and opportunities for synergistic therapy. J Clin Med 2021; 10: 1609.

9 Ruarus A, Vroomen L, Puijk R, et al. Locally advanced pancreatic cancer: a review of local ablative therapies. Cancers (Basel) 2018; 10: 16.

10 Venkat S, Hosein PJ, Narayanan G. Percutaneous approach to irreversible electroporation of the pancreas: Miami protocol. Tech Vasc Interv Radiol 2015; 18: 153–8.

Further reading

• Månsson C, Brahmstaedt R, Nilsson A, et al. Percutaneous irreversible electroporation for treatment of locally advanced pancreatic cancer following chemotherapy or radiochemotherapy. Eur J Surg Oncol 2016; 42: 1401–6.

• Martin RCG 2nd. Use of irreversible electroporation in unresectable pancreatic cancer. Hepatobiliary Surg Nutr 2015; 4: 211–15.

• Ruarus AH, Vroomen LGPH, Geboers B, et al. Percutaneous irreversible electroporation in locally advanced and recurrent pancreatic cancer (PANFIRE-2): a multicenter, prospective, single-arm, phase II study. Radiology 2020; 294: 212–20.

• White SB, Zhang Z, Chen J, et al. Early immunologic response of irreversible electroporation versus cryoablation in a rodent model of pancreatic cancer. J Vasc Interv Radiol 2018; 29: 1764–9.

33 Pancreatic cancers: post-intervention complications and management

Govindarajan Narayanan, Jacklyn Garcia, Ashwin Mahendra, Jonathan Eyshi

Case history

A 53-year-old man with no relevant medical history presented with epigastric pain, bloating and early satiety. Following endoscopic ultrasound with biopsy, he was diagnosed with TNM stage II (cT2cNXcM0) pancreatic ductal adenocarcinoma (PDAC), acute pancreatitis and biliary obstruction; his CA 19-9 level was 137.6 U/ml. He commenced neoadjuvant chemotherapy with folinic acid, fluorouracil, irinotecan and oxaliplatin (FOLFIRINOX).

An MRI scan 4 months after his initial diagnosis showed a lesion measuring 2.1×1.4×1.7 cm in the pancreatic head and uncinate process abutting the right postero-lateral superior mesenteric vein and right lateral aspect of the superior mesenteric artery (Figure 33.1). It encased the right hepatic artery which arose from the superior mesenteric artery, causing stricture of the main pancreatic duct (Figure 33.2).

Eight months after diagnosis and 12 chemotherapy cycles, the mass measured 1.6×1.1 cm; it was deemed borderline resectable and referred for irreversible electroporation (IRE). IRE was performed with two probes under CT guidance; the ablation zone showed coverage of the tumour on imaging (Figure 33.3). Following IRE, the patient had moderate abdominal pain and elevated levels of amylase and lipase. He was managed for pancreatitis and discharged 3 days later. One month after IRE, the lesion measured 1.2×1.1 cm and maintenance chemotherapy was resumed. Three months after IRE and 15 chemotherapy cycles, the lesion continued to abut the replaced common hepatic artery (Figure 33.4).

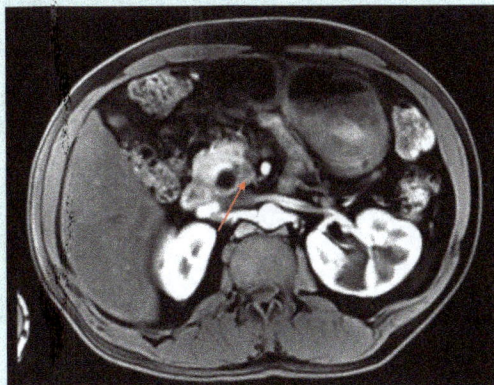

Figure 33.1 MRI axial view showing pancreatic tumour prior to ablation.

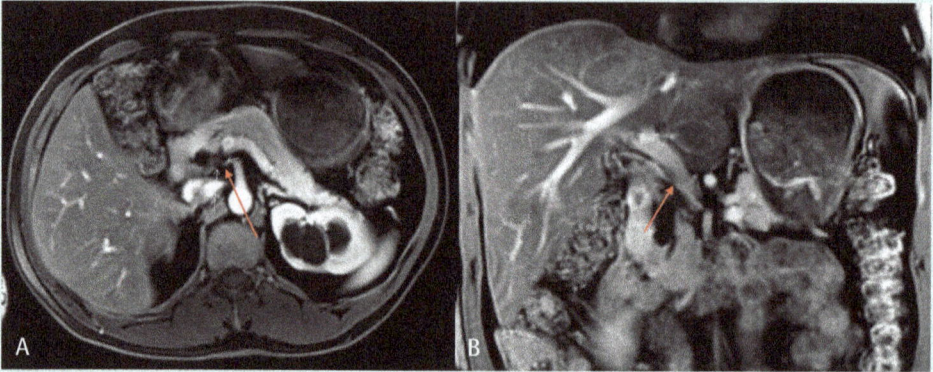

Figure 33.2 (A) MRI axial view and (B) MRI coronal view showing replaced hepatic artery.

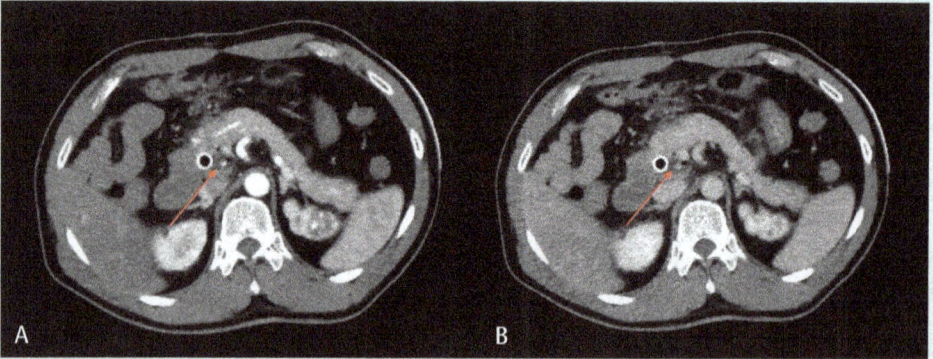

Figure 33.3 (A) Post-ablation arterial phase and (B) venous phase axial CT images showing tumour and ablation zone.

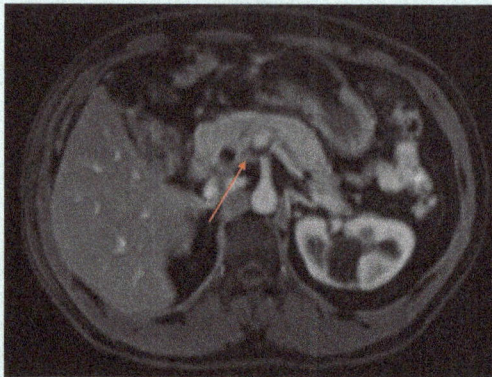

Figure 33.4 MRI axial view showing tumour and ablation zone at follow-up 3 months after the procedure.

A Whipple's procedure was attempted, but the superior mesenteric portal vein trunk could not be separated from the pancreas, as significant arterial anatomic variants complicated the separation from the pancreatic neck. Staging laparoscopically was attempted but converted to open when the lesion was unresectable. After surgery, the patient showed signs of acute respiratory failure. A CT scan showed airspace opacities in the lung bases and patchy ground-glass infiltrates in the upper lobes. Acute thromboembolic disease involving bilateral pulmonary artery branches was found; the right ventricle to left ventricle ratio measured 0.8. He was placed on a heparin drip and given oxygen at a flow rate of 2 l/min.

The patient improved during admission and was discharged to recommence systemic chemotherapy. Radiation was deferred because his CA 19-9 level was normal and the lesion had decreased to a stable size. His CA 19-9 level is currently normal at 19 U/ml and he remains under active surveillance.

What was the rationale for adding local treatment?

What is the protocol for post-procedural management for IRE of the pancreas?

What are the potential complications of IRE?

What was the rationale for adding local treatment?

The patient's tumour was considered borderline resectable and he had received induction chemotherapy. Follow-up imaging after chemotherapy indicated that his tumour was still borderline resectable; therefore, local treatment was added in an attempt to proceed to surgery. If downstaging were not possible, IRE would act synergistically with systemic chemotherapy and help prolong survival with preservation of quality of life.

What is the protocol for post-procedural management for IRE of the pancreas?

The post-procedural protocol involves pain management using a patient-controlled analgesic pump with hydromorphone at a loading dose of 1 mg followed by 0.2 mg every 10 min to a maximum of 1.2 mg/h. Ondansetron is used to treat nausea. The patient is kept *nil per os* except for ice chips; the nasogastric tube is left in place and connected to a wall suction. If amylase and lipase are elevated, the patient is kept *nil per os* with symptomatic management. Typically, the levels of amylase and lipase revert to normal within 48 h. Once the amylase and lipase levels have normalized the nasogastric tube is removed and the patient is started on a clear liquid diet which is advanced as tolerated throughout the day. The average length of hospital stay following the procedure is between 1.5 and 2 days.[1]

What are the potential complications of IRE?

Complications of IRE include bleeding, pancreatitis, injury to the pancreatic ducts, infection, arrhythmia, possible pseudoaneurysm, portal vein thrombosis and pancreatic ascites.[2,3] There are protocols in place to manage these complications intraoperatively including medical management and use of telemetry for monitoring of arrhythmias. Postoperative vital signs and laboratory values are obtained to monitor stability. Appropriate symptomatic management is put in place for pain and nausea.

Conclusion and learning points

- IRE is an adjuvant management technique for locally advanced PDAC to help downstage the tumour and preserve the vasculature to optimize the outcome of a Whipple's procedure.
- The role of IRE in borderline resectable pancreatic cancer is still not established, compared with its recognized role in stage III locally advanced pancreatic carcinoma.
- Post-procedural complications of percutaneous IRE of the pancreas are managed medically and symptomatically; most patients are discharged within 2 days after the procedure.
- Complications of IRE include bleeding, infection, arrhythmia and pancreatic duct injury.

References

1 Venkat S, Hosein PJ, Narayanan G. Percutaneous approach to irreversible electroporation of the pancreas: Miami protocol. Tech Vasc Interv Radiol 2015; 18: 153–8.

2 Dollinger M, Beyer LP, Haimerl M, et al. Adverse effects of irreversible electroporation of malignant liver tumors under CT fluoroscopic guidance: a single-center experience. Diagn Interv Radiol 2015; 21: 471–5.

3 Narayanan G, Daye D, Wilson NM, et al. Ablation in pancreatic cancer: past, present and future. Cancers (Basel) 2021; 13: 2511.

Further reading

- Ha HI, Kim MJ, Kim J, et al. Replaced common hepatic artery from the superior mesenteric artery: multidetector computed tomography (MDCT) classification focused on pancreatic penetration and the course of travel. Surg Radiol Anat 2016; 38: 655–62.
- Narayanan G, Bhatia S, Echenique A, et al. Vessel patency post irreversible electroporation. Cardiovasc Intervent Radiol 2014; 37: 1523–9.
- Zhao J, Wen X, Tian L, et al. Irreversible electroporation reverses resistance to immune checkpoint blockade in pancreatic cancer. Nat Commun 2019; 10: 899.

Index

www.ingramcontent.com/pod-product-compliance
Lightning Source LLC
Chambersburg PA
CBHW081808200326
41597CB00023B/4190